In *Warts and All* the good and credible information has already been sorted out. Dr Margaret Stearn has paid particular attention in referencing where information comes from. She has sourced medical and scientific journals, as well as reliable websites, making this an interesting book backed by good resources.

This book is an articulate, commonsense guide to all those ailments that you might find particularly difficult to talk about with your doctor. No time is wasted on trying to explain weird and wonderful syndromes or life-threatening diseases; Dr Margaret Stearn gets straight into tackling life's most common and embarrassing health issues: from acne and anal pain to warts and wind. Trained at Oxford University and St George's Hospital Medical School in the UK, she has gained a wealth of experience that translates effortlessly into the pages of this book.

Having spent nearly a lifetime studying medicine from complex, bland and boring medical textbooks, it was a treat to read *Warts and All*, with its straightforward and refreshingly easy-to-read style. By integrating information on useful health contacts and organizations where you can follow-up on what has been read, you have a helpful support tool for your ongoing health education, so that you have a better idea of what a particular health problem might be and will be able to seek the best health professional to speak to about it.

The answer to a long and prosperous life isn't an easy one, but if you can take responsibility for your own wellbeing, then you are well on the path to a life of good health, even if there are a few warts and all along the way.

Dr Andrew Rochford MBBS (Hons) BMedSc

Contents

WARTS AND ALL

STRAIGHT TALKING ADVICE ON LIFE'S EMBARRASSING PROBLEMS

DR MARGARET STEARN

Foreword

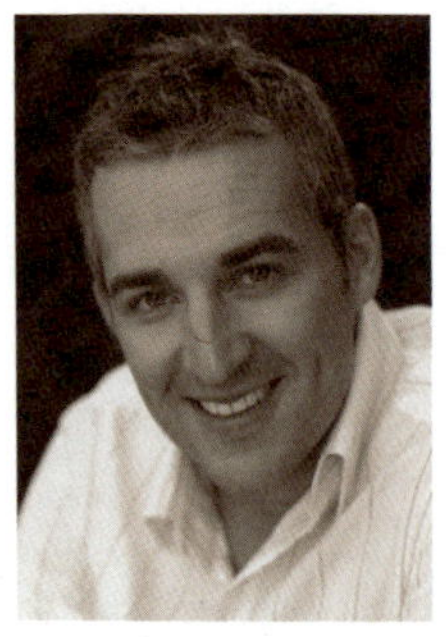

We all would prefer to be in good health and live a long and prosperous life. But how do we make sure that this happens?

When I first decided that I wanted to become a doctor, I was driven by a sense of self-fulfilment and satisfaction of being able to help sick people get better; the chance to pursue research into diseases, and hopefully to identify a possible cure. I was very much an advocate for the medical model of health. In other words, when the human body is afflicted with an illness it should be fixed through diagnosis and effective treatment. I was driven by my constant aspirations that when I finally became a doctor it was going to be me who did the fixing. It wasn't until I had graduated and left the sheltered walls of my university that I was forced to deal with more than just a section of a patient's anatomy, and I started to be aware of how naïve I really was.

My very first position as a doctor was in a busy cardiology ward – the perfect place to start fighting disease and 'fixing' broken hearts. Unfortunately, my role in the team was reduced to being a glorified secretary instead of a doctor: scribing notes, getting coffees and answering telephone, all of which did my ego no favours. However, this experience did offer me the chance to be the middle man; I was forced to be a line of communication between the experienced doctor and the scared patient. Within a short time I realized that the most important thing for a healthcare professional is not a CT scanner or a surgeon's scalpel – it is the patient.

A doctor can perform surgery, prescribe the right drugs, and use highly advanced medical equipment to monitor a patient's progress towards recovery, but once the patient is discharged, the most important thing they take with them is responsibility for their own health. I finally began to appreciate the concept of the social model of health, which places emphasis on changes that can be made within a society and to people's lifestyles to improve the health of the general population. This includes public health screening initiatives, such as pap smears and mammograms, as well as to provide good health information and public education so that people can begin to make informed decisions about their health.

As a doctor, I found that the most cooperative patient is one who has been given good, accurate information that they are able to grasp and understand. But there are only so many answers that a doctor can give you, so the next step is to try to educate yourself. The internet has fast become a powerful resource tool for this purpose. However, it is difficult for a layperson to qualify which information is good and credible and which is suspect and unreliable.

Author's preface

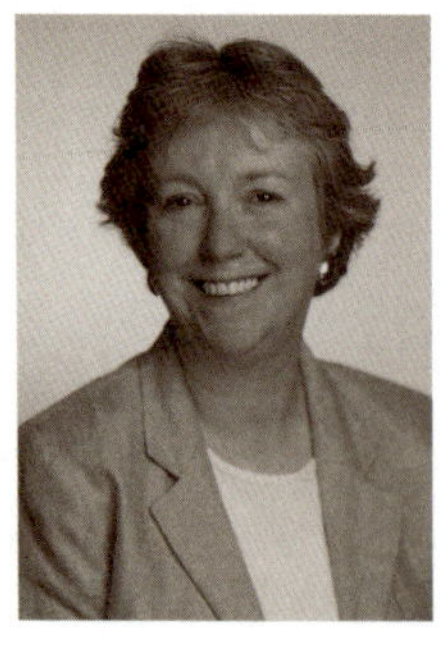

The aim of this book is simple – to help you deal with health problems that worry you and that are difficult for you to discuss with anyone. Almost none of the problems in this book are life-threatening in any way. Most are not painful. Yet they are not frivolous or trivial, because they can profoundly affect your happiness and your perception of yourself. In the following pages, I try to explain each problem, and tell you how you can deal with it yourself and what health professionals (such as your doctor) have to offer. Each section has lists of 'useful contacts' for further information and advice.

There is a lot of 'health information' around and much of it is unreliable, because it is not based on proper research. When I read health articles I always ask myself 'What evidence is this based on?'. So this book has an unusual feature that you will not find in many other health books – I have included 'references', which tell you the source of my information. If you do not believe what I have said, or you want more information, you can check it out by using the references; otherwise, just ignore them. Here is an example of a reference: *British Medical Journal* 2005;330:1194–8. This means that the information came from an article in the *British Medical Journal* in 2005. The volume number that year was 330, and the article was on pages 1194 to 1198. Your local library should be able to help you find the article mentioned in the reference, or you may be able to find it on the internet.

Finally, while I have tried to make this book as helpful and informative as possible, if you have any suggestions to make it even better, email problems@healthpress.co.uk.

Margaret Stearn FRCP

Acne & spots

What is a spot?

The skin contains millions of sebaceous glands that secrete a grease, sebum, through the skin pores onto the surface of the skin. Normally sebum simply helps to keep the skin healthy. A spot forms when a pore becomes blocked by a plug of dead skin cells mixed with sebum. This tends to happen when the sebaceous gland produces more sebum than usual.

- A whitehead is a skin pore that is blocked by a plug deep down.
- A blackhead is a pore that has become plugged at its opening. The black colour is a build-up of the normal skin pigments from dead cells (the same pigment that is responsible for a suntan) – it is not dirt.

The bacteria that normally live on the surface of the skin move into the blocked pore. This can result in pus formation, leading to yellow spots, redness and inflammation. In some people, these inflamed spots can become large and lumpy.

The worst ages for spots are 16–18 years for women and 18–19 years for men, but people of any age can get them

What is the difference between spots and acne?

There is no real difference, it is just a matter of quantity. If you have a few, they are usually referred to as 'spots', 'pimples' or 'zits'. But if you have quite a lot of whiteheads, blackheads or angry-looking inflamed spots, it is referred to as acne.

Why some people get acne

Normal hormone changes at puberty. No one knows why some people's skin secretes more sebum (grease) than others. The sebum-producing glands become particularly active soon after puberty, around the age of 11–14 years, and this is when acne usually starts.

Acne was more severe in teenagers 20 years ago than it is now

Heredity. Acne tends to run in families. If your parent, brother or sister was (or is) an acne sufferer, you are 3–4 times more likely than average to have it yourself. According to a report in the *New Scientist* (21 December 2002), studies of twins have shown that acne is 80% genetic; everything else is relatively unimportant.

Smoking. Smokers have more and worse spots than non-smokers.

Medications. Some drugs can cause acne. The best-known example is anabolic steroids taken by body builders, but phenytoin (for epilepsy), rifampicin (for tuberculosis/TB), vitamin B12 (for anaemia) and lithium (for mood swings) can also produce acne. Occasionally, chemicals in the workplace, such as industrial oils, are responsible.

Contraceptive pill. Most oral contraceptives contain both oestrogen and progesterone. Oestrogen usually improves acne, whereas progesterone can make it worse, so it is not surprising that the pill worsens acne in some people and improves it in others. There are various different types of progesterone, so check the label on your pill packet: 'gestodene', 'desogestrel', 'norgestimate' and the pill containing 'drospirenone' (Yasmin) are good choices.

Polycystic ovary syndrome. If you are a woman, and your periods have become irregular and you have noticed an increase in hairiness of your skin as well as acne, you might have polycystic ovary syndrome (see page 168). This can be treated, so see your doctor if you suspect it.

Environment. Chefs and sauna masseurs find that their hot, humid working environment worsens acne – perhaps by causing further blockage of the pores. Similarly, acne may worsen if you move to a hot country. For this reason, the armed forces are reluctant to enlist individuals who have moderate/severe acne, in case they have to be posted to the tropics.

Common beliefs – true or false?

'Acne is caused by not washing properly'

False. Washing is irrelevant (though over-washing can sometimes make the skin too sensitive to use anti-acne medications).

'Stress worsens acne'

Probably true, though some experts think it is because we fiddle with our skin more when we are stressed. A study of students found that acne was worse at exam time (*Archives of Dermatology* 2003;139:897–900).

'Eating chocolate, sweets or fried foods gives you spots'

False. There is no scientific evidence for this.

'Drinking lots of milk worsens acne'

Possibly true, at least for women (*Journal of the American Academy of Dermatology* 2005;52:207–14). (But remember that milk is good for building strong bones.)

'Masturbation, too much sex or too little sex worsens acne'

False – total myths!

'You can "catch" acne by skin contact, or by using the same flannel or towel as someone with acne'

False. Acne is not infectious.

'Greasy hair causes spots'

False. The hair is greasy for the same reason that the spots are present (which is overproduction of sebum).

'Acne is worse premenstrually'

True. Many women notice their spots are worse during the week before a period. Some women find acne improves during pregnancy, while others find it gets worse.

'Acne runs in families'

True. You are more likely to get it if one of your parents had acne.

'Acne affects only the face, chest and back'

False. Although these are the most common sites, acne can affect almost any part of the body.

'Acne usually clears up on its own'

True. In most people, acne will clear up on its own after 7 or 8 years. But there is no need to wait that long, as effective treatments are available.

'Acne always disappears in the late teens/early 20s'

False. Many 40-year-olds have acne and, in a few people, acne can persist into their 50s and 60s (*Journal of the American Academy of Dermatology* 1999;41:577–580).

'Adults do not get acne'

False. Some adults develop acne for the first time in their 30s, or women may develop it as part of the hormone changes at the menopause. In the past 30 years, severe acne has become less common in teenagers and more common in adults – no one knows why.

'Taking drugs causes acne'

Partly true. The drug ecstasy can cause an outbreak of acne; the spots last for several days. Inhaling solvents can produce spots around the mouth and nose.

'If you are a male with teenage acne, you are more likely to have a heart attack in later life'

False. In fact you are probably slightly less likely to have heart disease than men who have never had acne (*American Journal of Epidemiology* 2005;161:1094–1101).

How you can improve your skin

Be patient. Improving acne takes a long time, even with the most powerful treatments from your doctor. Do not expect much improvement in the first few weeks of any treatment.

Do not squeeze! Discipline yourself not to squeeze or fiddle with your spots, because this encourages scarring. Relaxation techniques may help you break the habit (cassettes, videos or books may be useful).

If you have a large yellow spot containing pus that you feel you really must get rid of, pierce it with a needle and gently squeeze the pus out using a tissue. Wash your hands and sterilize the needle in a flame beforehand.

For blackheads, you can buy a 'comedone spoon'. It has a hole in it, which you press onto the blackhead to release it from the pore; abandon the attempt if the blackhead does not come out easily.

Wash carefully. Wash the affected area twice a day with a pH-balanced, unperfumed soap. Antibacterial soap is no better than ordinary soap, and harsh soaps can irritate some skins. Alternatively, use a gentle antibacterial facewash; a variety of brands are available, and can usually be found alongside the anti-acne products in pharmacies and supermarkets. Avoid facial scrubs and abrasive cleansers, which might increase the inflammation of the skin and make scarring more likely.

Spot creams, gels and lotions. Do not waste your money on anti-acne preparations that simply describe themselves as 'medicated'. Most have very little effect. They are also expensive, and you are likely to need to continue your anti-acne treatment for months or even years. Similarly, expensive creams containing alpha hydroxy acids (also called AHAs or fruit acids) are sometimes advertised for treating acne, but there is little scientific evidence in their favour. The Acne Support Group (see Useful contacts on page 15) says that some cosmetic companies are preying on the vulnerability of acne sufferers, and wants tighter regulation of the cosmetic industry.

Tea tree oil has antibacterial properties, and might be worth trying if your acne is only mild. Apply a small amount of the 5% strength twice a day after washing, taking care to avoid your eyes.

Nicotinamide gel (available from pharmacies) may be helpful if the spots are inflamed, but not very severe.

Benzoyl peroxide. Your best bet is to ask the pharmacist for 2.5% benzoyl peroxide. This zaps skin bacteria, and is available as a cream or gel. The gel releases its active ingredient more effectively than the cream, but is more drying. Before using benzoyl peroxide, draw a diagram of your face on a sheet of paper. Mark in the areas where your spots are, and roughly how many. This will help you later to decide whether the treatment works.

Apply the treatment thinly twice a day after washing, avoiding the lips and eyes. Its main action is to prevent new spots, so apply it over the whole area – do not just dab it on individual spots that are already there. After a week or two, upgrade to the 4% and then the 5–10% strengths, unless you have excessive peeling and redness; some slight peeling is usual. If your skin feels very dry, use the treatment every other day, and use an oil-free moisturizer (for example, Neutrogena Clear Pore, Johnson & Johnson's Clean & Clear) on the alternate days. Keep benzoyl peroxide away from your clothes as it has a bleaching effect; you may also find bleach marks on coloured bed-linen.

After about 2 months, decide whether your spot count has improved by about a third. If it has, continue with the benzoyl peroxide. You may need to continue it for several months. If there has not been improvement, see your family doctor for some stronger treatment.

In 60% of people with acne, their back as well as their face is affected. Applying a cream or gel to the back can be tricky. Acne specialist Professor William Cunliffe suggests applying the cream on your back as far as you can, putting an old T-shirt on, sitting on a hard-backed chair and rubbing your back up and down.

Pore strips. Be cautious with pore strips. These are not really a treatment for acne; they do more harm than good if used on red, inflamed spots. But they can lift out blockages at pore openings (blackheads) and may prevent an inflamed spot developing, in addition to improving the appearance of the skin. The problem is that the adhesive is powerful and can damage sensitive skin. So:

- do not use pore strips more than once a week
- peel the strip off very carefully
- if pulling the strip off is painful, dampen it with water before continuing
- after use, wash your face with a gentle antibacterial wash.

Avoid greasy make-up. If you wear make-up, avoid heavy and greasy make-up; 'oil-free' make-up is available in some ranges. Remove it at night with a gentle cleanser before washing. To disguise an individual spot, use a medicated spot concealer stick or cream a couple of shades lighter than your normal skin tone to counteract any redness. Apply it with a tiny brush to just cover the spot, removing any excess by tapping the area gently with your finger. Do not apply it to a large area or you may make the skin sensitive.

More people in their 20s and 30s seem to have acne these days

Check your contraceptive pill. The label will tell which progestin it contains. The newer progestins – gestodene, desogestrel and norgestimate – are least likely to worsen acne. The pill containing drospirenone (Yasmin) also seems to be a particularly good choice for women with acne. In the USA, the Food and Drug Administration has approved a contraceptive pill containing norgestimate (Ortho Tri-Cyclen) for treating acne in women.

Consider a zinc supplement. One study has shown that zinc may be beneficial in acne that is inflamed (*Dermatology* 2001;203:135–140).

What your doctor can do

Doctors can now offer some effective treatments which was not the case a few years ago.

Seeing your doctor about acne

- Do not feel shy about seeing your doctor. Most doctors are now sympathetic and helpful to people with acne, and recognize how much psychological distress even acne that is not very severe can cause. Tell your doctor how much your spots are upsetting you.
- Getting prompt and effective treatment will lessen the chances of being left with scars. This is really important – acne is usually a temporary problem, but the scars can be permanent.
- Do not expect an immediate miracle from the treatment your doctor will prescribe. Expect a 20% improvement in 2 months, 40% in 4 months and 80% in 8 months.
- Acne treatments usually control rather than cure the condition. This means that if you stop the treatment the acne often reappears, so you may have to continue the treatment for several years.

Tretinoin cream/lotion/gel is an effective treatment if blackheads and whiteheads are the main problem, because it unblocks the pores by removing the build-up of dead skin cells. Apply it thinly at bedtime, because it is partly inactivated by light. There is usually a 60% improvement after 3 months' treatment. In some people, the acne worsens during the first few weeks of treatment, but then improves.

Some peeling and irritation of the skin may occur. If this happens, use a smaller amount or use it less often (for example every other day), or apply it for an hour and then wash it off. Tretinoin can also make your skin sensitive to sunlight, so you should always use an oil-free sunscreen (at least SPF 15) during the day and avoid strong sunlight. Do not apply skin toners, astringents or aftershave to the area. Tretinoin should not be used by women who are pregnant or may become pregnant.

Adapalene and tazarotene are cream or gel treatments that are similar to tretinoin. Like tretinoin, they work for mild-to-moderate acne in which there are blackheads, whiteheads and inflamed spots. The effectiveness of adapalene is similar to tretinoin (60% improvement after 3 months), but it needs to be applied only once a day before bed, and is less irritating than tretinoin. Tazarotene may be slightly more effective, but can be more irritating.

Antibiotics. Antibiotic creams may contain tetracycline, clindamycin or erythromycin. Some antibiotic creams also contain zinc, benzoyl peroxide or tretinoin, which improves their action. Do not go clubbing with tetracycline cream on your face – it fluoresces under ultraviolet light! Unfortunately, acne bacteria are starting to become resistant to these antibiotics (especially erythromycin).

For moderately severe acne, and especially if the spots are inflamed and angry-looking, the usual treatment is antibiotic tablets (usually tetracyclines, but sometimes erythromycin). Unfortunately, to be effective, some tetracyclines have to be taken several times a day, which can be inconvenient. If you think this will be problematic, ask your doctor if a once-daily tetracycline (such as lymecycline, doxycycline or minocycline) would be suitable for you. If you are taking doxycycline, avoid sunlight or you may get a skin rash. A low dose of doxycycline (20 mg twice a day) is effective (*Archives of Dermatology* 2003;139: 459–464).

Antibiotics have to be taken for at least 6 months; the acne will improve gradually over this period. Benzoyl peroxide should be used at the same time. The treatment may need to continue for 2 years or more until the acne improves of its own accord. Do not stop taking antibiotics suddenly as this may cause a flare-up.

Antibiotics can interfere with the contraceptive pill, so women need to use an additional method of contraception. Also, tetracyclines must not be taken during pregnancy, while breastfeeding or by children under 12. Some women develop thrush while taking antibiotics.

At 40 years of age, 5 women in 100 and 1 man in 100 have acne

Azelaic acid cream is another possibility for mild acne. It discourages bacteria, and has some anti-inflammation and anti-blackhead effects.

Hormonal treatment. Women have the option of using hormonal treatment for acne such as Dianette (ethinyloestradiol with cyproterone acetate). This is usually stopped 6 months after the acne has gone. It is a contraceptive pill that blocks the action of the hormone called testosterone (testosterone can encourage the overproduction of sebum). Although it is usually thought of as the 'male' hormone, testosterone also occurs in women's bodies. Diannette carries a higher risk of thrombosis than ordinary low-dose contraceptive pills, so is usually reserved for severe acne.

Ultraviolet (UV) light therapy. Although this may be recommended to you, I advise you not to consider it. It gives only a temporary improvement and, in the process, your skin will start to age and develop wrinkles. When you stop the treatment, the acne is likely to return, leaving you back at square one. And dermatologists are concerned that UV light therapy could increase your risk of skin cancer.

Isotretinoin tablets are the best treatment for severe acne, particularly if it is lumpy. For this, your family doctor will need to refer you to a dermatologist. Isotretinoin is usually very effective as it reduces sebum production, clears the build-up of the dead cells that block the pores and reduces inflammation. It is usually given for 4 months. Around two-thirds of people who use it are then permanently cured; in the others, acne will reappear over the next 18 months (*Clinical Medicine* 2005;5:569–72).

Isotretinoin has some side effects, such as reddening and scaling of the skin, lip soreness, and aching muscles and joints. There have been rumours that isotretinoin might cause severe depression. This is possible, but has not been proved (*Current Problems in Pharmacovigilance* 2006;31:8–9). More research is needed; meanwhile, be aware that depression could be a possible effect of isotretinoin.

Freezing/steroid injection. Lumpy cysts can sometimes be treated by freezing with liquid nitrogen or injecting triamcinolone steroid.

Laser treatment with a 'pulsed-dye' laser (N-Lite) is being used by some dermatologists, though it is not provided by the NHS in the UK. A scientific study (*Journal of the American Medical Association* 2004;291:2834–9) has concluded that it does not improve acne.

The ancient Egyptians relied on a spot cream made from bullocks' bile, ostrich egg, olive oil, salt and plant resin, mixed to a paste with flour and milk

Acne and pregnancy

If you are pregnant or intend to get pregnant, you and your doctor will have to consider your treatment options carefully, because many of the usual anti-acne treatments are not suitable for use during pregnancy.

- Isotretinoin tablets are completely banned if you are pregnant or intending to become pregnant, as isotretinoin can cause abnormalities in the developing fetus. The UK government is now insisting on a 'pregnancy prevention programme' for women prescribed isotretinoin; you should have a pregnancy test before treatment, monthly during treatment and 5 weeks after stopping it, and you must also continue to use contraception for at least a month after stopping it. The US government has similar regulations.
- Tretinoin cream must not be used for the same reason; although it is applied to the skin, a small amount will be absorbed into the bloodstream and could reach the fetus in the womb.

- Tetracycline antibiotics should also not be taken by women who are pregnant or intend to become pregnant. They can damage the developing teeth and bones of the fetus.

Benzoyl peroxide cream or gel is the usual option for treating acne during pregnancy. Another possibility is a solution containing salicylic acid. Erythromycin is the only antibiotic regarded as being safe in pregnancy, but it may not be very effective as many skin bacteria are now resistant to it.

Scarring

Severe acne can leave scars, which will fade with time. Various treatments are available, but none is completely satisfactory.

Laser. If the scars are extensive but not too deep, and the acne has burnt out, laser treatment is a possibility. In the UK, it is difficult (but not impossible) to obtain laser treatment under the NHS, but it is available from private clinics. It is claimed to be particularly effective for flat, 'tissue-paper' scars and for pitted 'ice-pick' scars, but not as good for thick, lumpy scars. However, there is little evidence that it is really effective (*British Journal of Dermatology* 2000;142:413–23), and it is costly in private clinics. If you are considering it, discuss it with your doctor first.

Collagen injections. Some specialist clinics use collagen injections to plump out flat 'tissue-paper' scars and pitted 'ice-pick' scars.

Liquid nitrogen/steroid injection. Lumpy cysts can sometimes be treated by freezing with liquid nitrogen or injecting with triamcinolone steroid. These are not treatments for scars.

Dermabrasion, 'planing down' of the skin using a high-speed wire brush, used to be a common method of dealing with acne scars. It is no longer used very often because of the risk of infection.

Silicone sheets. You can buy silicone sheets ('silicone skin') from pharmacies. You may have to ask your pharmacist to order them. You apply the sheet to your skin like a face mask. It is claimed that this can help lumpy scars, but its effectiveness is questionable.

Surgery. Scars which are deep and disfiguring can sometimes be cut out by a plastic surgeon.

Americans spend $100 million a year buying acne treatments

The future

There is a lot of ongoing research into acne, focusing on the bacteria that cause inflammation. One possibility is to use viruses to kill the bacteria; a virus commonly found on human skin (a type of bacteriophage) can damage acne-producing bacteria and could be used as a treatment in the future. Other researchers have looked at the genetic code of the bacteria, and found the genes responsible for producing enzymes that break down the skin. The next step would be to find a therapy against these enzymes.

Useful contacts

The Australasian College of Dermatologists is the medical college responsible for the training and professional development of medical practitioners in the specialty of dermatology. Its website contains basic information about various skin diseases and problems. It also lists details of individual dermatologists in each State and Territory.
www.dermcoll.asn.au

Health*Insite* is an Australian government initiative aimed to improve the health of Australians by providing easy access to quality information about human health. Follow the link to find information about acne, including causes and treatments.
www.healthinsite.gov.au/topics/Acne

The Acne Support Group is an excellent source of accurate and helpful information. They also raise money for research into acne.
www.m2w3.com/acne

The Acne Support Group also has a website specially for teenagers which provides tips and advice on common problems and reviews of other acne websites.
www.stopspots.org

The National Library of Medicine in the US provides an acne website. It consists mainly of links to other websites dealing with acne.
www.nlm.nih.gov/medlineplus/acne.html

AcneNet is an informative US website containing tips, facts and questions about acne, which is produced in collaboration with the American Academy of Dermatology.
www.skincarephysicians.com/acnenet/

Facefacts is the website of Roche Pharmaceuticals, the company that makes isotretinoin. This is an entertaining and informative site. Look at the 'thingamajig' section, which allows you to make a picture of your face with spots, by 'dragging' various sorts of spots onto the image of a face similar to your own. You can save this picture, and use it to check your progress.
www.facefacts.com

Dermatology in the cinema. Look at this website for stories and images of actors and musicians with acne and other skin problems.
www.skinema.com

www.dermatology.co.uk is a website covering common skin problems. Their acne section is at:
www.dermatology.co.uk/acne/index.asp

US government isotretinoin sheet. The US government Food and Drug Administration has an information sheet about isotretinoin on its website.
www.fda.gov/cder/drug/InfoSheets/patient/IsotretinoinPT.htm

Ageing skin

It is sad that natural changes in the skin as we grow older are often considered unacceptable and embarrassing. In the US alone, more than $12 billion is spent each year on cosmetics to disguise or prevent the signs of ageing. We might think this is due to our youth-fixated western society, but throughout history anti-ageing potions (many of them very bizarre) have been applied to the skin.

How skin ages

Old skin is wrinkled, dry and saggy, and has a mottled colour. In fact, these changes are more to do with exposure to sunlight than with simply getting old. This is why the exposed areas on the hands, face and neck seem to age faster and look less attractive than the smooth and even skin on the tummy.

Skin ages in two ways, through:

- sun damage, which is probably responsible for 80% of skin ageing
- normal ageing – but without sun damage we would probably not develop wrinkles until we were in our 80s.

The sun is very bad for the skin. It makes it thinner and damages its important proteins, such as collagen, which acts as scaffolding to give skin its strength, and elastin, which gives skin its bounce. Even young complexions develop fine wrinkles after sunbathing, giving the skin a coarse, grainy appearance. Collagen also supports the tiny blood vessels in the skin. Weakening of the collagen means the blood vessels show up as broken thread veins ('farmer's face') and bleed more easily; these tiny bruises end up as mottled discoloration. Brownish patches, known as liver spots, gradually develop on sun-exposed areas such as the hands and sides of the forehead.

The French call brown age spots 'les médaillons de cimetière' (cemetery medals)

Looking after your skin as you get older

Skin produces its own natural grease to protect the skin, and to prevent it from losing moisture. As we get older, our skin becomes more fragile, especially in sun-exposed areas, so it desperately needs the greasy protection. Unfortunately, older skin produces less grease, and every time we wash with soap we strip away the natural oils. Bubble baths contain detergent to make the foam, so they also remove oils from the skin.

Here are some hints to keep your skin in good condition.

- Use a sunscreen every day. This will prevent further ageing of your skin.
- Give up smoking.
- Avoid overwashing. As your skin does not sweat as much when you are older and does not produce as much grease, body odour is not such a problem as in younger people.

Obviously, you want to be hygienic, but consider bathing or showering on alternate days instead of daily.

- Use a 'cream bar' or 'cream body wash', rather than a soap.
- Avoid foam baths (bubble baths).
- After bathing or showering, apply a body cream. This is better than using a bath oil, which can make the bath or shower dangerously slippery.

For more information, look at the section on itching on page 183.

In the UK, £545 million is spent on skin care each year (Mintel 2004)

Preventing skin ageing

Stop smoking. One study found that wrinkles are five times more likely in smokers than non-smokers. The skin on the face of a smoker aged 40 resembles that of non-smokers in their 60s. Researchers in Japan have discovered that cigarette smoke reduces the ability of the skin to renew itself, so that less new collagen is produced by skin cells and the breakdown of existing collagen is encouraged (*New Scientist,* 15 April 2000).

Avoid sun exposure. Staying out of the sun as much as possible, wearing a hat that shades the face and using sunscreens will prevent further damage and may also help the skin improve – there is evidence that the skin can repair itself to some extent, if given half a chance.

Check that your sunscreen filters out both UVA and UVB light – look for 'broad spectrum' on the label. UVB light is the most important in causing skin cancer. Both UVB and UVA cause the skin to age, but experts are still arguing about which is more important. The SPF (sun protection factor) number on the bottle indicates the amount of UVB protection a product provides, but it is difficult to know how much UVA protection there will be. Most manufacturers use a star system, with four stars meaning maximum UVA protection.

Ideally, apply a sunscreen every day, not just on holiday or on sunny days, because even quite low but repeated doses of UVA and UVB can wreak havoc on collagen and elastin. Unfortunately, there is no such thing as a safe tan – a tan is a sign that the skin has already been exposed to too much light and is desperately trying to protect itself against further damage. Use fake tans and sunscreen instead.

Improving your diet may help to prevent wrinkles. According to *New Scientist* (14 July 2001), researchers in Australia studied 450 elderly people to see if there was a link between what they ate and how wrinkly they were. The least wrinkly people had been eating lots of vegetables, beans, fish, low-fat milk and tea. The most wrinkly had been eating lots of soft drinks, cakes, pastries, red meat and full-fat dairy produce.

Treatment

Moisturizers cannot prevent or really get rid of wrinkles. They coat the skin with a very thin layer of oil or silicone, which prevents it drying out. If skin is dry, wrinkles are more noticeable, so by keeping the skin moist and plump, moisturizers help to blank out smaller wrinkles. It is best to apply a moisturizer after washing in the morning, while your skin is slightly damp.

Do anti-ageing creams work? It is very difficult to get reliable facts about treatments for ageing skin. Most of the research is done by cosmetic companies, who often keep the results of their research secret. According to Anita Roddick, founder of the Body Shop, anti-ageing skin-care products (except moisturizers) are 'complete pap'. She said 'there is nothing on God's planet that will take away 30 years of arguing with your husband and 40 years of environmental abuse. Anything which says it can magically take away your wrinkles is a scandalous lie' (*The Times* 19 October 2000).

In 1998, the Consumers' Association magazine *Which?* selected 12 ordinary moisturizers and 12 anti-ageing creams. Four women tested each product, according to the manufacturers' instructions, for 4 weeks without knowing which product they were using. Most of the women did not notice any difference in the look or feel of their skin. Ten of the 48 women using anti-ageing creams reported an improvement, but even more of those who had used moisturizers – 18 out of 48 – noticed the same thing. Three-quarters of all the women thought that they had been using a simple moisturizer. *Which?* concluded that 'some of the claims made for the ingredients of anti-ageing creams can be substantiated but, in the low concentrations used in the creams, they are unlikely to do more than moisturize your skin'.

However, cosmetic companies are doing a lot of research, so some of the recent products may help. Nevertheless, it is hard to know whether claims are justified.

Fewer British women use anti-wrinkle cream than French, Spanish or German women (Mintel 2004)

Oestrogen makes skin look younger. Doctors in Germany guessed the ages of women around the menopause and then measured their oestrogen levels. The higher their oestrogen level, the younger they appeared. The women with the highest levels looked 8 years younger than they really were, whereas those with the lowest levels were guessed to be 8 years older than their true age. Oestrogen makes the skin thicker and increases its collagen and water content, making it less dry and flaky. So hormone replacement therapy (HRT) containing oestrogen will probably help to minimize skin ageing. However, the risks of HRT (such as breast cancer and stroke) mean that it should not be taken for cosmetic reasons.

Retinoids, such as tretinoin and isotretinoin, are chemicals that are related to vitamin A. They make the skin produce new cells more quickly, so it becomes thicker and more compact. The skin also produces more collagen but less pigment (melanin). After a month or two of using retinoids, the skin becomes smoother, fine wrinkles are repaired, age spots fade and the skin colour becomes more even, but it does not produce totally wrinkle-free skin. If you carry on using the cream, the skin continues to improve for a few more months, but after 6 months of use there is no further change. If you stop using it, the skin gradually goes back to how it was before. Retinoids do not have any effect on very noticeable wrinkles, such as the deep lines that appear between the nose and mouth, or on thread veins.

Some anti-ageing creams contain retinoids ('retinol'), but to obtain the most effective concentrations, you need a doctor's prescription. However, doctors cannot prescribe tretinoin for sun-damaged skin under the NHS in the UK, so you will have to ask your doctor for a private prescription. For the first 2 weeks, you apply it every other night, for the next few weeks you apply it every night and, after a few weeks, two or three nights a week is enough. If there is no improvement after 6 months, there is no point in continuing.

Retinoids irritate the skin, so that there may be dryness and flakiness, sometimes with itching, soreness, redness and a tight feeling. You have to avoid the sun and use a sunscreen. Some specialists worry that retinoids could increase the risk of skin cancer.

How effective is tretinoin cream?

A study of 251 people, aged 29–50 years, with sun-damaged skin showed that tretinoin cream used once a day for 6 months (*Archives of Dermatology* 1991;127(5):659–65):

- produced some type of improvement in 79%; however, 48% of people who used only sunscreen and moisturizers also showed improvement
- made the skin 29.3% less rough
- faded age spots by 37%
- improved wrinkles by 27.1% (measured by taking silicone impressions of the skin).

Verdict: in spite of the hype, tretinoin will not change your skin radically, but it may produce some improvement.

Alpha hydroxy acids (AHAs) are chemicals found in fruit juices (thus their name 'fruit acids'), wine, sugar cane and milk. They may be the 'magic ingredient' of skin ancient recipes containing milk, lemons or wine. AHAs improve the appearance of the skin by speeding up the shedding of dead cells from the skin surface. AHAs have very little effect on wrinkles, though some researchers claim that they make the skin thicker, help it to hold moisture and improve the elastin.

Many face creams now include AHAs. When buying such a cream, check the concentration of AHAs. Any cream containing less than 5% is not very effective, but the safest to use. A cream containing 5–10% AHAs is probably more effective, but scientists worry that, in the long term, this concentration might damage your skin, and you might end up with more wrinkles rather than fewer. For the first few weeks of use, AHAs may make the skin slightly flaky. If the cream is very acid, it may cause more irritation, so look for a pH of 3.5 or higher (the higher the pH, the lower the acidity).

So are AHAs safe? The US Food and Drug Administration (FDA) is concerned about them and is doing more research (see Useful contacts on page 23) and the European Commission (EC) is looking into the matter. So at the moment, we simply do not know. The main worries are that:

- they damage the skin by penetrating its defensive barrier; if you find that products containing AHAs cause irritation, stinging, burning, redness or swelling round the eyes, stop using them immediately

- because they make the skin sensitive to sunlight, they could increase the risk of further skin damage and of skin cancer; so they might actually speed up skin ageing.

If you use an AHA product, use a SPF 15 sunscreen as well, every day, even if the weather is overcast, and choose a cream with a low AHA concentration.

Cleopatra used red wine, now known to contain alpha hydroxy acids, on her face

Beta hydroxy acids (BHAs) are similar to AHAs, but may be less likely to irritate the skin. The most common is salicylic acid.

Labelling of skin-care products

Check for these words on skin cream labels – they mean alpha or beta hydroxy acids:

- mixed fruit acids
- triple fruit acids
- tri-alpha hydroxy fruit acids
- L-alpha hydroxy acids
- malic acid
- citric acid
- glycolic acid
- lactic acid
- hydroxycaprylic acid or alpha-hydroxycaprylic acid
- glycolic acid + ammonium glycolate
- alpha-hydroxyoctanoic acid
- sugar cane extract
- salicylic acid.

Vitamin C is essential for the production of collagen. It also encourages the renewal of skin cells and is an antioxidant, which means that it mops up free radicals. Free radicals are molecules produced by the body's metabolism, particularly when it has to deal with pollution in the environment. Free radicals can be harmful and may contribute to skin ageing. Vitamin C is a very unstable vitamin that is broken down by light and does not penetrate the skin readily, so cosmetic companies have had great difficulty making skin preparations containing it. However, they seem to have cracked the problem, and skin preparations containing vitamin C are now available. Whether they really do reduce ageing changes in the skin remains to be seen.

Botulinum toxin (Botox) injections have become a well-known anti-wrinkle treatment. Botulinum toxin is actually a powerful poison that blocks the action of nerve fibres. This causes a mini-paralysis of the muscles used for facial expression that crease the skin. By pinpointing a specific area, such as 'crow's feet' and frown lines, the specialist can smooth out the skin –

you do not have frown lines because you cannot frown. The effect is not immediate (it may take a week or two to show) and is mainly gone in 4 months.

Like any other procedure, it has some risks. If it is not done properly you could end up looking rather expressionless, or one side of your face could look different from the other. As with any cosmetic procedure, it is important to find a good doctor (see page 339 for general advice).

Fillers, such as collagen, injected into the skin fill in hollows and can help smooth out lines, including deep wrinkles such as nose-to-mouth grooves and frown lines. Collagen is absorbed by the body, so the effect does not last and the treatment has to be repeated every 3–6 months. It can be painful, and may cause bruising; there is often some redness and swelling on the day of the injection, which fades by the following day. Some people develop hard, red blotches as a result of an allergic reaction. The collagen comes from cattle, and there have been concerns that it could trigger an autoimmune reaction (in which the body attacks its own cells), but there is no evidence that this has ever happened to anyone.

Collagen is not the only type of filler – about 40 other substances are used (*New England Journal of Medicine* 2004;350:1526–34).

Chemical peeling with AHAs (glycolic peel) is another treatment provided by some private clinics. It went out of fashion for a while (when laser resurfacing seemed more promising), but is now regaining popularity. Chemical peeling works by producing a chemical burn on the surface of the skin. As the skin heals, some of the smaller wrinkles and irregularities are smoothed out and there is some improvement in the appearance.

Laser resurfacing of the skin removes part of the outer layer of the skin (the epidermis). This regrows in 3–6 weeks from the remnants left in the hair follicles and sweat glands. During this time, you will look as if you have severe sunburn, as your skin will be red and there may be some weeping. The repair process alters the skin collagen, 'lifting' mini-wrinkles from the skin during the subsequent 4 months. Afterwards, you must always use sunscreen to protect your skin.

There may be side effects, such as lightening or darkening of the skin. In people whose skin tends to form keloid scars (see page 224), laser treatment is risky. There is also a risk of reactivating herpes (cold sores).

Because these skin techniques are so new, discoveries are still being made about the best methods, and what they can and cannot do, and their long-term effects. As with all cosmetic operations and procedures, try to choose a reputable clinic and a well-known doctor; your family doctor may be able to advise you (see page 339). Ask to see 'before and after' photos, and check that the procedures were carried out by the person you are talking to, and are not simply promotional material supplied by the laser manufacturer.

Plastic surgery was the only option before retinoids became available. It can produce a big improvement in lines at the sides of the eyes and in sagging skin (which retinoids will not help), but will not improve the overall texture of the skin. As with all plastic surgery, make sure you choose a reputable clinic (see page 339). Ask to see 'before and after' photos, and check that the doctor you are talking to actually did the work shown.

Skin tags

As we get older, we often develop small skin tags. About 50–60% of people over the age of 50 have them. Sometimes they run in families. Their medical name is *fibro-epithelial polyps* or *achondrochordons*.

Skin tags are soft lumps attached to the skin by a stalk. They are the same colour as your skin, and are usually under 0.5 cm in size. They tend to occur in the armpits, neck and groin. You may have only one, but usually there are several.

They do not turn into cancer and they are not dangerous. However, they look unsightly and they can be a nuisance (catching on clothing or jewellery), so you may wish to get rid of them.

There is no way of preventing new skin tags developing, but your family doctor can deal with those that you already have. There are various ways of doing this, such as snipping them off (but do not try this yourself) or freezing with liquid nitrogen.

The Ebers papyrus, an ancient Egyptian papyrus from 1550 BC, has a recipe to cure wrinkles, made from pistachio nuts, wax, poppy seed oil and grass

'Liver spots' ('age spots')

'Liver spots' are like large freckles on the backs of the hands. They are sometimes also called 'age spots', but the medical term is *solar lentigines*. They may be up to 1 cm across in size. They are very common after middle age and are caused by exposure to the sun, which accounts for the word 'solar' in their medical name).

Preventing age spots. To prevent age spots, you need to use an SPF 15–20 sunscreen on the backs of your hands, but by the time you are bothered by them, it is too late. However, using sunscreen should help to prevent new ones occurring.

Selenium is an antioxidant chemical found in Brazil nuts, fish and kidney. Some people think that selenium prevents age spots, but there is no scientific evidence for this.

Getting rid of age spots. If you are very self-conscious about age spots on your hands, you could try 0.1% tretinoin cream (related to vitamin A), for which you need a doctor's prescription. It can cause irritation. If it does, use it less frequently (every other day, or every third day), or ask your doctor for a weaker cream. However, tretinoin will probably not make the age spots disappear completely; a study published in the *Archives of Dermatology* (1991;127:666–72) showed that it faded them by about 37%. More information about tretinoin is given on page 19.

Some anti-ageing hand creams now contain retinol, a natural form of vitamin A, similar to tretinoin. The concentration in these creams varies, and they are likely to be less effective than the 0.1% tretinoin cream, but less likely to irritate your skin.

Occasionally, large age spots can be treated by laser or chemical peels.

Suspicious-looking spots

Ask your doctor to check any dark spot that enlarges, changes colour, becomes itchy or bleeds. This is to make sure that it is not a melanoma cancer.

Useful contacts

The Australasian College of Dermatologists website contains basic information about various skin diseases and problems. It has a helpful section on cosmetic dermatology under 'A–Z of skin'.
www.dermcoll.asn.au

The Cancer Council Australia website has a range of evidence-based position statements under 'SunSmart' that communicate key cancer issues on skin protection. The organization also offers a comprehensive range of high quality, affordable sun protection products, which are available for purchase online or from State and Territory Cancer Council shops.
www.cancer.org.au

Health*Insite* is an Australian government initiative aimed to improve the health of Australians by providing easy access to quality information about human health. Follow the link to find information on cosmetic treatments, including plastic and cosmetic surgery, cosmetic dentistry and tattooing.
www.healthinsite.gov.au/topics/Cosmetic_Treatments

New Zealand Dermatological Society website is an excellent source of information about many skin problems. Its section on cosmetic dermatology deals with anti-ageing creams and wrinkle treatments.
www.dermnetnz.org/dna.cosderm/index.html

US Food and Drug Administration is a US government organization. Its website has detailed information about the safety of AHAs.
www.cfsan.fda.gov/~dms/cosbhaha.html

British Association of Aesthetic and Plastic Surgeons (BAAPS) will send you a fact sheet on cosmetic surgery and a list of their members. The list is also on their very informative website, which also gives details of common cosmetic surgery procedures, including facelifts and Botox, and tells you the risks and limitations of each.
www.baaps.org.uk

The American Society for Aesthetic Plastic Surgery can provide the names and qualifications of surgeons in all areas of the USA. Its website has information about botulinum toxin ('injectables') and chemical peels.
www.surgery.org/public/procedures.php

Lasercare are a chain of clinics providing laser treatments in the UK. They are private, but some are based in NHS hospitals. Their website has a page on lines and wrinkles.
www.lasercare-clinics.co.uk

Anal bleeding

Bleeding from the back passage is something that you should always see your doctor about, even if you are convinced it is piles (see page 212) or an anal fissure (see page 30). The reason you need to be checked is that bleeding from the back passage can be a symptom of bowel (colon or rectum) cancer. If you are worried about being examined in that area, look at the section on seeing your doctor about an anal problem on page 338.

In general, if the bleeding is bright red and you have anal pain, especially when you pass a stool, it is probably a non-serious condition such as anal fissure or piles – but your doctor needs to make sure.

What do you know about bowel cancer?

A survey by BUPA, a private healthcare organization in the UK, showed that people do not know much about bowel cancer. When prompted with a list of eight possible symptoms, only 57% of men and 70% of women in the UK named rectal bleeding as one of the main symptoms of bowel cancer. In 2006–2007, the UK Government is spending £37 million sending home-testing kits for blood in the faeces to people aged 60–69 years. The aim is to detect bowel cancer early. So if you receive a kit, use it and return according to the instructions.

If the bleeding is dark red, or in clots, or mixed with a lot of slime, or mixed in with the faeces, it could be a more serious condition (such as colitis, diverticular disease or cancer of the rectum or colon) that needs prompt treatment. Other symptoms that might be serious are a decreased frequency and/or hardness of the faeces, or an increased frequency and/or looseness of faeces.

Useful contacts

Colorectal Surgical Society of Australasia has some very useful information on diseases of the colon and rectum on its website under 'Patient info'. Brochures may also be purchased through their online order form.
www.cssa.org.au

The Cancer Council Australia website has an evidence-based position statement on 'Bowel cancer'. There is also an informative section on the website on cancer prevention and early detection.
www.cancer.org.au

Health*Insite* is an Australian government initiative aimed to improve the health of Australians by providing easy access to quality information about human health. Follow the link to find resources that provide an overview about bowel cancer, with further links to topics such

as prevention, treatment and risk factors for bowel cancer.
www.healthinsite.gov.au/topics/Bowel_Cancer

American Academy of Family Physicians have two detailed articles on 'Common Anorectal Conditions' on their website. The articles are intended for doctors, and explain how doctors examine the anus. They discuss itching, pain, bleeding, lumps, constipation and incontinence of faeces.
www.aafp.org/afp/20010615/2391.html
www.aafp.org/afp/20010701/77.html

Digestive Disorders Foundation is a UK non-profit organization that provides reliable information about all gut problems. They supply a range of leaflets, which are available on the 'Patients info leaflets' section of the website.
www.digestivedisorders.org.uk

National Digestive Diseases Information Clearinghouse is a US government organization. Its website has pages on piles (haemorrhoids/hemorrhoids), constipation and other gut problems.
www.digestive.niddk.nih.gov/ddiseases/a-z.asp

The American Gastroenterological Association is an organization for doctors who specialize in the gut. Look in the Patient Center of the website for excellent information about various gut problems including piles (haemorrhoids) and constipation.
www.gastro.org/clinicalRes/brochures/hemorrhoids.html

The Imperial Cancer Research Fund is a UK organization. Its website has a section on bowel cancer.
www.cancerhelp.org.uk/help/menuforthistopic.asp?page=2786

Beating Bowel Cancer is a UK non-profit organization that provides information about all aspects of bowel cancer, Its lively website is worth a look.
www.beatingbowelcancer.org

Colon Cancer Prevention is a US non-profit organization that provides information about screening and prevention. Not all the information applies to all countries.
www.coloncancerprevention.org

Anal itching

Anal itching may be just an annoyance, or may be so troublesome that it dominates your life. It is usually made worse by warmth, and is often most troublesome in bed. The skin round the anus easily becomes irritated and inflamed. This is because it is difficult to keep the area round the anus clean and dry; the skin is crinkly and traps tiny faecal particles. It is also sweaty and airless, and it may be moist from an anal or vaginal discharge. When it becomes irritated, scratching is a natural reaction, but this damages the skin further – the itch/scratch cycle. Ointments and creams can cause further problems by keeping the area damp.

Although it is very unpleasant, anal itching seldom means anything serious. If you have pain as well as itching, look at the section on anal pain (see page 30).

Causes of anal itching

Washing too much or not enough. Poor hygiene can be responsible for anal itching, but so can excessive cleaning, especially if you use harsh soaps or a brush.

Leakage of faeces can lead to itching around the anus. Look at the section on faecal incontinence (see page 123) for more information.

Pre-moistened toilet tissues (wipes), bought from chemists and supermarkets, can sometimes cause anal itching. The reason is probably perfume, alcohol or a preservative in the wipes.

Sensitivities and allergies to other chemicals, such as bubble baths and perfumed soaps, may be responsible.

Ointments and creams are notorious causes of anal itching. If you have itching, it is a natural reaction to buy an anaesthetic gel for the anal area. Most of these are labelled 'for haemorrhoids' and contain lignocaine, tetracaine, cinchocaine, pramocaine or benzocaine with other ingredients. At first they help, but then the itching may return because you have become sensitive to one of the ingredients in the cream or ointment and they are keeping the area moist. Do not use them for more than a week.

Skin conditions, such as psoriasis or eczema, can affect the skin round the anus and cause itching. Piles (see page 212) can sometimes be itchy, partly because of the slimy discharge they produce.

Fungal infections, similar to thrush or athlete's foot, are another common cause. Fungi love warm, damp and damaged skin, so if you have an itchy anus for any reason and then damage the skin by scratching, fungi can take hold and make it worse.

Sexually transmitted infections are what many people worry about, but are not usually the reason.

- Genital warts (vulva or penis), caused by papillomavirus, thrive in warm, moist conditions such as the skin near the anus and can be very itchy (see page 135).
- Genital herpes (caused by herpes virus) can also infect the anus, and causes itching just before the sores appear and also during the healing stage (see page 131).

Both these viruses are easily transferred on the fingers to the anal skin, and can therefore occur round the anus in anyone. The anus may be the only site of infection; the fact that you do not have genital warts or herpes elsewhere does not rule them out.

Threadworms (pinworms) are tiny worms, about 13 mm long, which live in the lower part of the bowel. They are very common – an estimated 40 million cases in the US alone. The female worms creep out of the anus at night – how they know it is night, and why they come out only at night, is a mystery. They lay thousands of eggs on the skin of the anus, causing intense itching at night. When you scratch, the eggs lodge under your fingernails, and it is easy to transfer them to your mouth and reinfect your gut by swallowing the eggs.

Certain foods can irritate the anus during defecation. Beer and curry are obvious examples. Some people find that citrus fruits, grapes, tomatoes, coffee or tea can cause problems.

Anxiety tends to make the brain hyper-alert to body feelings that we may otherwise be able to ignore. If you are going through an anxious period, a symptom such as itching can become magnified.

Pleasure. It is worth asking yourself whether you are deriving a perverse, almost erotic, pain/pleasure from scratching the itchy area, which is keeping the irritation going.

How you can help yourself

- Wash the anal area after you have had your bowels open, but not more than three times in a day, using an unperfumed soap and water. Some doctors recommend using aqueous cream (available from pharmacies) as a cleanser. Apply the cream, massage it gently over the area and then rinse off. If you are somewhere where you cannot wash, clean the area with wet tissues (but not with pre-moistened wipes). If you use shower gel to wash your body, make sure you rinse it off very thoroughly so that none remains between the buttocks.
- Dab gently with a soft towel to dry – do not rub. If drying is difficult, use a hairdryer on cool setting.
- Do not put any disinfectant on the skin or in the bath water – this can irritate the skin. Do not use bubble bath – the perfume can irritate. Instead, put a handful of kitchen salt in your bath.
- Keep a cottonwool ball, dusted with powder, against the anus, inside your underpants or panties. Use baby powder (not perfumed talcum powder) to dust it. Change it each time you wash.
- Wear loose cotton underwear. Avoid tights and elastic 'shapewear' underwear, because they encourage sweating and moistness in the anal area. Avoid anything that keeps the buttocks close together.
- Do not use biological (enzyme) washing powders for your underwear, or perfumed fabric softeners. Instead, use a detergent labelled 'for sensitive skin'.
- Do not scratch. If you scratch, you damage the skin more and then you itch more. If you feel you really must scratch, try pinching the skin near the anus between your thumb and forefinger through your clothing; this is less damaging than actual scratching. People

often scratch at night and do not realize they are doing so. If you think you might be scratching at night, talk to your doctor about taking an antihistamine, keep your fingernails short, wear cotton gloves at night for a while and ask your doctor to check for threadworms.

- Do not use any greasy creams (such as Vaseline) on the area. Greasy creams keep the skin soggy and make the problem worse.
- Be very cautious about anaesthetic creams or ointments. Sometimes they can help by relieving the itch/scratch cycle, but use them only for a short period (about a week).
- Similarly, be very cautious about steroid creams. In the UK, it is possible to buy weak steroid cream (containing hydrocortisone 1% or less) from pharmacies. In the short term, the steroid reduces inflammation and therefore relieves itching but, in the long term, it can make the skin thinner and worsen the problem. Resist the temptation to keep on using a steroid cream. Use it for just a week, then throw the tube away.
- Try witch hazel – an old-fashioned remedy available from pharmacies. Dab it on twice a day, but stop immediately if it seems to be making the problem worse instead of better.
- Dr James Le Fanu has a column in the UK *Daily Telegraph* that acts as a forum for readers' solutions to health problems. Readers have reported that the inside of a banana skin can relieve itchy skin, including anal itching.
- Feel round the anus for lumps. This may not be easy, because the skin round the anus is normally puckered. A lump might be a wart, a pile or a skin tag alongside an anal fissure.
- Avoid foods that cause excessive flatulence (see page 331).

How your doctor can help

If you are anxious about being examined by your doctor, look at the section seeing your doctor about an anal problem on page 338. Your doctor can check to see whether you have any conditions such as piles (haemorrhoids), anal fissure, warts, psoriasis, eczema, fungal infections or other infections that need treatment.

If you scratch at night, an antihistamine taken before you go to bed can help. Antihistamines relieve itching and some also tend to make you drowsy.

Discuss with your doctor whether you might have threadworms (pinworms). These can be eliminated with mebendazole. You may need several treatments at monthly intervals, because the eggs can persist for several weeks in the environment (*Prescriber* 2006;17(15):24–32). The other members of your household will also need to be treated, and you should also wash your hands and scrub your nails before eating and after each visit to the toilet, and wash the anal area in the morning to get rid of any eggs deposited during the night.

An ointment containing a chemical found in chilli peppers (capsaicin) is an effective treatment for very troublesome anal itching (*Gut* 2003;52:1233–5), but the researchers used a special very dilute ointment (0.006%) that is not generally available.

If nothing helps, your doctor might consider referring you to a specialist for injection of a chemical called methylene blue into the anal area. So far, research has involved only a small number of patients, but it worked in 80% (*Surgery* 2006;24(4):145–7). More research is awaited to find out how long the relief will last.

Useful contacts

Colorectal Surgical Society of Australasia has some very useful information on diseases of the colon and rectum on its website under 'Patient info'. Brochures may also be purchased through their online order form.
www.cssa.org.au

Health*Insite* is an Australian government initiative aimed to improve the health of Australians by providing easy access to quality information about human health. Follow the link below to find information relating to rectal diseases, including haemorrhoids.
www.healthinsite.gov.au/topics/Rectal_Diseases

American Academy of Family Physicians have two detailed articles on 'Common Anorectal Conditions' on their website. The articles are intended for doctors. They explain how doctors examine the anus. They discuss itching, pain, bleeding, lumps, constipation and incontinence of faeces.
www.aafp.org/afp/20010615/2391.html
www.aafp.org/afp/20010701/77.html

Bowel control. This website is provided by St Mark's Hospital, UK, which is a hospital specializing in bowel problems. The site covers faecal leakage, constipation and wind. It is a first-rate site that is very practical and informative.
www.bowelcontrol.org.uk

Digestive Disorders Foundation is a UK non-profit organization that provides reliable information about all gut problems. They supply a range of leaflets, which are available on the 'Patients info leaflets' section of the website.
www.digestivedisorders.org.uk

Pfizer, the manufacturers of Anusol, have a very pleasant website about piles.
www.pilesadvice.co.uk

Wyeth Pharmaceuticals, the manufacturers of Preparation H for piles, have an informative and entertaining website. Look at the symptoms section, which includes a page on 'Doctor's examination' (rectal examination).
www.preparationh.co.uk

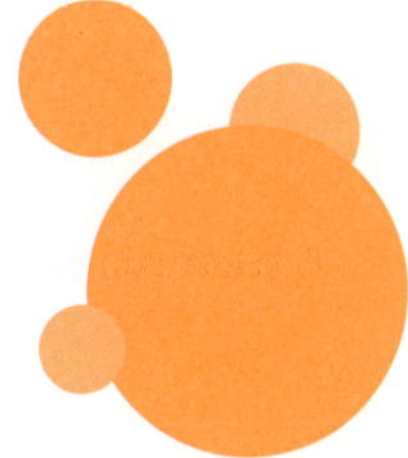

Anal pain

Pain coming from the bottom area is not something that we are used to feeling and, as a consequence, anal pain can cause a lot of worries.

What sort of pain is it?

- A knife-like pain when you have your bowels open, and which may last for 10–15 minutes afterwards, is probably caused by an anal fissure. Some people describe it as like 'passing glass'. In addition to the pain, you may notice some bright red blood on the toilet paper.
- A similar knife-like pain can be caused by herpes simplex virus.
- A nagging, aching discomfort made worse by defecation could be due to piles.
- A throbbing pain, worsening over a few days, and bad enough to disturb your sleep, is likely to be caused by an abscess.
- An occasional, severe, cramp-like pain deep in the anal canal, lasting about half an hour, is probably a condition called proctalgia fugax.
- A continuous aching pain in the anus needs to be sorted out by your doctor. It is most often caused by a back problem (when a part of the spine presses on a nerve).

Anal fissure

An anal fissure is a split in the anal skin, just inside the anus, usually towards the back. The pain of an anal fissure feels like being cut with glass when you have your bowels open and afterwards. It is worse when you have had a hard bowel motion. You may notice some bright red blood on the toilet paper at the same time. You may be able to feel a small lump alongside the crack; this is a 'skin tag'.

Anal fissures are most common in teenagers and young adults, and there has often been a period of constipation beforehand. Sometimes they follow childbirth. They usually heal on their own, but this often takes several weeks and the scar may split again.

What you can do. Do not feel anxious about the fissure. Although it is horribly painful, it is not a dangerous condition.

- Avoid constipation – this is very important. Keep your faeces soft by eating lots of bran cereals, fruit and vegetables.
- Smear some painkilling gel around the area just before you have your bowels open. You can buy a suitable painkilling gel from a pharmacy; they are sometimes labelled 'for piles' or 'for haemorrhoids'. It will prevent the anus going into a spasm, which can make the problem worse. Do not use the gel at any other time, or for more than a week, because you can easily develop an allergy to its ingredients. If you notice soreness and itching, in addition to the sharp pain, it is quite likely that the gel is responsible.

- Warm baths twice daily can help, if you have the time. Put a handful of ordinary kitchen salt into the bath.

How your doctor can help. You should see your doctor if the problem is not improving after 3 weeks. If you feel anxious about this, look at the section on seeing your doctor about an anal problem (see page 338). For some treatments, your doctor will need to send you to the 'rectal clinic' at your local hospital. Some treatments your doctor may use are listed below.

- Glyceryl trinitrate ointment, applied several times a day for 6 weeks, seems to heal the fissure in 60–70% of cases. However, about 50% of the people using this treatment get a headache as a side effect.
- A gel containing the drug diltiazem is being tried in some hospitals. It can help people who do not respond to glyceryl trinitrate.
- Some specialist hospitals have been using injections of botulinum toxin (Botox) into the muscle of the anus. Botulinum toxin prevents spasm of the muscle, because it blocks transmission of nerve impulses to the muscle. This treatment is not widely available. Healing rates are about 69–90%, but it needs more research to see how effective it is in the long term.
- The most common treatment (before glyceryl trinitrate ointment came on the scene) used to be a small operation under a general anaesthetic. The operation is designed to overcome the spasm of the anal muscle. The pain relief is dramatic and instantaneous. In the past, this operation could leave you less able to control wind, but a new type of operation (tailored sphincterotomy) does not have this drawback (*British Journal of Surgery* 2005;92:403–8).

Unfortunately, the fissure comes back within 3–4 months in about one-third of people treated with glyceryl trinitrate or diltiazem, and in about 40% of people after treatment with botulinum toxin (*Gastroenterology* 2002;123:112–7). Surgery seems to be the best long-term cure and is effective in about 90% of cases.

Herpes virus infection

A herpes virus infection can produce a pain similar to an anal fissure. Herpes can infect the anal area, either spread by the hands from a cold sore on the face, or transmitted as a sexual infection (see page 131). It can occur in homosexuals or in heterosexuals by spread from the genital area. At the anus, herpes often forms a crack rather than the small ulcers that tend to occur elsewhere. It can occur in individuals who have never had herpes elsewhere. The soreness occurs in episodes, each lasting for a few days. A sexual health clinic will be able to take a swab to check for the virus if you visit the clinic as soon as an episode starts; if you are worried about the thought of visiting a clinic, take a look at the section on visiting the clinic on page 335, otherwise see your family doctor.

Abscess

An abscess close to the anus produces a throbbing pain that worsens over a few days, and is usually bad enough to disturb your sleep. You may be able to feel a tender swelling in the skin beside the anus, or the abscess may be hidden inside. This is unlikely to go away on its own; it needs to be lanced by a doctor.

Proctalgia fugax

Proctalgia fugax is a severe, cramp-like pain, deep in the anal canal. It usually lasts for less than a minute, but can sometimes last for up to half an hour. Most sufferers have only 5 or 6 attacks a year. You may feel a need to defecate urgently, but nothing happens. It may even make you feel dizzy, or give you a headache. It occurs in both men and women. The pain often wakes sufferers at night, and men may have an erection at the same time. Some men experience it after sex. It is a mysterious condition; no one knows what causes it, but it is probably a spasm of the rectal or pelvic floor muscles and does not mean that you have anything seriously wrong. There are various methods of relieving the pain.

- Try putting pressure on the perineum (the area between the back passage and the vagina or base of the penis) by sitting on the edge of your bath or on a tennis ball.
- Sit in hot water or, alternatively, apply some ice.
- Two paracetamol tablets and a hot drink may give some relief.

The problem with medications for proctalgia fugax is that the episode is likely to be over before the drugs become active. They might be worth trying if your attacks last a long time. Possible treatments are glyceryl trinitrate spray or under-the-tongue tablets (as used for angina), glyceryl trinitrate cream applied to the anal area, or the asthma drug salbutamol (inhaled from a puffer at the start of the attack). These treatments are only available on prescription, for which you would need to see your doctor.

Bad breath

Most people worry about having bad breath, which is also known as halitosis, as shown by the huge sales of breath fresheners. However, it is not easy to tell whether you have it or not.

There is actually a psychological condition called delusion of halitosis or halitophobia, in which people have an unshakeable belief that their breath smells, although in fact it does not. Their lives are totally dominated by their 'bad breath' and they are not amenable to reason.

How to decide whether you have bad breath

If you think that you have bad breath, it is worth finding out what the true situation is. 'Fresh breath centres' have been set up in some cities in the UK, where the smelly chemicals in your breath are measured by a 'halimeter'. But there are other ways of deciding whether you have bad breath, such as the following.

- If you find your gums bleed when you brush or floss your teeth, it is almost certain that you have bad breath as well.
- Inspect your gums to see if they look red and swollen in places; if they do, it is likely you have bad breath.
- If you are a smoker you probably have smoker's breath.
- It is sometimes suggested that you can detect your own bad breath by breathing out through your mouth into a paper bag, and then breathing in rapidly from the bag through your nose. You might catch a whiff by this method, but usually it does not work because your nose is so used to your own breath smell.
- Put your tongue out as far as you can; lick your upper arm, or the inner surface of your wrist, wait 4 seconds and smell where you licked.
- Buy a BreathAlert device. You breathe into the battery-operated device and it gives a reading in terms of one of four grades from 'none' to 'strong'.
- Put a piece of gauzy cloth on your tongue, as far back as you can, for a few moments. Take it out, let it dry and then sniff it.
- Ask your dentist or dental hygienist; they are very used to being asked this question.
- Ask your partner or a close friend.

Many chemicals cause the smell in bad breath including hydrogen sulphide, methyl mercaptan and putrescine.

What causes bad breath

'Morning breath'. Almost everyone has bad breath first thing in the morning. During the day, movement of the tongue and cheeks dislodges food debris and dead cells, and these are washed away by saliva. While we are asleep our tongue and cheeks do not move much, and the flow of saliva is reduced. The food residues stagnate in the mouth, and mouth bacteria rapidly break them down, releasing an unpleasant stale smell. Breathing through the mouth when sleeping tends to make this worse. Morning breath normally disappears after breakfast, cleaning the teeth or rinsing the mouth with water. Get your saliva going with a drink of water and lemon.

Temporary bad breath is the lingering effect of cigarettes or something you have eaten or drunk in the past 24–48 hours. Alcohol, onions, cabbage, broccoli, radish, durian, garlic, curries and other highly spiced foods, cured foods such as salamis, and smoked foods such as kippers are particularly likely to remain on the breath. The problem is not simply that the smells stay in the mouth. These foods are digested and then broken down in the body, and the breakdown products of some, particularly alcohol, onions and garlic, are expelled in the breath for hours or days afterwards. (This is the basis of the 'breathalyser test' for alcohol.)

Smoking also reduces the flow of saliva, which makes its smell linger even longer.

Traditional remedies (such as eating parsley) can help, and mouth fresheners disguise the smell. Clean your mouth by rinsing it thoroughly with warm water, giving it a good brushing with toothpaste and then rinsing thoroughly again.

Bad breath can even result from not eating. When no food is available, the body starts breaking down fat. Waste products from fat breakdown, called ketones, are expelled in the breath, and smell like stale apples.

Garlic rubbed into the soles of the feet can be detected later in the breath.

Persistent bad breath

Gum disease, according to dentists, is the usual cause of persistent bad breath. Gum disease is not always painful, so we may not know we have it. The gum is likely to bleed when you brush your teeth. It will look very red, but goes pale for a moment if you press on it, and will be slightly swollen where it meets the teeth. Gum disease is caused by 'plaque', the sticky film of bacteria that naturally forms on the teeth of everyone every day. These bacteria tend to lodge between the teeth and where the teeth meet the gum. The waste products of the bacteria have a foul, stale smell. Apart from bad breath, gum disease can eventually cause loosening of the teeth.

Poor oral hygiene is an obvious cause. If you do not clean your teeth, you will soon develop bad breath.

Bacteria on the back of the tongue are one of the most common causes of bad breath. Food particles, postnasal drip and stagnant saliva build up in the 'fur' at the back of the tongue, providing a breeding ground for bacteria. These bacteria produce many nasty-smelling chemicals.

Postnasal drip can cause bad breath. This is mucus that trickles down the back of the throat. The reason for the mucus is inflammation in the air passages behind the nose because of allergies or a sinus infection. It often causes a ticklish cough, particularly when lying flat at night. This type of bad breath is worst when the person is speaking.

Anything that dries the mouth makes bad breath worse, because saliva cleanses the mouth. Tricyclic antidepressant drugs (such as amitriptyline) reduce saliva. Alcohol, alcohol-containing mouthwashes, heavy exercise and fasting can all result in a dry mouth and worsen a bad breath problem.

Isosorbide dinitrate, a drug for angina, sometimes produces an objectionable smell in the mouth.

Gut problems used to be blamed, and enemas and laxatives were often given as cures, but in fact these have very little to do with bad breath. Your stomach is shut off from your throat and mouth by a tight ring of muscle at the base of the food pipe (oesophagus), so it is normally a closed tube. Therefore no odour escapes from the stomach, except if you belch, or regurgitate food (vomit).

Chest problems, such as obstructive airways disease (chronic bronchitis), can cause bad breath.

Bad breath in a small child may mean that the child has inserted a small object (such as a seed or small toy) into the nose, where it has stuck and caused an infection. For this reason, small children with bad breath should be seen by a doctor.

What to do about bad breath

A dental check-up is the first priority. The British Dental Association suggests that you explain in advance that you will be asking for advice about bad breath. Tell the receptionist when you make an appointment, and ask that it is noted down and that the dentist is told. Ask the dentist for a thorough scale and polish, and ask if there are any defects where plaque and food debris might be building up.

On average, people in the UK clean their teeth 13 times a week
*(*Observer *20 June 2004)*

Clean your teeth properly. A dental hygienist (make an appointment via your dentist) will show you how to clean your teeth properly, and how to use floss to clean between the teeth.

- Give your teeth a thorough cleaning for 3 minutes twice a day to remove the plaque, and use floss.
- Also, clean your teeth after eating protein-rich foods.
- An electric toothbrush is 11% better at removing plaque (deposits of bacteria) than an ordinary brush. If you use an electric toothbrush regularly, instead of an ordinary brush, you reduce your chances of developing gum disease by 17% (*Journal of Dentistry* 2004;32:197–211).
- Use floss for cleaning between the teeth, or miniature 'interdental brushes', which you can buy from your dentist.
- Use disclosing tablets (which you can buy from pharmacies); these dye the plaque on your teeth, showing the areas you have not been cleaning properly.
- Use a toothpick after meals to remove large food particles from between the teeth and, if possible, rinse your mouth out after meals.

How to clean your teeth with a brush

- Use a brush with a small head, about the diameter of a 5c coin.
- Use only a pea-sized blob of toothpaste. Toothpaste is abrasive and too much can wear the teeth.
- The British Dental Association recommends the 'gentle scrub' method. Place the brush at the neck of the tooth where it meets the gum and use very short horizontal movements, at a 45 degree angle, to dislodge the plaque. The brush can be held like a pen to avoid excessive force.

Buy a tongue cleaner. This is a curved plastic scraper like a miniature garden hoe. Stick out your tongue and place the cleaner onto the tongue as far back as possible. Then pull forward while gently pressing against the tongue surface. Do not scrape too much, because if you scratch the tongue, bacteria will get into the cracks and make the problem worse. You can buy tongue cleaners from most dentists and some pharmacies.

If you cannot obtain a tongue scraper, brushing the tongue with a soft toothbrush once a day may be helpful. The most important part to clean is the back of the tongue, if you can do this without gagging. Wet the brush with mouthwash, then stroke from the back of the tongue in an outwards motion. Do not overdo the brushing; the idea is to dislodge any bacteria and flush out stagnant saliva.

Politicians, lawyers, judges and teachers have the worst breath – they talk a lot, so their mouths dry out (Professor M Rosenberg)

Do not skip meals (especially breakfast). You need to eat regularly to keep the saliva flowing.

Eat plenty of fruit. Pineapple is especially good, because it contains an enzyme that helps to clean the mouth.

Drink black tea (tea without milk). Researchers at the University of Illinois, US, found that chemicals in tea can stop the growth of the bacteria responsible for bad breath, and may suppress the bad-smelling chemicals they produce. However, to get the most benefit, the tea must be drunk without milk.

Chewing sugar-free gum can be helpful because it stimulates the flow of saliva and involves movements of the jaw and cheeks. Both these factors help to remove food debris and cleanse the mouth.

Stopping smoking will get rid of 'smoker's breath'.

Mouthwashes, deodorizing mouth sprays or tablets will mask bad breath temporarily – useful after eating onion or garlic. Modern mouthwashes also contain antibacterial chemicals so, in theory, they should improve gum disease and mouth odour. Before bedtime is the most effective time to use the mouthwash. Gargle with the mouthwash, sticking your tongue out at the same time, and then spit the mouthwash out. There are several types of mouthwash.

- Sarakan is a herbal mouthwash available from health shops. It contains extract of Salvadora persica, a bush grown in Africa and known locally as the 'toothbrush tree', because twigs from it are used to clean the teeth. Chemicals from the plant dissolve plaque. It has a pleasant taste, flavoured with oils of peppermint, clove and geranium, and does not contain alcohol. Tom's of Maine is another non-alcohol mouthwash made from natural ingredients, but has a stronger mint flavouring.
- You can make your own mouthwash by dissolving half a teaspoon of bicarbonate of soda (baking soda) in half a cup of warm water.
- A two-phase mouthwash (Dentyl pH) contains three antibacterial agents – natural essential oils, triclosan and cetylpyridinium. These absorb, lift and remove bacteria, debris, food and dead cells, which cause bad breath. (See the result when you spit out.) The oil phase absorbs smelly gases. The effect is said to last for 18 hours.
- A mouthwash and lozenge system (Colgate Neutralize) contains compounds that neutralize the bad-smelling chemicals.
- Chlorhexidine gluconate (as in Corsodyl, Colgate Chlorohex) is the most effective antibacterial wash, but tastes nasty and darkens teeth slightly for a few days.
- Phenolic mouthwashes (such as Listerine) are almost as effective as chlorhexidine in reducing gum disease, but are too 'zingy' for some people.
- Cetylpyridinium chloride (as in Search, Reach, Listermint, Macleans Mouthguard) is an effective antibacterial, but it does not remain in the mouth for long after rinsing.
- Povidone-iodine (as in Betadine) can cause irritation, and must not be used by pregnant women or children, or for longer than 14 days.
- Chlorine dioxide rinses (such as Retardex) are claimed to eliminate some of the bacteria and the sulphur chemicals that are partly responsible for the bad smell of halitosis.
- Peroxide (as in Colgate Peroxyl) is also an antiplaque agent.

At present, many mouth rinses are acidic, and dentists worry that they might damage tooth enamel. There is also a possibility that the bacteria they eliminate could be replaced by more harmful types that can withstand the effects of mouthwashes. Look at the label to check if the mouthwash contains alcohol. Alcohol can dry the mouth and make the problem worse.

Herbs may help. Chamomile and myrrh are said to have antibacterial properties. Peppermint, rosemary, sage and cloves have a pleasant smell, which helps to mask bad breath. Pour 0.5 litres (1 pint) of boiling water onto 75–125 g (2–4 oz) of herb or 30 g (1 oz) of cloves. Leave to cool for an hour, then strain and use as a mouthwash (that is, swish around your mouth and then spit out). Do not use herbs if you are pregnant.

If you have dentures, remove them at night and soak them in a solution of hypochlorite or chlorhexidine. A pharmacist will be able to advise you.

Shakespeare mentions breath smell – sweet or stinking – more than 100 times. In his day, most people had bad breath (Professor M Rosenberg)

Useful contacts

Australian Breath Clinic is a specialized dental clinic based in Sydney, NSW. It has developed a professional treatment for bad breath and sour taste. The clinic began life in 1997 as BreezeCare; a company that sold other people's bad breath solutions. Visit the websites for more information on products and services.
www.badbreath.com.au
www.breezecare.com

The Fresh Breath Centre is a private clinic for bad breath. The website has a 'Do I have bad breath' questionnaire and a FAQ section.
www.freshbreath.co.uk

Bad Breath Research is an excellent site from a world expert on bad breath, Professor Mel Rosenberg. It contains lots of questions and answers about bad breath, a list of 'Ten top tips for good breath' and links to other sites.
www.melrosenberg.com/research/

American Dental Association. The website has a list of frequently asked questions about bad breath.
www.ada.org/public/topics/bad_breath.asp

The American Dental Hygienists' Association has a factsheet on oral health.
www.adha.org/downloads/bad_breath.pdf

Bed-wetting

Bed-wetting is common, and it affects many teenagers and adults as well as children.

BED-WETTING IN CHILDREN
What is normal?

Of course babies wet their nappy any time they feel like it. Becoming 'dry' is a complex process. The urine-producing system has to develop its ability to produce less urine at night, coordination has to develop between the maturing nerves and muscles controlling the bladder, and the ability to wake up when the bladder is full also has to develop. All this takes time. This happens quite quickly in some children, but is slower in others. Boys tend to be slower than girls, so bed-wetting is three times more common in boys than in girls.

- By the age of 2 years, most children are dry during the day (if a toilet is nearby when they need it, and their clothing is easy to undo).
- By the age of 3 years, 3 out of every 4 children are dry most nights.
- By the age of 5 years, most children are dry at night. However, 1 out of every 10 children still wets the bed at least once a week.
- By the age of 10 years, about 1 out of every 15 children wets the bed several nights a week.
- By the age of 15 years, only 1 out of every 100 children is still wetting the bed several nights a week.

These facts and figures show that most children gradually grow out of bed-wetting, and it is certainly nothing to worry about in a child younger than 5 years. The medical term for bed-wetting is *enuresis*, and this is usually defined as wetting the bed at least three nights a week in a child over 5 years of age.

Babies pass urine in the womb.

Important points about bed-wetting

- Your child cannot help wetting the bed.
- Your child is not wetting the bed out of spite, or to attract attention, or by being too lazy to get out of bed.
- Try not to get irritated, and do not criticize your child for bed-wetting. Punishing a child for bed-wetting certainly will not help, and may make it worse.
- You and your child may feel depressed about the bed-wetting, and may feel it will never stop. Keep reminding yourself that most children grow out of it – think of it as a temporary problem.

Causes of bed-wetting

The exact reasons for bed-wetting are not very well understood, but here are some possibilities.

- Bed-wetting seems to run in families – the likelihood of a child wetting the bed is 40% if one parent suffered, and 70% if both parents suffered. So there is often a genetic element.
- One of the most common reasons for bed-wetting is the bladder muscle contracting and emptying the bladder when it is only half full of urine. This is because the child is just being slightly slow in developing the necessary nerve and muscle control – there is nothing wrong.
- Some children produce a lot of urine at night, because the mechanisms that reduce urine production at night are slow to develop – again, there is nothing actually wrong.
- There is very little scientific evidence to back up the idea that bed-wetting is a psychological problem. Some children do wet the bed if they have anxieties at home or school, but more often bed-wetting is a cause (rather than a result) of unhappiness.
- Parents often think that their child has a different, deeper sleep pattern than other children. There is no scientific evidence for this. The problem is more a difficulty with waking – the sensation of a full bladder is not enough to wake the child.
- Occasionally, a medical condition such as a urine infection is responsible.
- According to a report in *New Scientist* (2 August 2003), breathing problems caused by the roof of the mouth being narrow may result in bed-wetting. This is why bed-wetting often improves after children have their tonsils and adenoids removed. More research on this is needed, but doctors are trying a special device, similar to a brace, to widen the roof of the mouth.

In Victorian times, children who wet the bed were allowed only plain and boring food. It was thought that cakes and pastries made bed-wetting more likely by causing 'irritating' urine (Of course, this is not the case)

What you can do

Do not worry about bed-wetting if your child is 6 years old or under – just be patient.

Help your child not to feel bad about bed-wetting. Smelly bedrooms and lots of sheets to change and wash are annoying, but try to keep a calm, matter-of-fact attitude and not to fuss about it. It is important not to make your child feel guilty about something he or she can not control. Bed-wetting is a great worry to children – they often feel that they are being babyish or dirty. To punish a child for a wet bed will not help and is not fair.

Explain bed-wetting to your child. Explain how common it is, and that there will certainly be other children of the same age in his or her class with the same problem. Explain that he or she will grow out of it in time, and that you are finding out ways to make this happen faster. (In fact, it is not strictly true that all children grow out of it (see page 44), but most do.) If you used to bed-wet, tell your child about it.

How to explain bed-wetting to your child

The US National Kidney Foundation suggests you explain bed-wetting in the following way.

Tell your child it is the kidneys' job to make urine, which goes down tubes into the bladder. The bladder is like a water balloon that holds the urine. There is a muscle gate that holds the urine in. When the bladder is full, it sends a message to the brain and the brain tells the gate to open. Tell your child that, in order to be the boss of his or her urine at night, all the parts need to work together.

- The kidneys must make just the right amount of urine.
- The bladder must hold it and tell the brain when it is full.
- Then the brain must either tell the gate to stay closed until morning, or tell the child to wake up to use the toilet.

Bed-wetting affects 5–7 million children in the US and 500 000 children in the UK

Deal with practical problems. Think up ways of dealing with practical problems. Obtain waterproof mattress covers, for example (see Useful contacts on page 46).

Children who bed-wet are fearful of sleeping at other children's houses. To deal with this difficulty, buy your child some pyjamas and a washable (polyester) sleeping bag for sleepovers. Ideally, look for a child-sized bag (easier to wash) with a waterproof exterior. Tell your child to put his or her day clothes close by at night then, in the morning, it is simple to kick off the wet pyjama bottoms into the damp sleeping bag, quickly get dressed without anyone noticing the problem, and roll up the sleeping bag with the pyjamas inside ready for washing at home.

Consider using disposable padded absorbent pads (see Useful contacts on page 46). They are designed to be worn under baggy pyjamas or a nightdress, and do not look like nappies (diapers). They obviously will not solve the problem, but are useful for holidays or if you are becoming very stressed by wet beds.

Make access to the toilet easy. Make it easy for your child to get to the toilet. Pyjama bottoms should be easy to get off. Provide a plug-in night light to guide your child to the bedroom door. Leave a landing light on – your child may be afraid of the dark. Provide a potty in the bedroom if the bathroom is far away. And remember, sleeping in a top bunk makes getting to the toilet difficult.

'Lifting' your child to the toilet, and encouraging him or her to pass some urine, before you go to bed (for instance, at about 11pm) will not prevent a wet bed. However, it will slightly reduce the amount of urine that is released.

Encourage your child to drink plenty during the day – at least six drinks. This helps train the bladder to hold larger quantities, and will prevent excessive drinking in the evening. Check that the school provides access to drinks during the day.

Do not restrict drinks in the evening – this does not help. If your child seems to be drinking a lot in the evening, it may be because he or she is not drinking enough in the day, so the best approach is to encourage daytime drinking. It makes sense to restrict cola drinks, because they contain caffeine which can make bladder control more difficult.

Help your child to train his or her bladder. Explain that the bladder is like a balloon, and needs to be stretched. This will help to make it strong, so that urine is easier to control. Once a day (twice a day at weekends), encourage him or her to drink a lot, and then hang on until bursting and then a few minutes more if possible. This will only work if your child understands what he or she is trying to do, and if you have an encouraging and slightly laid back attitude. Do not get angry if your child finds hanging on difficult.

Try a 'star chart' if your child is 9 years or older. You will need some stick-on stars, and a calendar that has a large space for each day. If you do not have a suitable calendar, make a chart, or obtain one from ERIC (see Useful contacts on page 46). Each morning, your child sticks a star on the calendar if the bed has been dry. If the bed was wet, leave the space blank. If the bed has been dry for 3 nights in a row, he or she can add a special coloured star (such as red or gold).

Think of the star chart as a way of rewarding successes (even if they are very few), rather than a record of failures. So do not make any fuss about the 'wet' mornings, but praise your child on a 'dry' morning when the star can be applied. If after a few weeks there are no dry nights, stop using the chart – if you continue, your child may start to feel a failure. Simply tell him or her that you will start the chart again in a few months' time.

In an average class of thirty 10-year-olds, there will be two who wet the bed

Discuss the problem with your doctor. You should see your doctor if:

- the problem is really getting to you, and you are starting to feel angry with your child
- your child seems upset about the bed-wetting or about other problems, such as school
- your child is aged 7 or over – at this age a bed-wetting alarm may be helpful
- your child also wets during the day, or seems to have a feeble urine stream
- your child has any other health problems, or is not growing as quickly as other children.

What your doctor can do

Are any tests needed? If your child seems healthy apart from the bed-wetting, it is very unlikely that there is a serious cause. The only necessary test is a urine check. Your doctor will send a sample to the laboratory to check for infection, and will also do a simple 'dipstick' test to make sure the urine is not abnormal in any other way.

Bed-wetting alarms (enuresis alarms) ring or buzz when your child begins to wet the bed. These are the most effective treatment. They wake the child, and this gets him or her into the habit of waking up when urine needs to be passed. There are two main types of alarm. In the UK, you can buy them from ERIC (see Useful contacts page 46), or your doctor or practice nurse can arrange for you to borrow one. Even if you decide to buy one, it is important that the practice nurse shows you how to use it properly. Using an alarm requires lots of patience and commitment, but is worthwhile. There are two main types of alarm.

- 'Pad and bell alarms' have a plastic mat that you put into the middle of the bed, where wetness usually occurs. The mat has an electrical circuit within it that is connected by a flex to a bell or buzzer alarm. You place the alarm out of reach so that your child has to get out of bed to switch it off, and then go to the toilet.
- 'Mini-alarms' are neater. They clip onto the child's nightwear, near the collar. A thin flex connects the alarm to the sensor, which you attach to the underpants or panties. Wetness activates the alarm. It can be switched off temporarily, but the child has to change into dry clothes to prevent it going off again.

Using a bed-wetting alarm

- For at least the first 10 nights, you will probably have to wake your child when you hear the alarm, so that he or she can switch it off and go to the toilet. You will need to help your child change the sheets and reset the alarm. A 'baby alarm' system will help you to hear the bed-wetting alarm when it goes off.
- After about 10 days, many children will have learned to wake up promptly to 'beat the buzzer', so there will be a smaller wet patch. This is progress, so tell your child how pleased you are.
- If your child does not wake with the alarm, make it louder by placing the sound box in a tin.
- Be patient. Some children become dry after about 2 months of using the alarm, but many need 4 months.
- If your child becomes completely dry using the alarm, carry on using it for a further month.
- Bed-wetting alarms do not work for all children. The overall success rate is about 68%. If after about 6 weeks, there is no progress at all (such as a smaller wet patch, or the alarm going off later in the night), it is best to stop using it, and try again after a few months.

Medicines for bed-wetting can be very helpful, but they do not really cure the problem. When the child stops taking them, bed-wetting often occurs again. But they are a useful stopgap, for example, to use during a school trip. You require a doctor's prescription for these medicines.

- Desmopressin helps the kidneys make less urine. It can be taken as tablets or as a nose spray. On average, taking desmopressin gives 2 dry nights a week, and about one-third of children will be completely dry.

- Oxybutynin and tolterodine are medications that calm overactive bladder muscle. Either may be helpful if your child has daytime wetting as well as bed-wetting, and has to rush to get to the toilet (urgency). They can cause side effects (dry mouth, constipation, blurred vision), but these are minimized by taking the medication at night.
- Imipramine is a medication that somehow helps the bladder hold more urine. On average, taking imipramine gives 1–2 dry nights a week. It used to be popular, but is not used much now. It has some side effects and is very dangerous if too much is taken. It is not as effective as desmopressin.

TEENAGERS AND ADULTS

Wetting the bed at night (the medical term is enuresis) is more common in adults than you might think. It affects about one person in every hundred, mainly men. More than 100 000 teenagers in the UK wet the bed – some only occasionally, while others may never have experienced a dry night. Many feel so embarrassed that they hide it from their families and can find it a barrier to forming close relationships. It can be especially difficult when staying away from home. If you also have difficulty holding your urine during the day, look at the section on urinary incontinence on page 283.

Causes of bed-wetting in teenagers and adults

Adults who wet the bed at night often have problems in the daytime as well, such as having to rush to the toilet (urgency). It is not really known why this occurs. It may be a mixture of reasons. If you have always suffered from bed-wetting, you may:

- lack the necessary muscle and nerve control
- produce a lot of urine at night.

If you have only recently started to wet the bed, it could be caused by:

- urine infection
- alcohol, coffee or diuretic medicines
- sleeping tablets
- diabetes
- stress, anxiety or other conditions.

Lack of necessary muscle and nerve control. Your bladder may not have developed the necessary nerve and muscle control, so the bladder muscle contracts and empties the bladder when it is only half full of urine. If you are a teenager, your bladder may soon learn – it is just being a bit slow.

Producing a lot of urine at night. You may be producing a lot of urine, because the mechanisms that reduce urine production at night have not developed. Again, if you are a teenager, the problem may solve itself in time.

Urine infection. A urine infection can irritate the bladder, and make it more difficult to hold urine.

Alcohol, coffee or diuretic medicines. Diuretics are medications that are used to treat high blood pressure and some heart problems. They encourage the kidneys to make more urine. It is best not to take a diuretic at bedtime, because you will need to pass urine in the night and, if your bladder control is poor, this could cause bed-wetting. Alcohol and coffee have a similar effect, so avoid them within 3 hours of bedtime.

Sleeping tablets can make you sleep so soundly that you do not wake up when your bladder is full. If you take sleeping tablets, discuss with your doctor whether you really need them, or try reducing the dose.

Diabetes is a disease in which the blood sugar is too high. The kidneys try to lower the sugar by making lots of sugary urine, so you pass more urine in the day and during the night (you are also thirsty). If your bladder control is poor, this could cause bed-wetting. The problem goes away when the diabetes is treated.

Stress and anxiety can cause bed-wetting.

Other conditions, such as expansion of the prostate gland, neurological problems and sleep apnoea can result in bed-wetting.

What you can do

Do not blame yourself. Remind yourself that it is not your fault. There is no need to feel guilty or dirty. And remember that no one can tell just by looking at you that you have this problem.

Cut down on alcohol. Trial and error will show you if this helps. Similarly, try cutting down on coffee in the evening.

Use an alarm clock to wake you a couple of hours or so after going to bed, and a couple of hours before your usual waking time. Vary the time every few days, to avoid getting into the habit of emptying the bladder at the same time each night.

Try sleeping in a different bed or moving to a different room or even just moving your bed into a different position – some people find this helps.

Visit your doctor if you have not already done so. You may be so embarrassed that you feel this is impossible for you – and in fact 1 in every 6 adults and teenagers who wet the bed never seeks help. Resolve to be one of the brave people who gets it sorted. Your doctor will not be surprised or embarrassed, and will be pleased to help (refer to the section on talking to your doctor on page 335). But you must explain clearly to the doctor that your problem is wetting the bed. Do not pretend you have cystitis or some other urine problem, hoping the doctor will guess what is wrong, because he or she probably will not. For 2–3 weeks before you see the doctor, keep a diary detailing when you wet the bed.

What your doctor can do

Check that there is nothing seriously wrong. Your doctor will ask you questions, especially about whether you have wet the bed since childhood, or whether it is a new problem. He or she will do simple urine tests for infection and for diabetes. Your doctor will also check that there is nothing physically wrong with the bladder system – this may require a hospital referral to a consultant urologist and/or a bladder X-ray or ultrasound scan.

Bed-wetting alarms (enuresis alarms) are used for children who wet the bed (see page 42), but they can also work for teenagers and sometimes for adults. Modern types are worn between two pairs of pants, so they are small and discreet. If you have a partner, they will obviously have to be understanding and as motivated as you are. Your family doctor can advise you about obtaining an alarm or, in the UK, you can buy one from ERIC (see Useful contacts below). If the alarm has not produced any improvement after 3 months, talk to your doctor about combining it with desmopressin (see below).

Medications are available on prescription from your family doctor.

Desmopressin is the best medication and is taken as a tablet or nose spray. It works by concentrating your urine so that there is not such a large volume to cope with. It is especially useful if you stay away from home, or if you have a bed partner. Although it stops bed-wetting completely in less than one-third of people, most find it reduces the number of wet nights. It does not cure the problem – when you stop taking it, the bed-wetting often recurs – but it is safe to take it over a long period.

Imipramine is a medication that somehow helps the bladder to hold more urine. It used to be popular, but is now used only if desmopressin has not helped. It has some side effects and is dangerous if too much is taken.

Tolterodine and oxybutynin calm overactive bladder muscle. They may be helpful if you have daytime wetting (see page 283) as well as bed-wetting, and have to rush to get to the toilet (urgency). They can cause side effects, such as dry mouth and constipation, but these can be minimized by taking the medication at night. If desmopressin has not worked, they may be useful in combination with imipramine.

Useful contacts

Bedwetting Cured provides a useful fact sheet on bed-wetting and bed-wetting alarm systems.
www.bedwettingcured.com.au

Bedwetting Australia.com is a directory of available services, products and clinics dealing with bed-wetting issues Australia wide.
www.bedwettingaustralia.com

Health*Insite* is an Australian government initiative aimed to improve the health of Australians by providing easy access to quality information about human health. Follow the link to find information relating to bedwetting, or nocturnal enuresis, alarms.
www.healthinsite.gov.au/topics/Bedwetting_Alarms

The Enuresis Resource and Information Centre (ERIC) provides information on all aspects of bed-wetting and daytime wetting in children, teenagers and adults. Their excellent website has a special section for teenagers. ERIC also produces a range of very helpful publications, including *Bed-wetting: A Guide for Parents* and *Daytime Wetting,* which can be ordered through their website.
www.trusteric.org (for teenagers)
www.eric.org.uk

The National Enuresis Society and the National Kidney Foundation are American organizations which have good general information about bed-wetting in children and younger adults.
www.kidney.org/patients/bw/index.cfm

Canadian Paediatric Society compares the various treatments for bed-wetting on their website. It was written in 1997, but is still relevant. It is intended for doctors, and is quite detailed. They also have a question-and answer fact sheet on bed-wetting, with cartoon drawings to help you explain bed-wetting to your child on their 'Caring for Kids' site.
www.cps.ca/english/statements/CP/cp97-01.htm
www.caringforkids.cps.ca/behaviour/Bedwetting.htm

American Academy of Family Physicians have a fact sheet on their website and a link to a detailed article on enuresis (intended for doctors).
www.aafp.org/afp/20030401/1509ph.html

Disposable absorbent pads (e.g. Dry Nites) are available in supermarkets and pharmacies.

Belly button discharge

The belly button can easily become infected by *Candida*, or other fungi – it is just the sort of warm, moist crevice that fungi like. If you have a fungal infection, the belly button will look red, and the redness may extend to the surrounding skin for a few millimetres. It may be itchy.

Bacteria may also infect the belly button, often taking advantage of the damage already done by the fungi. This leads to scabbing and a yellowish discharge.

Redness may not be an infection at all – it may be caused by psoriasis, a skin disorder. On the arms and legs psoriasis causes scaly patches but, in moist areas like the belly button, there is no scaliness – it just looks red and shiny. Usually, but not always, you will have psoriasis somewhere else on your body.

What you can do

- Resist the urge to pick or scratch.
- Do not try to turn your belly button inside-out to clean it properly – just wash it gently using water to which you have added enough salt to give it a salty taste (about a tablespoonful in a bowl, or two handfuls in the bath). If you have a shower, use the shower head to rinse it well. Carefully dab it dry.
- Do not dab on any antiseptics, or add antiseptic to your bath water. This could irritate the skin and make it worse.
- Stop applying any creams from the chemist – they could be making it worse.
- If it does not start improving within a few days, or there is a yellowish discharge, see your doctor. You may need an antibiotic cream.

Blushing & flushing

Flushing and blushing are two words for the same thing – flushing is the word used by doctors. Flushing is almost never a serious medical condition. The only exception is a rare disorder called 'carcinoid syndrome' in which there are episodes of bright red flushing of the face lasting about 20 minutes with sudden diarrhoea and stomach cramps. The usual cause of carcinoid syndrome is a tumour.

If your face is too red most of the time, look at the section on red face (page 216).

Why do we blush or flush?

Flushing of the cheeks and nose (and sometimes the forehead and chin) is a normal emotional response. This is why it is annoying and can be embarrassing. Without our permission, our body is giving away emotions which we may prefer to keep secret – we may not want the world to know that we feel anxious, excited or ashamed.

In an experiment, people watched a video of shoppers who, by mistake, toppled a display of toilet rolls. The shoppers who looked embarrassed and tried to replace the rolls were rated more highly by the viewers. So psychologists think that blushing acts as a sort of unconscious public apology when we do something wrong, showing that we are upset and making people more likely to forgive us.

In the 18th and 19th centuries, women who blushed were regarded as very attractive

Flushing caused by anxiety

There is no magic drug to prevent the normal flushing caused by anxiety, but there are things that you can try.

Decide not to mind it. Your face is probably not as red as you think it is, and your blushing is probably less noticeable than you imagine. Think carefully about whether it really matters if other people know that you are nervous. Everyone knows that giving a speech, meeting new people, asking someone out, being complimented or having an argument (or any other situation that makes you blush) are circumstances that make everyone nervous, whether or not they are prone to blushing.

Control your anxiety. If you think that you tend to be overfearful or apprehensive, relaxation therapy or cognitive therapy (which helps you to see situations in a different light) may help. Your doctor will be able to give you advice about these, or look in your local library for self-help books (look also at the section on shyness on page 241).

Surgery. Consider surgery if your blushing is so bad that it is really affecting your life. Ask your doctor about an 'endoscopic transthoracic sympathectomy' operation. This destroys the nerves that dilate the tiny blood vessels in the face. A survey of 244 patients 8 months after the operation suggested that 85% were pleased with the result (*British Journal of Dermatology* 1998;138:639–43). The operation is similar to the operation for excessive sweating of the palms and armpits (see pages 261 and 256), and requires a general anaesthetic. It is not something to undertake lightly; like all surgery, it has risks and has even caused deaths (*British Journal of Surgery* 2004;91:264–9).

Flushing caused by drugs, chemicals or foods

A few drugs can cause flushing, so it is worth checking whether you are taking any of the following:

- chlorpropamide (for diabetes), which can cause flushing if you take it with alcohol
- glyceryl trinitrate, isosorbide dinitrate (for angina)
- tamoxifen (for breast cancer and some other conditions)
- buserelin, goserelin, leuprorelin and triptorelin (for prostate tumours in men)
- raloxifene (for osteoporosis)
- calcitonin (for some bone disorders)
- calcium-channel blockers (for angina or high blood pressure).

Monosodium glutamate (MSG) is a flavour-enhancing chemical sometimes added to foods (e.g. Chinese meals), which can cause flushing in some people. Alcohol and spicy foods can also be triggers.

In Victorian times, flushes at the menopause were treated by applying leeches to suck blood out of the skin

Flushing at the menopause

Most women experience flushes around the menopause. They can be the earliest sign, so you can have them while your periods are still quite regular. A survey showed that 41% of women whose periods were still regular, but who were over the age of 39, had flushes. They usually go on for 2–3 years, but 1 in 4 women has them for 5 years, and an unlucky 1 in 20 has them for the rest of their lives.

A flush is an unpleasant sensation of heat which begins in the face, head or chest. Often, there is sweating, visible redness of the skin, palpitations and a feeling of weakness. It usually passes after 1–2 minutes, leaving a feeling of coldness. Some women have just the flush without the sweating, while others sweat profusely, but hardly flush. Flushes may occur frequently, even several times an hour, or just occasionally. Some women find that any slightly stressful situation will bring on a flush, or that flushes are more likely to occur when they are warm (e.g. in bed, in an overheated room, on holiday in a warm place). The flushes and sweats disturb sleep – some women wake covered in sweat – and this results in lethargy and irritability during the day.

Common-sense ways to help menopausal flushing Remember that the flush may not be as noticeable as you think. You may be very aware of sweat on your forehead, but other people may not notice.

Wear suitable clothing. Avoid clothes made from synthetic fibres (acrylic, polyester, nylon) and clothes that will show sweat (such as plain-coloured silk shirts). Instead, choose natural fibres that will absorb and hide sweat (e.g. cotton T-shirts). A cotton bra (such as a sports bra) will absorb sweat better than a nylon one. Wear several layers of light clothing, instead of one thick item, so you can easily peel something off.

Avoid trigger foods and drinks. Alcohol, coffee and spicy foods can provoke flushes.

Keep your bedroom cool. Buy a summer-weight duvet and use it all year, or use sheets and a blanket. Choose pure cotton sheets.

Take exercise. Some research suggests that regular exercise reduces menopausal flushes.

Stop smoking and lose weight. The more you smoke and the heavier you are, the greater the likelihood of troublesome flushes (*Obstetrics and Gynecology* 2003;101:264–72).

Increase your intake of plant oestrogens. Some fruits and vegetables contain oestrogen-like substances known as 'phytoestrogens'.

Foods that contain phytoestrogens

Vegetables

- Alfalfa
- Broccoli
- Carrots
- French and green beans
- Peas
- Fennel

Beans and pulses

- Soy beans
- Tofu and miso (both made from soya)
- Lentils

Herbs

- Parsley
- Sage
- Garlic

Fresh fruit

- Apples
- Cherries
- Dates
- Pomegranates

Seeds and grains

- Linseed
- Sesame seed
- Oats
- Rye
- Wheat

Other

- Breads containing soya and linseed
- Liquorice

However, not enough research has been done on phytoestrogens, so we do not know exactly what they do, but it is possible that eating these foods could help menopausal symptoms such as flushing. Phytoestrogens are very much weaker than human oestrogens, so it is unlikely that they would deal with really troublesome flushing. You might find they help a bit.

The easiest way to take phytoestrogens is to add a pint of soya milk to your daily diet, or to switch to a soya- and linseed-containing bread (available from supermarkets).

Some women find that taking extra phytoestrogens makes their flushes worse. This could be because menopausal women still have some oestrogen, made from other hormones (androgens); the phytoestrogens might interfere with this conversion process.

Herbal remedies and vitamins are heavily promoted to menopausal women, but there is no good scientific evidence that they are effective.

- Black cohosh, which you can buy as tablets from health food stores, is a plant from the buttercup family, *Cimicifuga racemosa*, native to North America. A German study in the 1980s suggested that it can help menopausal symptoms such as sweating and flushes (*Therapeuticon* 1987;1:23–31), but a more recent study showed no effect (*Journal of Clinical Oncology* 2001;19:2739–45). It can cause gut symptoms, headache, dizziness and serious liver damage (*UK Committee on Safety of Medicines*, October 2004).
- Dong quai is a Chinese plant, *Angelica sinensis*. In one study it was given to some menopausal women, and while others were given a dummy tablet. There was no difference in effect between dong quai and the dummy tablet (*Fertility and Sterility* 1997;68:981–6). It can act like a blood thinner, so you should avoid it if you are taking anticoagulants, aspirin or similar drugs.
- Evening primrose oil was tested in a study in which some women were given dummy capsules and some were given the primrose oil. There was no difference in flushes and night sweats between the dummy capsules and the evening primrose oil (*British Medical Journal* 1994;308:501–3).
- Red clover is claimed to relieve the symptoms of the menopause, but good evidence for any effect is lacking. Some studies have shown no effect at all. Other studies claim to show an effect, but were flawed so cannot be relied on (*Menopause* 2001:8:333–7). It can act like a blood thinner, so you should avoid it if you are taking anticoagulants, aspirin or similar drugs.
- Ginseng is a herb from China and Korea. In a study, 384 women who had menopause symptoms were given either ginseng or a dummy tablet for 4 months. There was no difference between the effects of ginseng and the dummy tablet (*International Journal of Clinical Pharmacology Research* 1999;19:89–99). Ginseng can have serious side effects in some people.
- Vitamin E is a popular 'natural' treatment. The only proper scientific study found it reduced the number of flushes by just one per day, which was no better than dummy capsules (*Journal of Clinical Oncology* 1998;16:495–500).
- Sage is sometimes recommended, although it has not been assessed scientifically. It is taken by infusing some sage leaves in boiling water.

A famous Victorian doctor, Brown-Sequard, recognized that flushes at the menopause were caused by shutting down of the ovaries. He recommended that women should eat a daily sandwich containing two sheep's ovaries

What your doctor can do

Hormone replacement therapy (HRT) is the most effective treatment for menopausal flushing. It consists of oestrogen and (unless you have had a hysterectomy) a daily dose of progesterone for 14 days of the month. It may be a few weeks before the flushes disappear.

HRT can increase your risk of breast cancer and stroke, so you should take it only if your flushes (or other menopausal symptoms) are intolerable, and not long term. Unfortunately, when you stop taking HRT, the flushes will probably return.

*Sheep, primates and humans are the only animals that have menopausal flushes (*Financial Times *2003; August 9)*

Tibolone is a hormone drug that is being investigated as a treatment for menopausal flushes. It is not yet clear whether it increases the risk of breast cancer. It does not reduce the number of flushes that you experience, but they are much less severe (*British Journal of Obstetrics and Gynaecology* 2005;112:228–33).

Paroxetine and venlafaxine are drugs that can help if you prefer not to take HRT and have really troublesome flushes. They are mainly used to treat depression, because they change the way that cells in the brain handle transmitter chemicals, such as serotonin and noradrenaline. These chemicals may also be involved in hot flushes, so it is not surprising that these drugs reduce flushes by about 60% (*Lancet* 2000;356:2059–63, *Journal of American Medical Association* 2003;289:2827–34). However, they do not get rid of the flushes entirely and can have side effects.

Gabapentin is a promising treatment that is being investigated. It is normally used for seizures (epilepsy), but it has another effect – it halves the number and severity of hot flushes (*Obstetrics and Gynecology* 2003;101:337–45). Sleepiness is the main side effect.

Useful contacts

Health*Insite* is an Australian government initiative aimed to improve the health of Australians by providing easy access to quality information about human health. Follow the link to find information about health issues relating to menopause.
www.healthinsite.gov.au/topics/Menopause

Royal College of Psychiatrists provides leaflets to help with a range of emotional problems, including anxiety. These leaflets are also available on their website.
www.rcpsych.ac.uk/info/index.htm

National Phobics Society gives help with anxiety and panic attacks. It has a fact sheet on 'Blushing phobia' for people who worry about blushing.
www.phobics-society.org.uk

The Menopause Exchange provides an unbiased, reliable quarterly newsletter about menopause and female midlife issues to its members.
Email: norma@menopause-exchange.co.uk

Eat to Beat the Menopause is a recipe book by Linda Kearns for those wishing to increase their intake of phytoestrogens. It includes a 'menopause cake' recipe. Published by Thorsons. ISBN 0 7225 3922 3.

Breast problems

PAINFUL BREASTS

Almost all women have tender, painful breasts at some time during their life. If you suffer from regular pain, ask yourself these two important questions:

- is the pain related to the menstrual cycle (is it worse before your period)?
- are both breasts affected, or just one?

You can check these points by keeping a daily diary over 2 or 3 months. Every day, record whether or not you have any breast pain, whether it is mild or severe and which breast is affected. Also make a note of the days of your period.

Breast pain and breast cancer

If you have breast pain, you are probably worrying that it might be breast cancer. This is very unlikely. Breast pain is very common – about 70% of women have it at some time. Doctors at the Edinburgh Breast Unit have looked at the medical records of more than 8500 women who attended the unit simply because of breast pain. They found that less than 3% of these women – whose breast pain was probably quite severe – had breast cancer. And breast cancer is very, very unlikely if your only symptom is pain that varies with the menstrual cycle and both breasts are affected.

Breast pain related to the menstrual cycle (cyclical breast pain)

It is common to have painful, heavy, bloated breasts before a period. Both breasts are affected at the same time and you may also feel the discomfort in the armpit or upper arm. The breasts may feel generally lumpy but there is not one particular lump. If you are particularly unlucky, it may be so bad you cannot bear to be touched, are pain-free for only a few days each month and have to wear a bra at night because it is so tender when you lie on your side in bed. The problem usually starts in the 20s and 30s, and ends about the time of the menopause. It may go away for long periods and then return.

Causes. Cyclical breast pain affecting both breasts is not a symptom of breast cancer. It occurs because some women's breasts are particularly sensitive to hormone changes. Each breast is made up of a collection of glands for producing milk; these look rather like bunches of silky white grapes. The 'stalks' of the bunches are small milk ducts, which lead into larger and larger ducts for the milk to reach the surface of the nipple. The glands are supported and padded in 'packing tissue', which is mostly fat. Each month, the glands respond to the rise and fall of hormones. It used to be thought that the problem was caused by fluid retained in the packing tissue, but this has been disproved.

What you can do. There are a number of things that you can try to ease the pain.

- Wear a soft bra at night.
- Avoid jogging, aerobics or other high-impact exercises.
- Make sure your bra fits correctly – get properly measured by a specialist fitter (most department stores have one).
- If you are taking any hormones, such as the oral contraceptive pill or hormone replacement therapy (HRT), consider stopping them for a while to see if the breast pain lessens. Breast pain seems to be common in women who have recently started HRT.
- Try a low-fat diet. There is some evidence that high levels of saturated fats in the blood make the breasts more sensitive to hormone levels, so it may be worth changing your diet. Avoid fatty meat, cheese, full-fat milk, cream, butter and anything made of pastry. Instead eat oily fish, such as herring and mackerel, twice a week. Fill up with carbohydrates (bread, potatoes, rice, pasta), fresh fruit and vegetables.
- Try avoiding coffee and cola drinks for a few weeks to see if this makes any difference.
- Consider *Vitus agnus castus* (chasteberry), which is available from health-food stores. It affects various hormones, such as progesterone, and may help cyclical breast pain, though the scientific evidence is scanty (*American Family Physician* 2005; 72:821–4).

What your doctor can do. Most treatments for cyclical breast pain take several months to work, so you will have to be patient. Continue your diary when starting any treatment; this will help you decide whether it is having any effect. If any treatment works, it is best to continue it for about 6 months and then stop. In 50% of women, the pain will not recur; if it does, further treatment can be given.

Gamolenic acid. Try gamolenic acid, the active ingredient of evening primrose and starflower oils. You can buy this at a health store. Three to four capsules are usually taken twice a day for 8–12 weeks; it may take this long to have any effect and the improvement is usually gradual. If it works, the dose is then reduced. It can sometimes cause nausea and indigestion, but has no other side effects. Of women who take this treatment, 30–40% find their condition improves.

NSAIDs. A cream or gel containing an NSAID (non-steroidal anti-inflammatory drug) may help. NSAIDs are painkillers and also reduce inflammation. A research study found that gently massaging the cream into the breasts three times a day for 6 months totally relieved breast pain in almost half of the women in the study (*Journal of the American College of Surgeons* 2003;196:525–30). If this does not work, the next step is hormone treatment, such as danazol or bromocriptine.

Danazol has several different effects on the hormone system. In the breast, it may block the effects of hormones such as progesterone. It works in about 70% of women with breast pain, and works more quickly than the other treatments. It has some side effects such as irregular periods, weight gain, headache, nausea, acne, oily skin and sometimes deepening of the voice. These effects can be minimized by taking the drug for only the 7 days before a period. It interferes with the effectiveness of the contraceptive pill, so you will have to use a different method of contraception.

Bromocriptine reduces the level of the hormone prolactin, which stimulates breast tissue to grow. It works in about half of women, but is seldom used now because of its side effects – a third of those taking it develop nausea, headache, constipation or dizziness when they stand up suddenly.

Clinic treatments. If no treatments seem to help after 4 months, ask for a referral to a specialist breast clinic.

Testosterone. Some clinics prescribe drugs related to testosterone (the male hormone), such as Restandol. These can have some masculinizing side effects and would usually be prescribed for only a short period (e.g. 3 months).

Tamoxifen is another possibility. This drug counteracts oestrogen and is often used for breast cancer, but sometimes a low dose is used for breast pain not caused by cancer (though it is not officially licensed for this purpose at present). If the specialist suggests that you take tamoxifen, do not assume that you have cancer. It must not be taken during pregnancy, so effective contraception is essential. About 30–40% of those taking it experience side effects such as flushing, vaginal discharge and vaginal dryness.

Goserelin. If the pain is very severe, the specialist might suggest goserelin. This is a drug that works on the hormone system, and is effective in 80% of women with bad breast pain. However, it has to be given by an injection once a month and does have side effects.

Treatments to avoid. A few treatments do not really work.

- Diuretics do not work, because the pain is not caused by fluid retention.
- Vitamin B6 is sometimes prescribed if gamolenic acid does not help, before moving on to hormone treatment. Studies have shown that about 30% of women find that vitamin B6 helps; however, the same number reported an improvement with a placebo (dummy tablet), so its effect is probably psychological. Taking a dose of vitamin B6 of more than 10 mg a day over a long period may cause nerve damage.
- Antibiotics are pointless; there is no infection.
- Progesterone hormone has been tried in tablet form and as a breast cream, but there is no evidence that it does any good (apart from having a psychological effect).

Pain unrelated to the menstrual cycle (non-cyclical breast pain)

If your breast pain has no monthly pattern and occurs in just one breast, it is known as 'non-cyclical breast pain' and should not be ignored. Rather than a heavy, bloated, tender feeling, this pain tends to be sharp or burning. There is usually a very simple cause such as bruising from an injury, a sports strain, an infection such as shingles or a breast abscess, a viral infection of the muscles between the ribs (Bornholm disease), inflammation of the joint between the front of a rib and the breastbone (Tietze's syndrome), a lung problem such as pleurisy or even gallstones. However, there is a very faint chance that it could be related to early breast cancer, so you should check it out with your doctor. If no cause can be dealt with, it is usually treated with NSAIDs such as ibuprofen, or in the same way as cyclical breast pain, such as with gamolenic acid.

DROOPING BREASTS

It is natural for breasts to droop with age, particularly in women with large breasts who have had several pregnancies. Jogging causes saggy breasts. Research from the University of Portsmouth, UK, in 2006 found that when you jog your breasts move in a three-dimensional figure-of-eight. With the average 36C breast weighing 200–300 g, this puts a lot of strain on the fragile supporting tissue. A very supportive sports bra can reduce bounce by 765%, but does not eliminate it completely.

Treatments that do not work

Breasts do not contain any muscle, so there is no exercise that will improve matters. Cosmetic companies and private clinics have realized that huge numbers of women are self-conscious about drooping breasts, and offer dubious and expensive 'treatments'. For example, some clinics offer 'non-surgical breast lifts' using electrical (galvanic) stimulation to 'tone and lift the breast'; this cannot and does not work. Many 'firming' gels and lotions are available; these simply tighten the skin and so give a temporary sensation of breast firmness. Some claim that they contain elastin or collagen, the body's structural proteins. In fact, elastin or collagen applied to the surface of the skin will not be absorbed through it.

Surgery

Very droopy breasts can be tightened up by mastopexy surgery. The surgeon removes a wedge of skin and tissue from the loose, saggy upper part of the breast. The nipple and the breast tissue underneath are moved so that the nipple is positioned in the skin further up than it was. There will be a scar around the nipple area, a scar running from the nipple to the crease line underneath the breast, and sometimes a small scar in the crease line.

The breasts end up the same size as before, but have a more pleasing shape. If the nipple area has become stretched, the surgeon can make it smaller. As with all cosmetic breast surgery, it is important to choose a reputable surgeon (see choosing a cosmetic surgeon on page 339). For more detailed information about mastopexy, look at the British Association of Aesthetic and Plastic Surgeons' website listed in Useful contacts on page 67.

LARGE BREASTS

Disproportionately large breasts can make a woman self-conscious. They can cause backache, probably because of adopting a drooping posture to try to hide their size. After a few years, the pressure from bra straps may cause grooves in the shoulders. High-impact sports such as jogging or aerobics can be uncomfortable or impossible. Clothes that fit properly can be hard to find. The oral contraceptive pill may have to be abandoned because it makes the breasts even larger.

The first essential is a well-fitting bra. Women with large breasts often make the mistake of choosing a large size with too small a cup, rather than a smaller size with a larger cup. For example, a woman who needs a 34E often buys a 36C.

Choosing a bra

- If the straps dig into your shoulders, the bra back size is probably too big, as the main support for the breasts should come from the strap around your body and the cups.
- If your bra rides up your back, the bra is too big around your body – the strap should fit around your ribcage.
- Lift up your arms. Did everything stay in place? If your bra pulls up across your breasts you need a smaller size bra, probably with a larger cup size.
- If your bra wrinkles, your cup size is too big – the breasts should be in the cups with a smooth outline.
- If your breasts bulge out of the top or sides of your cup, and your bra looks lumpy under clothes, your cup size is too small.
- If wires poke out at the front or dig in under your arms, the cup size is too small – the wires should lie flat against your body and surround your breasts.
- Look for a bra with two or three fastenings or hooks – these give the best support
- Underwires give good support, but the upper end of the wire should not press into the breast tissue near the armpit.

Breast reduction surgery

Discuss the pros and cons of breast reduction surgery with your doctor. This does not commit you to anything, and may help you decide whether you can come to terms with your figure – and see it as an advantage – or whether you really would like surgery. In the UK, it is very unlikely that you would be able to have the operation on the NHS.

Breast reduction surgery is a more complicated operation than breast enlargement with implants, and takes 2–3 hours. Skill is needed to make both breasts look the same shape. The operation is more 'final' as it cannot be reversed. It is not surprising that far fewer breast-reducing than breast-enlarging operations are performed.

As with breast enlargement surgery, it is important to find a skilled surgeon (see choosing a cosmetic surgeon on page 339). Within reason, the surgeon can remove as much or as little as you want, so you should end up with breasts the size you want.

The surgeon removes a wedge of breast tissue and reshapes the remaining skin and tissue. The nipple will have to be moved to a new position. Usually you will end up with scars right round the nipple, in the crease line under the breast and along a line joining the nipple to the crease line. These scars take about a year to fade. The scars around the nipple fade first.

Problems. A number of problems can occur after breast reduction surgery.

- There is often some loss of feeling from the nipple – often touch can be felt, but there may be loss of erotic feeling.
- Breastfeeding may not be possible afterwards.
- The incisions may take a long time to heal, especially round the nipple and the central part of the incision in the crease line.

- The scars from the incisions usually fade in 6–12 months, but can become thickened and unsightly.
- As with all operations, there is a risk of infection and internal bleeding.

SMALL BREASTS

In an ideal world, we would be judged only on our personality, and not on our appearance. Unfortunately, we live in a culture which suggests that impossible standards and physical beauty are the norm. Most of us are too fat, too thin or too blemished to conform with the images churned out by the media. Many of us feel self-conscious and dissatisfied as a result.

Breast size is a prime example. Breast enlargement operations are becoming much more common and sales of push-up bras are booming. This is despite the fact that small breasts are as functional as large breasts for breastfeeding, do not go droopy with age, are a kilo less of flesh to carry around, are better for sports and look good.

The Independent newspaper has pointed out that women who have implants to please men may be wasting their time. 'Men are far less discerning than women take them for,' Phil Hilton, editor of *Men's Health* magazine, told the newspaper. 'Men think all breasts are good and are delighted to have access to any at all. The idea that they are connoisseurs is inaccurate. There's no need for operations and scars and that kind of thing.'

Breast enlargement operations are increasingly popular. In the UK, 5646 were done in 2005 – a 50% rise since 2004 when 3731 were done.

Boob booster pads

Boob boosters might be the answer. Department stores sell gel-filled breast enhancers that you tuck into your bra, and which feel like real breasts. Or look for gel-filled bras.

Exercises, creams and pills

Exercises can increase the size of the muscle beneath the breast, but will not increase the actual breast tissue. There is no scientific evidence that electrical stimulation, non-hormonal creams or massage treatments have any effect.

Women with large breasts often find that they become much larger with hormone treatments, such as the oral contraceptive pill or hormone replacement therapy, or during pregnancy. This does not usually happen if the breasts were small to start with.

'Natural' pills to boost breast size are available in some health food stores. These often contain 'phytoestrogens', which are substances from plants that have an oestrogen-like effect on the body. The pills contain very large amounts of phytoestrogens (compared with the quantities we would eat as part of our normal diet). The effect of phytoestrogens on the breast needs a lot more study. Experts worry that they could encourage breast cancers, although some studies have suggested that phytoestrogens might protect against breast cancer. Whether or not these pills increase breast size is debatable.

Breast implant surgery

Breast implant surgery (breast augmentation) is the only method of making breasts larger. It is obviously essential that the surgeon is reputable. Talk to your doctor about it. In the UK, it is very unlikely that you can have the operation on the NHS – this is normally possible only if the breast is being reconstructed after breast cancer surgery, or if one breast is very underdeveloped compared with the other. If it is to be done privately, here are some things to think about.

- Look at the very informative website from the UK Government's Medicines and Healthcare products Regulatory Agency (MHRA); (see Useful contacts on page 67). This site explains the pros and cons very clearly, and has a list of points to discuss with your surgeon.
- Check that the surgeon is a Fellow of the Royal College of Surgeons and a member of the British Association of Aesthetic Plastic Surgeons (see the sections on choosing a cosmetic surgeon on page 339 and Useful contacts on page 67); other countries have similar organizations.
- Ask the surgeon to explain all the possible risks and, if you do not understand the explanation, ask for a clearer explanation.
- Take a notebook with you, so you can write down important points.
- After your discussion with the surgeon, go home and consider the information for a few days. In fact, the official recommendation is that there should be a 'cooling-off' period of several days between seeing the surgeon and having the operation, to give you sufficient time in which to change your mind.
- Bear in mind that your implant will not last forever. The average silicone implant lasts about 16 years, so it might need to be replaced at some time in the future.

Breast enlargement is more common than rhinoplasty (nose job). Only 172 420 rhinoplasties were done in the US in 2003

The operation. The implant is placed behind the breast tissue, between it and the chest wall muscle (although very occasionally, it is placed behind the chest wall muscle, between the muscle and the ribcage). It is never placed in the breast tissue, so it does not interfere with the function of the breast and you can breastfeed later on if you wish. The implants come in a great variety of sizes, so a correct-sized implant can be used to make your breasts look similar in size.

There will be a scar in the crease line under the breast. This will be red at first, but will gradually fade over 12 months. If a saline implant is used, some surgeons will be able to insert the bag of the implant by keyhole surgery (endoscopically) through an incision in the armpit. The bag is gradually filled with saline afterwards, and this technique means there is no scar on the actual breast.

For more detailed information about breast enlargement surgery, look at the British Association of Aesthetic and Plastic Surgeons' website listed in Useful contacts on page 67.

Problems. A number of problems can occur after breast enlargement surgery.

- After the operation, there will be some discomfort on moving your arms, but this wears off after 1–2 weeks.
- Occasionally, blood collects around the implant in the first 24 hours after surgery, and the surgeon may have to reopen the incision to remove the blood.
- Infections can occur and can usually be treated with antibiotics. However, if the infection is severe, the implant may need to be removed and replaced a couple of months later.
- The nipple may feel sore or there may be loss of feeling in the nipple area. This is only temporary.
- The scarred skin may become red and thick, and may stay like this for a year or two before starting to fade slowly. Tissue may tighten round the implant, squeezing it and making it feel much firmer. This used to be a common problem, but occurs less often with modern implants, which have a textured surface. If this happens, you may need another operation.

Types of implant

Silicone-gel implants produce the most natural-feeling breasts, and are still the most common in the UK, though they have had a bad press in recent years. In particular, some people thought leakage might cause 'auto-immune' diseases (arthritis-like diseases such as systemic lupus erythematosus or scleroderma). In fact, all the evidence shows this does not happen and that silicone-gel implants are safe.

- Silicone-gel implants stopped being used in the US in 1992 following the health scare. But now an independent panel of scientists convened at the request of Congress has concluded that silicone breast implants do not cause major disease, and has recommended that they should become available again (*Lancet* 2003;362:1384).
- Researchers in the US thoroughly re-examined data from 20 previous studies on silicone implants. The results, published in the *New England Journal of Medicine* in 2000, showed no connection between breast implants and connective tissue diseases.
- Swedish researchers have studied 3486 women with breast implants for an average of 18 years, and found no increase in breast cancer risk (*Journal of the National Cancer Institute* 2006; 98: 557–60).
- Leakage can, however, cause painful hardening of the breasts. In Europe, safety checks on implants were stepped up in 2003, and they now have a stronger casing to reduce the risk of leakage. If you have a silicone-gel implant, you should see your surgeon every year to try to detect leaks.
- Silicone-gel implants show up as a shadow on X-rays. This means cancer cannot be detected easily by mammography in a person who has had an implant, and the breast has to be screened from special angles. If you have an implant, mention it to the radiographer.

Saline implants may be safer than silicone gel implants and are the type used most frequently in the US, but they may leak (which will mean another operation); they may also produce a rippled effect under the skin. Saline implants cause the same difficulties with mammography as the silicone type. They do not have the same consistency as breast tissue, so can feel wobbly and strange.

Soya-oil implants were used between 1995 and 1999. They are no longer used because some leaked into the breast, and it is feared that aldehyde chemicals from the oil could encourage cancers (though there is no evidence this has actually happened).

Tissue grown from our own bodies may be used as implants in the future. Researchers in the US have taken fat cells from the thighs and buttocks, and grown them on breast-shaped polymer mesh. When the mesh is full it dissolves, leaving a piece of breast-shaped fatty tissue that could be implanted.

LOPSIDED BREASTS

One in 20 women has one breast bigger than the other – it is just as common as having one foot bigger than the other. Sometimes the difference is very noticeable, as if one breast has hardly developed at all. When it comes to breastfeeding, this is not a problem – the small breast usually produces milk normally – but if you feel self-conscious about it, you may consider surgery. In the UK, it is possible to have the operation done on the NHS, but the waiting list is likely to be a year or two. Usually the small breast is enlarged by an implant, and sometimes the size of the larger breast is reduced as well.

REDNESS UNDER THE BREASTS

A red 'sweat rash' under the breasts is called intertrigo. It may be sore and itchy, and you may have it in your armpits as well. The rash has a definite edge, and there may be some whitish material on it. It is usually caused by skin-on-skin friction and by *Candida* fungus or *Corynebacterium* bacteria, both of which like to live in warm, moist places. If you are overweight as well as having large breasts, the skin crease underneath them is ideal for *Candida*. *Candida* also likes skin that has been slightly damaged; this makes it easier for the fungus to take hold.

What you can do

Get a supportive bra to lift your breasts up. Although underwired styles give good support, they tend to trap sweat under the breasts so choose a non-wired style. Cotton is better than a synthetic fibre, because it allows sweat to evaporate. Wash it in a non-biological (non-enzyme) detergent and do not use a perfumed fabric conditioner.

Wash carefully under the breasts with a non-perfumed soap (some perfumes can damage the skin). Do not put any disinfectants in the water. Rinse well to ensure no lather remains in the skin crease. Dry thoroughly but gently – pat dry with a soft towel or use a hairdryer. Do not wash your hair with shampoo in the shower – the shampoo may contain perfume that trickles down and irritates the area under your breasts.

Stop applying creams. If you have been applying creams from the chemist, stop using them, even if they say 'for *Candida*' on the label. You could have become sensitized to one of the ingredients, and the cream could be making it worse. Instead, simply follow the instructions for washing under the breast for about 2 weeks. If at the end of that time the rash is no better, see your doctor, who will be able to prescribe a different cream.

Lose weight, if you need to. If you are obese, you may find the rash difficult to eliminate completely unless you lose some weight.

See your doctor to check it is not eczema or psoriasis.

BREASTS IN MEN

The breasts can enlarge if you are overweight, simply because fat has settled there. They can also enlarge because the actual breast tissue is overdeveloped; this is called gynaecomastia.

To decide which it is, lie flat and grasp your 'breast' tightly between your thumb and forefinger. Then gradually move your finger and thumb towards the nipple. If you can feel a firm, rubbery disk-like mound of tissue which is more than 2 cm across, and which seems to be stuck to the back of the nipple and to the pink area surrounding the nipple (areola), it is likely that the breast tissue is overdeveloped. The area may feel tender. Usually both breasts are equally affected, but sometimes development of one is more obvious than the other.

If one breast is more enlarged than the other, ask your doctor to check it; breast cancer is rare in men, but it can occur. If there is no distinct mound of tissue under the nipple, it may simply be that you are too fat.

How breasts develop

Even a newborn baby has some basic breast tissue, which started to develop when it was a 6-week-old fetus. Before puberty, the breasts are the same in girls and boys. They consist of tiny branching tubes embedded in packing tissue. The glands for making milk have not yet formed.

At puberty, hormone levels start to rise. In females, the main hormone is oestrogen (the 'female hormone'). Oestrogen makes the tubes thicken, lengthen and become more branched, and also stimulates the development of glandular lobules.

In men, the main sexual hormone is testosterone. This is made mainly in the testicles. The level of testosterone rises at puberty to 30 times the level it was previously. Men normally also have a small amount of oestrogen; at puberty, it rises to only three times the level it was before. This often makes the breast tissue grow slightly in teenage boys (see below), but eventually the high levels of testosterone take over completely and prevent the oestrogen having any further effect on the breast. Therefore glandular lobules do not form in men. Instead, the breasts flatten out, and remain as a collection of tubes in packing tissue, just as they were before puberty.

Breast growth in teenage boys

Teenage boys sometimes notice that their breasts are enlarging and/or are tender. This is nothing to worry about, and happens to about half of all boys at some time. It does not mean you are changing sex! It can start anytime after the age of about 10, and the breasts may be quite large by the age of 13 or 14. In the mid-to-late teens, they start to become smaller again, and will usually have flattened out by age 18 or 19.

Results of some surveys of breast enlargement in normal teenage boys

Number of normal teenage boys examined	Percentage with breast enlargement
1865 American scouts, aged 10–16	39%
993 Turkish schoolboys, aged 9–17	7%
29 American schoolboys, at puberty	69%
681 Italian schoolboys, aged 11–14	33%
135 Swiss youths, aged 8½–17½	22%
377 American schoolboys, aged 10–15	49%

Source: *New England Journal of Medicine* 1993;328:490–5

Why it happens. At puberty, the testosterone level does not rise steadily. Over the first few teenage years, it continually fluctuates wildly and, on some days, the level will dip quite low. These dips in testosterone allow the small amount of oestrogen that circulates in the blood of all men, to have an effect on the breast. This stimulates the growth of the packing tissue and tubes, so that the breasts enlarge. In men over about 15 years of age, the testosterone settles at a more steady, high level. This prevents the oestrogen from having an effect any longer, and the breast tissue usually starts to shrink.

What if the breasts remain enlarged? In only a few men, the breasts remain enlarged at the end of the teen years. This is not usually because there is anything wrong with the male hormones, but because the enlarged breast tissue has remained hypersensitive to the tiny normal amounts of oestrogen, or else is not responsive to the 'shutting down' effect of testosterone. Occasionally, a rare medical condition may be responsible, so consult your doctor to check your hormone levels. If everything is normal (which it usually is) a surgeon can remove the excess breast tissue.

Breast enlargement in men

It seems that breast tissue is very sensitive to the balance between oestrogen and testosterone in the blood. If there is either a fall in the testosterone level or a rise in the oestrogen level, the breasts will be stimulated to grow.

Obesity is a common cause. If you are overweight, the breasts will of course be larger because they are more fatty. In addition, fat produces oestrogen which stimulates breast development.

Medications are the other most likely reason. Some drugs have an oestrogen-like effect on the breast, and some block the effect of testosterone. Oestrogens are easily absorbed through the skin; men have developed breasts after using anti-balding scalp creams containing oestrogen, and even by absorption through the skin of the penis from a partner using a vaginal oestrogen cream.

Drugs that can cause breast enlargement in men

Hormones
- Oestrogen
- Body-building steroids

Drugs for hypertension or heart problems
- Calcium-channel blockers (such as nifedipine, verapamil)
- ACE inhibitors (such as captopril, enalapril)
- Digoxin
- Amiodarone
- Spironolactone
- Methyldopa

Drugs for duodenal ulcer
- Omeprazole
- Cimetidine
- Ranitidine

Psychiatric drugs
- Phenothiazines (such as chlorpromazine)
- Tricyclic antidepressants (such as amitriptyline)
- Benzodiazepines (such as diazepam)
- Opiates

Drug misuse
- Alcohol
- Marijuana
- Heroin, methadone
- Amphetamines

Antibiotics and antifungal drugs
- Isoniazid
- Metronidazole
- Ketoconazole

Alcohol abuse upsets both sides of the oestrogen–testosterone balance. It stimulates the liver to clear testosterone from the blood, so testosterone levels fall. It probably also reduces the ability of the liver to break down oestrogens, so levels rise. Fortunately, the liver can often recover if alcohol intake is reduced.

Tumours are a rare cause of breast enlargement. Breast cancer can occur in the male breast, but is usually on one side only. Tumours in other parts of the body can sometimes produce hormones that make the breasts grow and may also cause erection problems and/or oozing of milk from the breast. If you have these symptoms, see your doctor immediaely.

Breast cancer in men

Breast cancer can occur in men. It kills about half the men who get it, whereas only about one-quarter of women with breast cancer die from the disease. This difference is because men with breast cancer do not go to their doctor early enough. Therefore men are dying from breast cancer because:

- they did not know about the disease
- they were too embarrassed to seek help.

And by the time they get treatment, the cancer has spread. This is a shame, because breast cancer is just as treatable in men as in women if it is found early enough. So if you have the slightest worry that you might have a lump in your breast, see your doctor straightaway so that you can have tests and treatment if necessary. Other signs of breast cancer include a sore or rash on the nipple, discharge from the nipple, the nipple turning in, or a change in shape of the breast. If you are a woman reading this, try to educate the men in your life about male breast cancer.

Old age. It is natural for men's breasts to enlarge in old age. This often seems to happen over a few months, after which no further enlargement occurs. The reason is partly that less testosterone is produced in old age. Also, in old age, the body often contains a higher proportion of fat, which produces oestrogens. In about 50% of people, the breasts will become smaller again in time.

What your doctor can do about breast enlargement in men

See your doctor if you think your breasts are enlarging, even if you have worked out the most likely cause. Your doctor will be able to:

- check whether the actual glandular breast tissue is overdeveloped, or whether the enlargement is simply fat
- check your testicles (because they make most of the testosterone)
- decide whether any drugs are likely to be responsible
- do blood tests to measure various hormones, including testosterone.

The treatment will depend on the reason for the growth. It may simply be a matter of losing weight or cutting down your alcohol intake. If the problem is a low testosterone level, testosterone can be given by injection or as a patch. Tamoxifen – a drug that interferes with the action of oestrogen – is used by some specialists to reduce gynaecomastia. Another possibility is danazol, a drug that promotes the effect of testosterone. Danazol can have troublesome side effects, such as weight gain, acne, muscle cramps and nausea. The excess breast tissue can also be removed by surgery.

Useful contacts

Australian Society of Plastic Surgeons (ASPS) website offers useful information on surgical procedures for breast augmentation, reduction and reconstruction. You can also contact the society for advice and ask for a list of State and Territory members. Society members are all fully qualified in both reconstructive and cosmetic surgery. All members are Fellows of the Royal Australasian College of Surgeons (FRACS).
www.plasticsurgery.org.au

The Cancer Council Australia website has an evidence-based position statement on 'Breast cancer'. The website has an informative section on cancer prevention and early detection.
www.cancer.org.au

Health*Insite* is an Australian government initiative aimed to improve the health of Australians by providing easy access to quality information about human health. For more specific information on the diagnosis, treatment and statistics of breast cancer, follow the link to the HealthInsite pages on those subjects.
www.healthinsite.gov.au/topics/Breast_Cancer

American Cancer Society has a web page about breast conditions that are not cancerous ('benign'). It also has information about breast cancer on its website. The information is provided in English and Spanish.
www.cancer.org/docroot/CRI/content/CRI_2_6X_Benign_Breast_Conditions_59.asp

Breast Cancer Care gives emotional support and practical information to people who have breast cancer, or fear they may have it, including men. The website has useful information on breast pain and on breast cancer, and a FAQ section.
www.breastcancercare.org.uk

Bravissimo specializes in mail-order lingerie and swimsuits for large-breasted women. They produce an excellent life-enhancing catalogue.
www.bravissimo.com

British Association of Aesthetic and Plastic Surgeons (BAAPS) have available on their website a fact sheet on plastic surgery and a list of their members. The most common operations to change breast size or shape are also explained on their website.
www.baaps.org.uk

The American Society for Aesthetic Plastic Surgery has some useful web pages giving American information (possibly not completely applicable to the UK).
Breast enlargement – www.surgery.org/public/procedures-breastaug.php
Breast reduction – www.surgery.org/public/procedures-breastreduce.php
Operations for drooping breasts – www.surgery.org/public/procedures-breastlift.php

The National Cancer Institute is a reliable US government organization. It has a website titled 'Understanding breast changes: a health guide for all women', with information that you need to know while waiting for your screening (mammogram) result. It describes common breast changes at various life stages, types of follow-up testing and types of biopsy. It will help you to understand your screening (mammogram) result, and emphasizes that not all breast changes mean cancer.
www.cancer.gov/cancertopics/understanding-breast-changes

MHRA (Medicines and Healthcare products Regulatory Agency) is a UK government website with an excellent section on breast implants for women considering the operation. It has a useful checklist of questions to ask your surgeon.
www.mhra.gov.uk

Cold sores

We all hate cold sores, because they are so ugly and noticeable. Cold sores start as tiny blisters on or near the lips. A cold sore is usually gone within a week or two, but is really upsetting while it lasts.

How do you know if you have a cold sore?

- The first sign is a burning, tingling or itching feeling in the skin where the cold sore will erupt. If you have had a cold sore before, you will recognize this feeling as soon as it starts.
- The tingling lasts for about 6 hours. Then you will notice a group of tiny blisters (usually 3–5) with some reddish swelling of the skin around them.
- After a day or two, the blisters become an open sore. This is the start of the ugly stage.
- Within a further day or two, a scabby crust forms over the sore.
- The sore gradually heals, and is gone about 7–10 days after it started.

What causes cold sores

Cold sores are caused by a virus called herpes simplex. (Herpes simplex viruses also cause genital herpes.) Most adults worldwide have been infected with this virus, usually when we were children and were kissed by someone with a tiny cold sore that they were not aware of. When a child first gets the infection, there may be no symptoms at all, or there may be a fever and a sore mouth that clears up after 2–3 weeks.

After the first infection, the virus often remains. We seem to have difficulty in getting rid of it completely. It travels away from the mouth using the nerves of the face as a pathway. When it reaches the clusters of cells at the end of the nerves (which are called ganglia), it stops. The herpes virus DNA then remains quietly in the ganglia. Fortunately, it does not damage the nerves or interfere with their function.

In some people (about 1 in 12), from time to time, the herpes virus travels back the way it came, along the nerve towards the mouth. This is called activation. But instead of going to the inside of the mouth, it takes a slightly different path and ends up in the skin of the lips or nearby. When it arrives in the skin, it causes a cold sore.

After the cold sore heals, the virus goes back up the nerve to the ganglion again, where it rests. But it can become activated again at any time, and travel down the nerves to the skin to cause another sore. The virus always travels up and down the same or nearby nerve pathways, which explains why cold sores always recur in roughly the same place.

How you get a cold sore

- Infection with herpes simplex virus causes sore mouth (or no symptoms).
- Herpes virus travels up nerves to the nerve ganglion where it remains.

- At a later date, herpes virus may travel down the nerves to the skin, causing a cold sore.
- The cold sore heals, and herpes virus retreats to the ganglion again.
- At a later date, herpes virus may travel down to the skin again, causing another cold sore (recurrence).

What activates the virus to cause a cold sore? No one really understands why the virus in the ganglion suddenly wakes up from time to time, and decides to go to the skin and cause a cold sore. But, in some people, there are definite triggers that make this happen, such as:

- bright sunshine
- wind
- other damage to the skin
- emotional stress
- physical stress, such as having another illness
- major dentistry, such as having a tooth removed
- menstruation.

What to do if you have a cold sore

Get early treatment. The earlier you treat a cold sore, the better. In fact, the best time to start treatment is as soon as you feel the telltale tingle. The standard treatment is aciclovir cream, applied 5 times a day for 5 days. It is an antiviral drug that prevents the virus from multiplying and speeds up healing. You can buy it from pharmacies without a prescription. (Another antiviral cream, penciclovir, is available, but requires a doctor's prescription in the UK, and needs to be applied more frequently than aciclovir.)

Do not expect miracles from the cream. If you start treatment early enough, it will shorten the attack from about 8 days to about 6 days (*Journal of Family Practice* 2004;53:923–4). If you often get recurrences, it makes sense to ensure that you have a supply of antiviral cream in readiness, so that you can start treatment promptly.

Dry the sore up or keep it moist? This is a dilemma, because a sore that is oozing does not look very nice. Some people like to dry it by dabbing on surgical spirit or witch hazel (from a pharmacy), or even gin or vodka. However, it is possible that cold sores heal better when they are kept moist. Of course, aciclovir cream will keep it moist as well as having a specific antiviral action. Tea-tree oil, or oil from a vitamin A or vitamin C capsule, are other methods of keeping it moist and may reduce inflammation slightly. A cream containing the herb melissa (lemon balm) is said to help cold sores to heal, and is available in the UK from the Herpes Viruses Association (see Useful contacts on page 71).

Be hygienic. Hygiene is important, because you do not want a bacterial infection to move in.

- Try not to touch the sore with your hands.
- If you apply any cream or oil to the sore, use a new cottonwool bud each time.
- To wash the area, dab it gently with a moistened tissue. Do not apply any disinfectant because this may be too harsh for the damaged skin.

Protect your eyes. Herpes simplex can cause a nasty eye infection, so take care.

- Be careful when applying eye make-up – it is easy to touch your cold sore without realizing it.
- Wash your hands very thoroughly before putting in contact lenses (this is one reason why you should never use saliva to moisten contact lenses).
- If your eye does become sore, see your doctor straightaway.

Do not infect anyone who is vulnerable. Although herpes simplex is not normally a damaging virus, it can cause serious problems in people whose immune system is poor.

- Keep away from babies.
- Do not kiss anyone who is unwell for any reason, or who is pregnant, old, or has eczema (herpes can cause a nasty infection in skin already affected by eczema).
- Do not share your toothbrush or eating utensils with anyone (because the virus can be passed in saliva).
- Do not give oral sex to anyone until the sore has healed completely, or you could be giving them genital herpes.

Preventing another attack

Keep out of wind as much as possible. If you ride a bike, wrap a scarf around the lower part of your face.

Use sunblock if you find sunshine provokes an attack. This really can work. Researchers tried it out on 38 people who suffered from recurrent cold sores and it stopped the problem. Then they supplied a fake sunscreen, and 71% of the people developed a cold sore. (This research was published in *The Lancet* in 1991.)

Choose a high-factor sunblock (such as those intended for skiers), and apply it to the area where your cold sores occur. Do not just dab on the exact spot – cover the surrounding skin also, because cold sores do not always recur in exactly the same spot. If you tend to get sores on the actual lip, use a lip balm that contains UV protection.

Do not waste money on special supplements. Some people think that taking a supplement of L-lysine (an amino acid) will prevent cold sores, or will help your cold sore heal rapidly. There is no scientific evidence that this works.

Eat healthily and do not exclude foods from your diet. Some people think that avoiding foods that are high in arginine (an amino acid) or low in L-lysine will help to prevent attacks. Therefore they avoid wholegrains, nuts, onions, green vegetables, coconut and chocolate. The problem is that all these foods form part of a healthy diet (yes, even chocolate), and there is no scientific evidence that cutting them out has any effect on herpes.

It makes sense to keep generally healthy, and this means eating a varied diet with plenty of fruit and vegetables and food containing iron. Although there is no scientific evidence for its benefits, there would be no harm in trying a diet that is high in L-lysine. Such foods include yoghurt, apples, pears, mangoes, tomatoes, beetroot, chicken and oily fish.

'Avoid stress' is a common piece of advice to cold sore sufferers, as cold sores do tend to occur when people are run down or stressed, but avoiding stress is more easily said than done.

See your doctor if you are having really bad or frequent attacks, or if you also have eczema or other health problems. Your doctor might consider prescribing an antiviral drug in tablet form as a preventive measure, or giving you a supply of tablets to take at the first sign of another attack.

Useful contacts

Health*Insite* is an Australian government initiative aimed to improve the health of Australians by providing easy access to quality information about human health. Follow the link to find out more information on cold sores.
www.healthinsite.gov.au/topics/Cold_Sores

Australian Herpes Management Forum has information and some colour photographs on its website. It is sponsored by two pharmaceutical companies, GSK and Novartis Pharmaceuticals; both of these companies make antiherpes drugs.
www.herpes.on.net/cold_sores

Herpes Viruses Association is a UK non-profit organization that gives information on all types of herpes infections to its members. Its website has a FAQ section (but mainly about genital herpes rather than cold sores) and gives information about joining the association.
www.herpes.org.uk

Herpes.com is a large US website with lots of information about all types of herpes, including cold sores. If you are keen on changing the balance of L-lysine foods in your diet, look at its nutrition section for a list of the lysine content of foods.
www.herpes.com

The Cold Sore Information Bureau has an excellent website. It is sponsored by GSK, the manufacturer of aciclovir, and advertises their product. It has a questionnaire to help you identify your triggers, a good 'Coping strategies' section and FAQs. You can also request a free copy of their booklet.
www.csib.co.uk

Condoms

What are condoms?

A condom is a stretchy tube of latex rubber or polyurethane. One end is closed. Most condoms have a small pouch at the closed end (the teat), which collects semen and holds it in the condom. Condoms are designed to fit over the erect penis, so put the condom on when the penis is erect. If you try to put it on to a soft penis, it will fall off.

How effective are condoms?

Latex condoms have a contraceptive failure rate of 3% per year. This means that if 100 couples having regular sex used condoms correctly every time for a year, 3 of the women would become pregnant. Of course, if you do not use condoms every time you have sex, or if you do not use them properly, they will not be as effective, and the 'failure rate' would be about 15%.

Condoms have an important advantage over other types of contraception – they give good protection against sexually transmitted diseases. As a result, many women who use the contraceptive pill for protection against pregnancy, still like their partner to use condoms.

Early condoms were made of linen or pig or sheep's gut, tied at the end with ribbon. After sex, they were rinsed out and reused!

Using a condom

Choosing a condom. The range of available condoms is bewildering. With so many sizes, shapes and thicknesses on offer, how do you know which to choose? Obviously, you are safest with a well-known brand bought from a pharmacist or brand vending machine. Always check the sell-by date and quality certification. Try several until you find one that is comfortable for you. The preferred shape – be it straight, flared or contoured – seems to be a matter of personal choice. Researchers at the University of Exeter gave a variety of condoms to over 400 young men and women, and asked them to complete a questionnaire rating each condom for comfort and sensitivity. The results showed that roughly equal numbers of people preferred each shape – there was no outright winner. So just because a friend recommends a certain type, do not assume it will be right for you.

Some people prefer a thicker condom because it may make intercourse last slightly longer. Thicker condoms usually have words such as 'ultra-strong' or 'super strong' on the packet. Anyone intending to have anal sex must use an 'ultra-strong' or 'super-strong' condom.

Most condoms are made from latex rubber. If you think your condom reduces sensitivity or you dislike the rubbery, latex smell, try a polyurethane condom such as Durex Avanti or eZ.on. Polyurethane condoms feel thinner than they actually are, because they conduct body heat better. Avanti is as effective for contraception as the latex type and eZ.on slightly less so (*Cochrane Database Systematic Review* 2004;3:CD003991). However, non-latex condoms are slightly more likely to break.

Some condoms contain casein, a substance derived from milk; however, vegetarian/vegan-friendly condoms are available (see Useful contacts on page 78).

An 18th-century illustrated condom, featuring three naughty nuns, was sold at a Christie's auction for £3300

'Dos and don'ts'

- Do buy your condoms from a pharmacist or reputable brand vending machine, or another reliable source, not from a street trader.
- Do check the sell-by date when you buy – the further ahead it is, the better.
- Do choose a reputable brand that has a quality certification mark on the pack and an expiry date of over 2 years from now. In the UK this is the British Standard Kitemark, which means the sheaths are properly tested. Expiry dates are usually 5 years after manufacture. Alternatively, choose a pack marked 'BS EN 600' – this is the European standard, which is similar to the British Standard.
- Do make sure you have several condoms with you, in case you damage one or it goes on wrongly.
- Do be careful as you unwrap the condom – they can be damaged by teeth, fingernails and jewellery.
- Do be careful not to unroll the condom inside out (except eZ.on, which can be put on either way).
- Do use a water-based lubricant if needed (see the section on lubrication below for more advice).
- Do put the condom on before your penis touches your partner's genitals. It is possible for a woman to become pregnant if any sperm are spilt near the entrance of the vagina even if you do not have full intercourse. Sperm can ooze out of the penis before ejaculation happens ('pre-cum').
- Do pull the foreskin back before rolling on the condom (obviously, this does not apply if you have been circumcised).
- Do hold the condom on after you have ejaculated, otherwise it may slip off as you go soft and spill sperm.
- Do remember that the more you use condoms, and the more familiar you are with them, the more comfortable and efficient you will become.
- Don't feel embarrassed at the thought of buying condoms. As the Planned Parenthood Federation of America says, "Be proud. Buying condoms says you are responsible and that you accept your sexuality as a normal part of living". If you really are embarrassed, get them from a slot machine in a pub/bar toilet.

- Don't use a condom that is past its sell-by date or which feels sticky or very dry.
- Don't rely on a gimmick condom (such as glow-in the-dark or musical condom) for contraception.
- Don't use Vaseline, hand cream, butter, baby oil or any other oils for lubrication with latex rubber condoms (see the section on lubrication below for more advice).
- Don't use a condom more than once; use a new one each time you have intercourse.
- Don't flush the condom down the toilet after use, because it could cause a blockage. Wrap it in tissue or toilet paper and chuck it in the bin.

There is no truth in the story that condoms were invented by a Dr Condom, physician to Charles II

Talking about using condoms. It can be very awkward talking to a new partner about condoms. For some really practical advice, look at the website of the Planned Parenthood Federation of America to get some ideas for responses to partners reluctant to use a condom (see Useful contacts on page 78).

Lubrication. Some people find that sex is more enjoyable for themselves and their partner if they use a lubricant. Condom manufacturers admit that the lubrication they put on the condoms may not be enough, but adding more would make packaging difficult. Lubricants are especially useful if your partner has vaginal dryness (see page 311), and will also help prevent wear and tear on the condom. Smear the lubricant on the outside of the condom after you have put the condom on.

Do not just use any old thing as a lubricant. Most condoms are made of latex rubber and oils can cause latex to break down, reducing the strength of the condom by up to 95% in 15 minutes.

Lubricants that should NOT be used with latex rubber condoms

- Baby oil
- Cooking oil
- Massage oil
- Body lotion
- Bath oil
- Hand cream
- Suntan oil
- Petroleum jelly (Vaseline)
- Hair conditioner

Choose a water-based lubricant, such as KY Gel, Sylk, Boots Lubricating Jelly, Durex Play Lubricant, Senselle or Replens. The packet should tell you whether a lubricant is water-based or not. If you are unsure, ask the pharmacist or family planning clinic. Spit is not a good idea, because it dries quickly and could theoretically transmit HIV or hepatitis.

Some condoms are made from polyurethane, not latex rubber. These are not damaged by oily substances.

Common problems with condoms

Allergy. If you notice irritation, redness or itching after using a condom, you may wonder if you are allergic to the condom. In fact, allergy to rubber (latex) condoms is very unusual, but it would be sensible to switch to a polyurethane type such as Durex Avanti. There have been no reports of allergic responses to the polyurethane material.

In fact, irritation is more likely to be due to nonoxynol-9 or nonoxynol-11, spermicides (substances that kill sperm) that are ingredients of some lubricated condoms; however, they are becoming less commonly used. So try avoiding condoms that are labelled 'spermicidally lubricated'.

Another possible cause of irritation is too much friction, so use extra lubrication. Put some of the lubricant inside the top of the condom so that it covers the surface of the penis as you roll the condom on.

Putting it on and taking it off. Condom manufacturers never mention this problem in their leaflets. They simply tell you to unroll it onto the hard, erect penis, and preferably to pinch the teat or closed end to keep it empty at the same time. To do this properly, you need three hands or the assistance of a cooperative partner. It is no wonder that a survey conducted by the University of Sydney, Australia, which asked men about what really happened when they used condoms, found that two-thirds of them sometimes or often lost their erection while trying to put the condom on, so it was then impossible to put it on properly. Many disliked using a condom because it drew attention to this wilting problem (*Reproductive Health Matters* 1994;3:55–62).

Although it has been suggested that condoms were used by the Ancient Egyptians, the earliest actual report of a condom was by the Italian anatomist, Fallapio in 1564. He claimed to have invented a linen sheath, made to fit the penis, as protection against syphilis

The researchers suggest that, to make things easier for yourself, you should not try to pinch the teat at the end of the condom as you put it on. They found that pinching the teat makes no difference to the likelihood of the condom breaking or slipping off during intercourse. Latex condoms are designed to stretch enormously, so there is no reason why the presence of 1 mL or so of air in addition to 3–5 mL of semen should 'burst' the condom. They also suggest that instead of rolling the condom on, as recommended by the manufacturers, you could try pulling it on like a sock with your thumbs or fingers inside. Using this method, you can put it on securely even if your penis is not fully rigid. Obviously you have to be careful not to damage it with your nails. In their study, the researchers found that people who used this method had less chance of the condom slipping off or breaking.

If the condom does not reach the base of your penis or is difficult to roll down, then it is probably inside out. Take it off and try again with another one.

Slipping off. If you find a condom slips off, you probably assume it is too large for you. In fact, it is probably too small. If the condom is too tight you probably aren't unrolling it fully down the penis. This means that, during intercourse, the ring at the base of the condom is entering your partner's vagina, where it can be dragged off. If the condom is the right size, the ring will be right at the base of your penis, and will remain outside the vagina during sex.

If you have difficulty putting the condom on properly try the 'pull-on' method (see above). Finding the right size may be a matter of trial and error, because only a few manufacturers clearly show the length and width on the pack. The consumer magazine *Health Which?* measured various brands; the lengths varied from 168–191 mm, and the circumference from 98–111 mm.

The other problem is that most men do not really know how the size of their erect penis compares with other men, so are unsure whether they need a large condom or not. And most men only consider length whereas, just like short fat legs in stockings, a short fat penis also needs a large condom.

After ejaculation, when the penis quickly becomes limp, the condom can easily slip off, spilling sperm into your partner's vagina. At this stage, you must hold the condom firmly round the penis so that it remains in place until you have withdrawn.

Splitting or breaking. Research has shown that condom breakage is not a myth – it can happen.

In England condoms are known as 'French Letters', while in Italy they used to be called 'English Overcoats'

How commonly do condoms split?

A few surveys have tried to find out how often condoms split, but have given wildly differing results. Here are some figures:

- The University of Sydney, Australia, ran a study of condom breakage in three brothels. They supplied the fresh condoms, together with forms to fill in if there was an accident and little plastic bags to put the torn condoms in so the researchers could analyse in the laboratory how and why they tore. Of the 1269 condoms the sex workers used, only 6 were broken. Next, they did a survey of ordinary men, and found that their breakage rates were far higher – about 7%, including breakages while putting the condoms on (*The Lancet* 1988;ii:1487–8)
- A USA study asked 92 couples to keep a sex diary, totalling 4637 condom usages. Six condoms split while being put on, and 13 split during sex – a total breakage rate of 0.41% (*Contraception* 1997;56:3–12)
- French researchers did a telephone survey of 20 000 people, asking about condom breakages. The breakage rate seemed to be 3.4% (*American Journal of Public Health* 1997;87:421–4)

Why condoms split

Damage from ripping the packet open with teeth, scissors, knives or pencils is a common cause of tears.

Inexperience. Practice with condoms makes perfect, which is probably why, in the University of Sydney's study, the sex workers had the lowest breakage rate. The study also found that men were most likely to break condoms if they did not use condoms often, and if they rolled the condom on rather than pulled it on (see above).

Lack of lubrication may be another reason for breakage. Prostitutes tend to use additional lubrication, which may be another reason for their lower breakage rate.

Penis size is a possible factor. Condom manufacturers say that condoms are designed to stretch enormously, so a large penis should not make a condom more likely to break. However, a study from Australia suggests that you are more likely to break a condom if you have a thick penis, but the length of the penis does not make any difference (*International Journal of Sexually Transmitted Disease and AIDS* 1998;9:444–7).

What to do if a condom slips or breaks. If a condom slips off during intercourse, or if it breaks, the woman should visit her doctor or a family planning clinic as soon as possible for emergency contraception.

Emergency contraception (previously called the 'morning-after pill')

- Emergency contraception prevents pregnancy after intercourse has occurred, so it is a back-up if another method fails (such as when a condom breaks or slips off, or you forget a pill).
- In fact, it can be taken up to 72 hours after intercourse, not just on the morning after, but the earlier the better.
- The main side effect is nausea (in 50%) and vomiting (in 20%).
- It usually consists of a single dose, or two smaller doses taken 12 hours apart.
- In the UK (not in Ireland), you can buy it from a chemist for about £20, but only if you are aged 16 or above. It can only be given to you by a trained pharmacist, who will try to check that you are 16 or over. You cannot simply pick it up from the shelf.
- You can also obtain it from your doctor, from a family planning clinic or in the UK from an NHS walk-in centre (see Useful contacts on page 78). If you are a college student, your college website may give advice about getting emergency contraception from the Student Health Centre. As a last resort, you could try a hospital Accident and Emergency (casualty) department.
- The next period is unpredictable – it might be earlier or later than usual.
- Emergency contraception does not always work, so if your next period is late you might be pregnant. Have a pregnancy test to check.

Useful contacts

Family Planning NSW has a 'Useful contacts' link on their website to other family planning and sexual health clinics in Australia. The website also provides fact sheets and FAQs under the section 'Sex matters'.
www.fpahealth.org.au/sex-matters

HealthInsite is an Australian government initiative aimed to improve the health of Australians by providing easy access to quality information about human health. Follow the link to find out more information on condoms.
www.healthinsite.gov.au/topics/Condoms

Condoms Australia is an online product site selling a range of condom packages and lubricants. The website also has some useful information from sources around the world in regards to safe sex, the use of condoms and background history of condom brands on the market.
www.condomsaustralia.com.au

Brook provides free, confidential advice on sex and contraception (as well as free condoms) for young people under the age of 25. Its website has a special section that lists Brook centres in the UK (click on the Go to Brook button) so that you can find one near you. You can write to Brook confidentially via the 'Ask Brook' section on the website.
www.brook.org.uk

Durex offers information about its contraceptives (and also about penis size). The site also has a question-and-answer section, and several health tips.
www.durex.com

Family planning clinics in the UK provide free condoms. Look in the telephone directory under 'Family Planning' for your local clinic.

Health Which? is no longer published, but back issues should be available in local libraries in the UK.

FPA (previously the Family Planning Association) provides free information on contraception and sexual health. The website has information about all types of contraception.
www.fpa.org.uk

The Planned Parenthood Federation of America has a very good website with lots of practical advice about using condoms, including pictures of how to put them on, as well as advice about lubricants. Check out this site before buying condoms or lubricants from internet sites.
www.plannedparenthood.org/bc/condom.htm

Sylk is a lubricant, made from kiwi fruit, that is safe to use with condoms. It is available by mail order and from some shops (see website for stockists).
www.sylk.co.uk

Condoms by Professor Adrian Mindel is a book that tells you everything that you could wish to know about the history, manufacture and use of condoms. It is published by BMJ Books.
ISBN 0 7279 1267 4

Marie Stopes International website has information on types of contraception and other sexual health topics.
www.MarieStopes.org.uk

Constipation

How the bowel and anus work

The colon (large bowel) is the lower part of the gut. It is more than a metre long. Its job is to store faecal material and remove fluid from it, so that the faeces are fairly solid and the body does not waste water. The colon may absorb 1 litre of fluid a day. The colon contains lots of helpful bacteria that break down food residues (turning some of them into wind) and manufacture some vitamins. The muscles of the colon gently contract and relax all the time, rolling the waste matter about like clothes in a washing machine. Several times a day, usually after meals, the colon makes some big muscular contractions to dump the faecal material in the rectum further down.

An average person on a typical western diet passes about 150 g of faeces each day. Faeces consist of about one-third solids and two-thirds water

The rectum and anal canal. The large bowel (colon) leads into the last part of the gut, which is called the rectum. It is about 12–15 cm long. The final 3 cm of the gut is called the anal canal.

When faeces arrive in the rectum, it sends a message to the nerve centres in the spinal cord, and these send a message to the sphincter muscles of the anal canal, making them relax to open the anus. If it is inconvenient for us to have our bowels open, the brain sends a message to the spinal cord to prevent the 'open anus' message being sent. We are not aware of this until the rectum becomes very full, when we have to make a conscious effort to keep the anus closed. When we allow the anus to open, the muscles in the wall of the large bowel and rectum contract to push the faeces out. The wall of the anal canal is very muscular. The muscles keep the anus closed, except when faeces ('stools') are passed.

- The ring of muscle at the top of the anal canal is called the 'internal sphincter'. This muscle is not under our conscious control.
- The ring at the opening of the anus is called the 'external sphincter'. This muscle is more like the sort of muscle that we have in our arms and legs, and we are able to control it (until the urge to pass faeces becomes overwhelming).

It is obvious that in babies the system of nerve messages that keep the anus shut is not in place – babies pass faeces as soon as the rectum fills. After about 18 months of age, the system develops, but in some children this can take a long time.

A network of small veins lies under the lining of the anal canal. These veins form a soft, spongy pad that acts as an extra seal to keep the canal closed until you go to the toilet. The lining of the gut is very slimy (so that faeces can pass along easily); the extra seal stops the slime (mucus) from leaking out. The spongy pads can become swollen. When this happens they are called piles (see page 212), also known as haemorrhoids.

Most of the waste matter from food is passed out in the faeces within 72 hours, but in healthy people up to 30% may remain in the colon for a week or more

ADULTS
Are you really constipated?

Constipation is difficult to define. What one person regards as constipation, another person may regard as normal for them. So try the following questions.

- Do you have to strain to pass faeces at least one time in four?
- Are your faeces lumpy or hard at least one time in four?
- Do you feel that you have not emptied your bowel completely, at least one time in four?
- Do you pass faeces only once or twice a week?

If you answered 'yes' to two or more of these questions, and you have had the problem for more than 3 months, then you do have constipation.

Alarm signals

Constipation is usually just a nuisance. There is no scientific evidence that 'toxins' from faeces in the bowel can affect your health. However, very occasionally it is a sign of serious disease such as cancer of the colon (large bowel). So it is very important that you see your doctor if any of the following applies to your symptoms.

- Your constipation is a new symptom, and there is no obvious reason for it.
- It is severe and changing your diet has not helped.
- The constipation alternates with diarrhoea.
- You have noticed other symptoms, such as bleeding (see page 24) from the back passage (even if you think this is caused by piles), passing slime from the back passage, tummy pain, weight loss, and/or pain in the back passage when you strain to pass faeces.
- Anyone in your family has had colon cancer.

If the idea of seeing your doctor worries you, have a look at the section on seeing your doctor about an anal problem on page 338.

In a UK survey, 6% of people said they had suffered from constipation in the past year, 13% had difficulty in passing their faeces at least once a month and 19% took laxatives at some time

Causes of constipation

To understand constipation, it helps to know how the lower part of the gut (colon, large bowel) works. As food moves through it, the colon absorbs water while forming waste products. The waste products are the faeces ('stools'). Muscle contractions in the colon push the stool towards the rectum, which is the last section of the bowel before the anus (back passage). By the time the stool reaches the rectum, it is almost solid because most of the water has been absorbed.

The hard and dry stools of constipation occur when the colon absorbs too much water. This happens because its muscle contractions are slow or sluggish, causing the stool to move through it too slowly.

The following questions will help you to work out the reason for your constipation.

- Are you really constipated? (See the checklist on page 80.)
- Are you taking enough fluids and fibre in your diet? In northern climates, dehydration is not usually a problem, but in hot climates, it can cause dry stools that are difficult to pass.
- Do you take enough exercise?
- Are you taking any medicines that can cause constipation (see below)?
- Are you allowing enough bathroom time to defecate?
- Has there been any change in your lifestyle? Has your job or have your personal relationships become more demanding?
- Are you depressed? Nerves link the brain to the gut and, if you are depressed, reduced activity of these nerves affects the muscle activity of the bowel and results in constipation in some people.
- Do you have a frequent desire to defecate, then strain to pass a few small pellets and leave feeling there is still more to come? This is typical of irritable bowel syndrome (see Useful contacts on page 87).
- After straining for some time, does the back passage seem to bulge as the stool comes halfway through? This feeling often occurs with piles (haemorrhoids, see page 212).
- Do you have a painful condition, such as piles (haemorrhoids, see page 212) or anal fissure (see page 30)? If passing faeces is painful, constipation is a likely result.
- If you are a woman, do you have to put a finger in your vagina to help pass the stool from the back passage? This probably means that you have a rectocele, a weakness in the supporting tissues between the vagina and rectum. This is not dangerous and it can be treated by a gynaecologist.
- If you are a woman, did the constipation start after childbirth or after hysterectomy? Hysterectomy may sometimes damage the delicate nerve fibres connected to the bowel.
- Have you gained weight and tend to feel the cold, and maybe have dry or thinning hair? You might have an underactive thyroid, which can also cause constipation.
- Do you have any other symptoms?
- Are you pregnant? About 1 in 3 pregnant women has constipation, probably because of the hormone progesterone. The best way to deal with it is to take extra fibre in your diet.

- Have you recently stopped smoking? Almost 1 in 10 quitters experiences constipation (*Addiction* 2003;98:1563–7).

In the USA, more than $800 million is spent on laxatives each year

Check your medicines. Some medicines can cause constipation. Common culprits are:

- painkillers or cough medicines containing codeine
- antacids (for indigestion) containing aluminium or calcium
- iron tablets
- some antidepressants (tricyclic and monoamine oxidase inhibitor types) and tranquillizers
- some drugs for Parkinson's disease and for epilepsy (Parkinson's disease can itself cause constipation)
- some diuretic drugs (for high blood pressure or heart failure).

Obviously, you should not stop a medicine that has been prescribed for you just because it is making you constipated – it could be an important medication for you, so discuss it with your family doctor.

About 4 500 000 people in the US say they are constipated most or all of the time (National Health Interview Survey)

Improving constipation

There are three main ways of dealing with constipation:

- eat more fibre (see page 83)
- drink more fluid
- take more exercise.

Your diet. The best way to deal with constipation is to eat plenty of fibre and drink plenty of fluid. Drink about 8–10 glasses of water a day (that is 2 litres). Fibre is not digested and absorbed in the intestines, so the stools are softer and more bulky, and it is easier for the bowel muscles to push them along. You may think you have a high-fibre diet, but in reality you may not be taking enough. In the UK, 100 years ago, we each consumed about 40 g of fibre a day, but most of us now have less than 15–20 g a day. Traditional African diets contain 50–150 g of fibre a day.

Aim for at least 30 g of fibre a day, which really means eating one fibre-rich food at every meal. If you suddenly increase the amount of fibre you eat, you may notice wind and bloating, so increase the amount slowly, over about 2 weeks, to allow your gut to adjust to the new diet.

A simple way of increasing fibre in your diet is to:

- change to wholemeal bread, and eat 2–4 extra slices a day
- eat 2–3 extra helpings of fruit and vegetables a day
- change to a wholewheat cereal (the packet will tell you)
- add some raw bran to your cereal or yogurt.

A high-fibre diet is healthy for most people, but if you are elderly and not very mobile it can make the constipation worse, so check with your doctor. Also some people find that a high-fibre diet worsens bloating without improving constipation. And if you have a medical condition, such as heart failure, it may not be advisable to take so much fluid. Again, check with your doctor.

Fibre checklist

High-fibre foods

Bowl of All Bran	9.8 g
Bowl of Bran Buds	8.0 g
Bowl of muesli	6.2 g
Bowl of Bran Flakes	5.2 g
2 slices wholemeal bread	4.1 g
½ large can red kidney beans	12.4 g
½ large can baked beans	7.6 g
Medium jacket potato	4.2 g
4 tablespoons peas	4.1 g
5 dried apricots	5.8 g
5 prunes	4.9 g
100 g Quorn	4.8 g

Medium-fibre foods

2 Weetabix	3.9 g
Bowl of Fruit'n Fibre	2.8 g
2 slices ordinary brown bread	2.5 g
2 slices white bread	1.1 g
3 tablespoons cooked sprouts	3.1 g
2 tablespoons cooked broccoli	2.3 g
3 tablespoons cooked carrots	1.9 g
½ avocado	3.4 g
Apple (with skin)	3.1 g
Orange	2.7 g
Banana	2.2 g
1 tablespoon peanuts	1.6 g
1 tablespoon mixed nuts and raisins	1.1 g

Source: *MeReC Bulletin* 1999;10 (No 9).

Think about your lifestyle. Exercise is important. Inactivity can make the bowels sluggish, so be as active as possible. Changing patterns of shift work can upset the rhythm of your bowels. Similarly, it is quite common to be constipated at the beginning of a foreign holiday, especially if you have crossed time zones and are also eating foods that are different from your normal diet.

Toilet training (for adults). Another reason for constipation is what doctors call 'poor bowel habit'. This means ignoring the urge to have your bowels open, perhaps because you are too busy or you dislike using a toilet away from home or near other people.

The problem with that is that, after a while, you stop feeling the urge. So do not ignore it when your body tells you that you are ready to open your bowels. And give yourself enough time for an undisturbed visit to the toilet, preferably half an hour after breakfast.

Humans are probably meant to open their bowels in a squatting posture – sitting on a toilet is not the optimum position. So, when you sit on the toilet, prop your feet up on a footstool.

Do not push and strain to pass a stool. This increases the likelihood of piles or painful anal cracks (fissure), and can be dangerous if you have high blood pressure. If nothing has happened after 10 or 15 minutes, go away and do something else, and try again later.

Dealing with painful anal conditions. If you have a painful anal condition, look at the sections on anal pain (see page 30), piles (haemorrhoids, see page 212) and anal fissure (see page 30).

Do you need a laxative? Laxatives should be a last resort; they are usually not necessary and can be habit-forming. Dozens of laxatives are available from pharmacies without a prescription, so if you have tried changing your diet and it has not worked, you may be tempted to try one. Before doing so, see your doctor. This is because constipation in most people is dealt with by increasing the fibre in the diet as suggested above, by increasing the amount of fluid you drink and by taking more exercise. If this has not worked for you, there could be a more serious reason, which your doctor needs to sort out.

If your doctor decides there is nothing seriously wrong, a laxative might be appropriate, particularly if:

- you have piles, and they bleed if you strain to pass faeces
- you have bad angina, and your doctor has told you to avoid straining to pass faeces
- you are elderly, and your tummy and pelvic muscles are weak, so passing faeces is difficult.

Types of laxative

Bulk laxatives (such as psyllium husk from health-food stores, bran, ispaghula husk, methylcellulose, sterculia) provide fibre in a concentrated form. They have to be taken with plenty of water, and it can be several days before they have an effect. They are the best type of laxative for long-term use.

Stimulant laxatives (such as senna, bisacodyl) work by increasing contractions of the bowel, and so they can cause tummy cramps. The effect occurs in about 6–12 hours, so they are taken at night to produce a morning bowel action. Some experts think that if you use these regularly for years, the contractions of the large bowel (colon) may eventually become weakened, making the problem much worse than before, so this type of laxative is inadvisable for long-term use. Glycerol suppositories that you insert into the back passage (rectum) act as a stimulant because they are slightly irritant to the bowel.

Osmotic laxatives retain fluid in the bowel, which then softens the faeces. Examples of this type of laxative are: Cream of Magnesia, which is magnesium hydroxide; Epsom salts or Andrews Liver salts, which are magnesium sulphate; and Movicol.

Lactulose and lactitol are types of sugars that the body cannot digest, so they remain in the bowel where they act partly like fibre and partly like an osmotic laxative. They often cause bloating, wind and tummy cramps and have to be taken regularly for up to 3 days before having an effect.

Faecal softeners, such as 'liquid paraffin' from a pharmacy, lubricate and soften the stool. They probably act by lining the bowel with a film of oil that stops water being absorbed into the body from the stool. Liquid paraffin is also a mild stimulant and is not suitable for long-term use.

Biofeedback. Some people, most often young women, have a problem coordinating the muscles of the bowel, anus and pelvic floor. For example, when they are trying to pass faeces, they contract the anus muscle instead of relaxing it. Special feedback training can overcome the problem. This treatment is available in only a few specialist hospitals, and is reserved for people with a severe constipation problem.

CHILDREN

Constipation in children is a common problem, and is not very easy for parents to deal with. The good news is that it usually clears up with time. Parents often worry that it means there is something seriously wrong, but this is very seldom the case.

What is normal?

Normal healthy children vary in how often they have their bowels open. Most children aged 1–4 years pass stools (faeces) once or twice a day. However, some children have their bowels open three times a day, whereas others have a bowel motion every other day. All this is quite normal. And a few perfectly healthy children have their bowels open once every 3 days.

The size and consistency of the stools will vary, depending on what your child has been eating and drinking.

How do I know my child is constipated?

Signs of constipation are:

- your child seems to be straining hard to have a bowel movement
- having a bowel movement is painful – suspect this if your child seems to be trying to hold the bowel motion in (for example by crossing the legs or sitting up on the heels) or if your child seems frightened of using the toilet
- the stools are very hard and dry.

Causes of constipation in children

Not enough fluid and fibre in the diet is probably the most common cause.

Anal fissure is another common cause (see page 30). An anal fissure is a crack in the skin at the edge of the anus, and this makes a bowel movement very painful. Often the problem will have started after the child was unwell with a viral infection. During the infection he or she might not have taken in enough fluids, so the stools became dry and difficult to pass. The hard, dry stools are then likely to have scratched the anus, causing the fissure.

Worries about using toilets, for example at nursery school or school where there might be a lack of privacy, can trigger a period of constipation.

A tummy upset, in which the child had diarrhoea that was difficult to control, can sometimes result in constipation afterwards. This could be because the child is worried about not being able to hold faeces in.

Emotional upset is another possible trigger if, for example, there has been a lot of family stress recently.

Medicines are not a common cause of constipation in children (unlike in adults), but some cough mixtures can have this effect.

Cows' milk allergy seems to be a fashionable diagnosis at the moment for all sorts of gut problems in children. In some, it may be the cause of constipation. If other people in the family have a tendency to asthma and eczema, it is worth considering. Constipation sometimes occurs when an infant is switched from breast milk to cows' milk or formula milk.

How to help your child

Talk to your doctor if your child is less than 1 year old. If your child is over a year old, here are a few things you can try.

Encourage the child to drink plenty of fluids. Avoid sweet and fizzy drinks because they are bad for teeth. Offer a variety of drinks, such as water, diluted fruit juices and milk. (In some children, too much milk can have the opposite effect, making constipation worse.) Prune, pear and apple juices contain a sugar called sorbitol that is particularly good at keeping stools soft. In cooler climates, children aged 4–6 years should drink about 1.5 litres in a day and children aged 7 years and older should drink about 2 litres in a day. Obviously, children in hot climates will need more.

Increase the amount of fibre in the diet. This can be difficult. A survey showed that 29–48% of children with constipation are 'fussy eaters', and 47% have a poor appetite. Eating often improves once the constipation has been dealt with. Meanwhile, you could explain to your child that you are changing the diet to make the stools soft and easier to pass, but do not make it into an issue. Give the whole family the same foods. Aim for five portions of fruit or vegetables a day. You will find a list of high- and medium-fibre foods on page 83. With luck, this list contains some foods that your child will like.

Do not exclude milk from the diet without talking to your doctor; it could result in nutritional deficiencies. About 50% of children with true cows' milk allergy are also allergic to soya protein, so changing to soya might not be a simple solution.

Provide breakfast, and serve it early. For many children, breakfast seems to trigger a bowel movement. (This is called the gastrocolic reflex.) If you serve breakfast early, there will be plenty of time for the child to go to the toilet. Otherwise, because of the rush to get ready for school, the child may hold the stool in and then be reluctant to use the toilet at school.

Provide a child's toilet seat (which fits over the normal seat), because it will make your child's hip bend at the optimum angle for having a bowel movement.

Do not give your child laxatives without talking to your doctor or health visitor. There are several different sorts of laxatives. Let your doctor or health visitor choose the most appropriate type if necessary.

When to see your doctor

You should see your doctor if your child is under a year old. If your child is older, you could try the measures outlined above for a couple of weeks, and then see your doctor if they have not solved the problem. Another reason for seeing the doctor promptly is if you find yourself becoming angry with your child about it. A child with constipation can make you feel very frustrated, but the constipation is not the child's fault, and is not being done deliberately. It is important to be patient.

The main reason for getting help is that constipation has to be sorted out, because if it continues for a long time the rectum enlarges. Then your child will miss a feeling that he or she needs to have a bowel movement, and the muscles of the bowel will not work properly to push the faeces out. Instead, liquid waste will dribble out from around the faeces, and there will be soiling of underwear. Then you will think that diarrhoea is the trouble, when in fact constipation is still the actual problem.

What your doctor can do

Your doctor will check that there is nothing physically wrong with your child. Your doctor might then decide that a laxative would be a good idea. Several types of laxative are available (see pages 84–85). It is usual to start with lactulose to make the faeces soft, but other types may be needed. The laxative is often continued for about 3 months, and then very gradually reduced.

Useful contacts

Colorectal Surgical Society of Australasia has some very useful information on diseases of the colon and rectum on its website under 'Patient info'. Brochures may also be purchased by completing their online order form.
www.cssa.org.au

Health*Insite* is an Australian government initiative aimed to improve the health of Australians by providing easy access to quality information about human health. Follow the link to find information relating to constipation.
www.healthinsite.gov.au/topics/Constipation

Bowel Control. This website is provided by St Mark's Hospital, UK, which is a hospital specializing in bowel problems. The site covers faecal leakage, constipation and wind. It is a first-rate site that is very practical and informative.
www.bowelcontrol.org.uk

American Academy of Family Physicians have two detailed articles on 'Common Anorectal Conditions' on their website. The articles are intended for doctors. They explain how doctors examine the anus. They discuss itching, pain, bleeding, lumps, constipation and incontinence of faeces.
www.aafp.org/afp/20010615/2391.html
www.aafp.org/afp/20010701/77.html

Children's Hospital of Iowa. This site has been checked for accuracy by the Children's Hospital of Boston. It provides straightforward factsheets about constipation in children.
www.vh.org/navigation/vch/topics/pediatric_patient_constipation.html

Digestive Disorders Foundation is a UK non-profit organization that provides reliable information about all gut problems. They supply a range of leaflets, which are on the 'Learn more about disorders' section of their website.
www.digestivedisorders.org.uk

National Digestive Diseases Information Clearinghouse is a US government organization. Its website has pages on piles (haemorrhoids), constipation and other gut problems.
www.digestive.niddk.nih.gov/ddiseases/a-z.asp

The American Gastroenterological Association is an organization for doctors who specialize in the gut. Look in the Patients/Public section of its website for excellent information about various gut problems including piles and constipation.
www.gastro.org/clinicalRes/brochures/constipation.html

The Mayo Clinic website provides information about all aspects of constipation and also has a slide show explaining how digestion works.
www.mayoclinic.com

Crab lice

Lice feed on human blood. There are three types: head lice (see page 171), which are common in children; clothing lice – sometimes called body lice – which are common in vagrants, live in clothing and only visit the skin to feed; and crab or pubic lice.

How crab lice are caught

Lice cannot jump, hop, fly or swim. Crab lice probably cannot be caught from toilet seats or even from bedclothes, but this is not 100% certain. They probably cannot survive for more than 24 hours away from a person. They are transmitted by close body contact, during which they are able to transfer their grip from one person's hair to that of the other before letting go entirely from the first person. Sexual contact is their ideal situation.

Lice have been found on 4000-year-old mummies

Where crab lice live

Crab lice cannot live in hair that is too dense, so they will not colonize the hair of the scalp (except at the hairline). However, they will live happily on armpit hair, eyebrows, eyelashes, chest hair and upper thigh hair as well as pubic hair.

How to tell if you have crab lice

Itching occurs, especially at night, in the pubic hair area.

Seeing the lice. The lice are small (up to 2 mm long), and can just be seen with the naked eye. They are squat in shape and, with a magnifying glass, you can see that all the legs emerge close together from the front of the body, and the middle and hind legs have large pincer-like claws giving the 'crab' appearance. They use their claws to grasp hairs close to the skin surface. They hardly move except at night, when they slowly transfer their grip from one hair to another.

Nits, which are the egg cases, can be seen attached to the hairs. The female lays the eggs in a hard brown shell, which she attaches to the hair on the surface of the skin. As the hair grows, the egg case will be further up its shaft, so the position of the nits on the hair gives you an idea of how long you have had them. After about 8 days the eggs hatch, and the empty egg case appears white and is easier to see.

Rust-coloured specks may be seen on the skin – these are louse faeces.

Blood specks may be seen on underwear.

What you can do

There is a choice of treatment. In the UK, you can buy 0.5% malathion lotion without prescription from the pharmacy (e.g. Prioderm, Derbac-M or Quellada-M). Prioderm contains alcohol, which can irritate the skin of the scrotum and any scratched areas. Derbac-M or Quellada-M are preferable because they do not contain alcohol.

A single application of either lotion is probably enough, but some specialists advise another application after 7 days to eliminate any newly hatched lice. Apply the lotion to the whole body from the neck down, even if you think only the pubic area is affected. A paintbrush is the best method. To be on the safe side, change underclothes and bedlinen after treatment.

Do not treat yourself, but go to a doctor, if:

- you are pregnant
- you think you have crabs on your eyelashes or eyebrows; do not try to treat these yourself with lotion.

The French used to call crab lice 'papillons d'amour', which means 'butterflies of love'

What your doctor can do

You can see your family doctor or go to a sexual health clinic. The advantage of the clinic is that the staff are expert crab spotters who will be able to confirm that your diagnosis is correct. Also, you can have tests to check you have not picked up any other infection at the same time, and the treatment will probably be free.

Useful contacts

Family Planning NSW has a 'Useful contacts' link on their website to other family planning and sexual health clinics in Australia. The website also provides fact sheets and FAQs under the section 'Sex matters'.
www.fpahealth.org.au/sex-matters

Health*Insite* is an Australian government initiative aimed to improve the health of Australians by providing easy access to quality information about human health. Follow the link to find information on a variety of sexually transmitted infections.
www.healthinsite.gov.au/topics/Sexually_Transmitted_Infections

The Society of Health Advisers in Sexually Transmitted Diseases has a page on pubic lice on its website, with photographs. The site also has information about visiting a sexual health clinic, a list of the clinics in the UK and Ireland, and a link to a list of clinics in the US.
www.ssha.info/public/infections/pubic_lice.asp

Cystitis

CYSTITIS IN WOMEN

Cystitis is inflammation of the bladder. There are two main types. The only sure way to tell the difference is by a urine test.

Bacterial cystitis is caused by bacteria (germs). These bacteria, mainly *Escherichia coli* (*E. coli* for short), normally live in and around the anus (back passage). In men, the urethra goes along the length of the penis and is about 24–30 cm long but, in women, it is only about 6 cm long. So in women bacteria on the skin can easily get into the bladder by using the short urethra as a ladder. This probably explains why cystitis is much more common in women than in men.

Interstitial cystitis (also called painful bladder syndrome, non-bacterial cystitis, urgency and frequency syndrome) is inflammation of the bladder without any bacteria being present. Most sufferers (90%) are women. It can occur at any age, but is most common in women in their early 40s.

Interstitial cystitis is a bit of a mystery – no one really knows what causes it.

- One theory is that a substance called glycosaminoglycan is deficient in the bladder. This substance is part of the slimy layer that covers and protects the lining of the bladder.
- Another theory is that it is a type of allergy, because cells common in allergy (mast cells) are present in the bladder wall in interstitial cystitis.

Every year, 1–3 women out of 10 have an attack of cystitis

Symptoms of cystitis

The symptoms of cystitis are:

- a burning, stinging or aching pain when you pass urine
- a need to pass water very frequently, often only a small amount each time
- bloody or cloudy urine (severe cystitis).

Not all urine problems are cystitis. For example:

- if you have soreness or itching around the opening of the urethra (pee hole) you might have a herpes infection (see page 131), thrush (see page 139) or a chlamydia infection (see page 127)
- if your only problem is having to pass urine frequently, you might have diabetes (especially if you are thirsty all the time), so see your doctor
- if your main problem is having to rush to the toilet, you may have a continence problem (see page 283).

Bacterial cystitis. With bacterial cystitis, you usually experience only the burning pain and frequent urination. However, it is possible for the infection to travel upwards to the kidney. Fortunately, this is unusual. Infection in the kidney needs proper medical treatment, so see your doctor straightaway if you also have:

- blood (or a smoky appearance) in the urine
- backache or stomach ache
- fever and weakness.

Interstitial cystitis. With interstitial cystitis the symptoms are diverse. You have to pass urine frequently, and maybe urgently, and passing the urine may be uncomfortable. You may notice discomfort in the lower abdomen when the bladder is filling (pelvic pain), which is relieved by passing small amounts of urine. Sex may be painful. Often, symptoms are worse in the week before a period.

At any time, about 1 in 20 healthy women has bacteria in her bladder, without any symptoms. Only 10% of these progress to cystitis symptoms

What you can do

Cystitis can come on very suddenly, and the last thing you want to do is go to the shops. So make sure you have paracetamol, long-life cranberry juice, potassium citrate cystitis remedy (available from pharmacists) and two hot water bottles available.

It is not necessary to see your doctor for every attack of cystitis – 60% of attacks of bacterial cystitis cure themselves within 4 days without antibiotics. The following measures will relieve the discomfort, and help you to get through the attack.

- Take painkillers such as paracetamol if you need them.
- Decide whether you need to see your doctor, for example, if this is your first attack (see below).
- Drink plenty of water. As soon as you feel an attack coming on, drink 300 mL (that is a glassful) of water straight away. Then continue to drink 300 mL of water or very weak tea every hour for 3 hours. Avoid coffee and alcohol because these can irritate the bladder.
- Make sure you empty your bladder completely each time, pushing out every last drop.
- Drink about 300 mL of cranberry juice twice a day, because it may help to shorten the attack
- Use a potassium citrate cystitis remedy according to the instructions on the packet. This neutralizes acidity in urine. It will not get rid of bacteria, but it can relieve symptoms. If you do not have potassium citrate, mix a teaspoonful of bicarbonate of soda with some water – this will do a similar job. Repeat it three more times, an hour apart. (But do not use bicarbonate of soda if you are on a low-salt diet for blood pressure.)
- Use hot water bottles, in a cover or wrapped in a towel, and put one on your lower back, and one between your legs, close to the opening of the urethra (pee hole).

Cranberry juice and blueberries

There is some evidence that cranberry juice is useful for preventing cystitis and possibly also for treating an attack.

- A study of 150 female students (*British Medical Journal* 2001;322:1571–3) showed that a daily drink of concentrated cranberry juice reduced the likelihood of bacterial cystitis by 20%, so it is good for prevention.
- Some studies have shown that cranberry juice will shorten an attack of cystitis, while other studies have shown no effect.
- Cranberry juice contains proanthocyanidin chemicals, which prevent *Escherichia coli* bacteria from sticking to the wall of the bladder and urethra. Therefore they can be flushed out before establishing an infection.
- The effect of cranberry juice lasts only about 10 hours, so it should be taken twice a day.
- Researchers have now found that blueberries also contain proanthocyanidins
- Apart from their benefits in preventing cystitis, blueberries and cranberry juice are good sources of vitamin C and antioxidants.

When to contact your doctor

Consult your doctor if:

- you have never had cystitis before
- you are having a bad attack, and after 24 hours it does not seem to be getting better
- you have other symptoms, such as stomach ache or backache
- you are feverish
- you are sore and/or itchy around the urethra. This could mean you have thrush (see page 139) or herpes (see page 131)
- you have vaginal discharge; this could mean you have a sexually transmitted infection
- there is blood in your urine or it looks smoky (which could mean that it contains blood)
- you are or may be pregnant
- you keep getting attacks and/or they last a long time
- you have other health problems (such as diabetes) or you have had kidney problems in the past
- you think you might have interstitial cystitis.

Doctors are very used to dealing with cystitis, but if you think you might have thrush or a sexually transmitted infection such as herpes you might prefer to go to a sexual health clinic instead.

What your doctor can do

Antibiotics. Your doctor can prescribe an antibiotic (such as nitrofurantoin or trimethoprim) if bacterial cystitis seems likely. Cure rates with antibiotics are about 85–95%.

Checking your urine for bacteria. Your doctor can check your urine for bacteria, but may not do this for an ordinary single attack of cystitis. It is only if you keep getting cystitis that you definitely need a urine check. Ideally, the doctor needs a urine sample when you are having an attack, and one that is not too dilute, which is problematic if you have started drinking lots of water. A way round this difficulty is for you to collect a special sample container from the surgery at the beginning of an attack so that you can pass some urine into it first thing next morning (because early morning urine is more concentrated). Contact your doctor's surgery and ask for their advice.

Interstitial cystitis. If no bacteria are present and your doctor thinks you have interstitial cystitis, there are several possible treatments (*Journal of Urology* 2003;170:816–7). They do not cure the condition, but can keep symptoms under control. There is a lot of interest in this condition, and many new treatments are being investigated, so the future is hopeful.

- Amitriptyline and similar drugs are often used. These drugsa are commonly used antidepressants, but they also have a pain-blocking effect. In interstitial cystitis, they are used as a pain blocker, not because your doctor thinks you are depressed or imagining your symptoms.
- Antihistamine medications (similar to hayfever treatments) have been tried, on the basis that interstitial cystitis might be a type of allergy.
- Pentosan polysulfate is used in the US, but is not available in the UK. It contains the glucosaminoglycans chemicals that some researchers think are deficient in the bladders of women with interstitial cystitis. Scientific studies to assess whether it works have given contradictory results.
- 'Hydrodistension' is stretching of the bladder with water. This is a specialist treatment and you would need an anaesthetic. No one knows how it works, but it helps 60% of people. The improvement lasts for several months.
- DMSO (dimethyl sulfoxide) can be squirted into the bladder to reduce pain and inflammation. It works in about 50% of people. For this treatment, you will need to be referred to a specialist. There have been worries that DMSO could affect the eyes and liver.

In the US, over 11 million women each year receive antibiotics for cystitis, costing over $1.6 billion

Preventing further attacks

Most women who have a urinary infection do not get another one, but some unlucky women seem to get them constantly. Here are some things you can do to lessen the chance of frequent attacks. They apply mainly to bacterial cystitis, but might also be helpful in interstitial cystitis.

- Drink cranberry juice or eat some blueberries every day.
- Wash thoroughly, using your hand to soap the anus and vulva (the area between the legs in women). Rinse well. Do not use a flannel or sponge to wash yourself. These harbour bacteria, even if you rinse them well.
- Do not use antiseptic wipes or perfumed soap, and do not put antiseptics or bubble baths in the bath water. Antiseptics, perfumes and other chemicals can irritate the vulva and the opening of the urethra, and make the problem worse.
- After you have passed a bowel motion, wipe your bottom from front to back. There is no need to wash the vulva after each bowel movement.
- Do not wear jeans that are too tight. The knot of seams can bruise the opening of the urethra, which might make infection more likely.
- If you have interstitial cystitis, check your diet. Some people find that caffeine, alcohol, chocolate, artificial sweeteners or acidic foods make it worse. Smoking may also make it worse.
- If you are at or have had the menopause, vaginal dryness (see page 311) can cause soreness and bruising of the urethra during intercourse. Use a lubricant.
- Ask your doctor about long-term, low-dose antibiotics (such as nitrofurantoin or trimethoprim) if bacterial cystitis is making your life a misery. Some women have taken these successfully for 5 years. You will need to try them for 3 months to find out whether they work for you. Alternatively, your doctor could give you a standby supply of antibiotics to keep at home and use when the symptoms start, continuing until 24 hours after the symptoms have gone.

In the UK, doctors write 5.5 million prescriptions for cystitis each year

Cystitis related to sex. Boisterous sex is a common cause of cystitis ('honeymoon cystitis'), partly because it can bruise the urethra slightly. It may also squeeze bacteria in the urethra upwards towards the bladder.

- Wash your genital area before and after having sex.
- Think about the contraception you are using. Spermicides are used with contraceptive diaphragms to increase their efficiency, and some condoms are manufactured with a spermicidal lubricant. Research at the University of Washington, published in the *Journal of Infectious Diseases* in 2000, showed that urinary tract infections were most likely in women who were most sexually active and who had contact with spermicides.
- Your doctor can prescribe an antibiotic for you to take just one dose of after you have sex.
- Ask your partner to wash his hands and penis before sex.
- Pass urine as soon as possible after sex, to flush out any bacteria – drink a glass of water beforehand so that you have something to pee afterwards.

CYSTITIS IN MEN

Cystitis means inflammation of the bladder, usually caused by an infection. It may not cause any symptoms at all, or it may cause pain or burning when you pass urine.

- In young men, true cystitis is uncommon. It may mean that the urinary system has some abnormality that is allowing germs (bacteria) to take hold. The abnormality could be a pocket-shaped pouch sticking out from the wall of the bladder, or a stone in the bladder.
- Young men sometimes think they have cystitis if urinating is painful, but the cause is more likely to be inflammation of the urethra (the tube that runs from the bladder, along the penis to the pee hole). Inflammation of the urethra is called urethritis. It is often caused by a sexually transmitted infection such as chlamydia (see page 127).
- Older men (in their 50s and older) are more likely to get cystitis than younger men. This is because the prostate gland often starts to enlarge in middle age. An enlarged prostate stops the bladder emptying efficiently, and bacteria can breed in the stagnant urine in the bladder.

What you can do

- If you have pain passing urine, the best plan is to go to a sexual health clinic, because they can do all the necessary tests very easily. They will check for sexually transmitted infections such as chlamydia and gonorrhoea that can inflame the urethra, and will give you the correct treatment. They will also do a urine test to see if you do have true cystitis (bladder infection). Alternatively, you could see your own doctor.
- If you do have a urine infection, you will need more investigations to look for abnormalities of your urinary system. Your doctor will arrange an X-ray and an ultrasound test, or an IVU (intravenous urogram).

Useful contacts

Australian Interstitial Cystitis Resource Centre provides extensive and effective support, research, current information, and a safe haven for IC patients too ill or too distant to attend local support group meetings. The AICRC offers the largest online support system for Australian Interstitial cystitis patients, located in the Community Centre.
www.icnaustralia.com

Health*Insite* is an Australian government initiative aimed to improve the health of Australians by providing easy access to quality information about human health. Follow the link to find information relating to cystitis.
www.healthinsite.gov.au/topics/Cystitis

WellBeing is a non-profit organization that funds research into obstetrics and gynaecology. It publishes helpful information leaflets, including 'Cystitis', which you can download from its website; go to the 'Reproductive health information' section of the site.
www.wellbeing.org.uk

National Kidney and Urologic Diseases Information Clearinghouse is a US government organization. It has clear information about cystitis and interstitial cystitis on its website.
www.kidney.niddk.nih.gov/kudiseases/pubs/uti_ez/index.htm

Cystitis and Overactive Bladder Foundation is a UK non-profit organization, which provides information and support to sufferers of bladder problems.
www.cobfoundation.org

Interstitial Cystitis Association (ICA) is a US non-profit organization that gives information and funds research on interstitial cystitis; its website is very comprehensive (and even includes a cookery section).
www.ichelp.com

The American Academy of Family Physicians has a fact sheet about interstitial cystitis on its website.
www.aafp.org/afp/20011001/1212ph.html

The Society of Health Sexual Advisers has information about visiting a sexual health clinic on its website as well as a list of the clinics in the UK and Ireland, and a link to a list of clinics in the US.
ww.ssha.info/public/clinics/locations.asp

BUPA, a UK private healthcare provider, has a good cystitis fact sheet on its website.
http://hcd2.bupa.co.uk/fact_sheets/html/cystitis.html

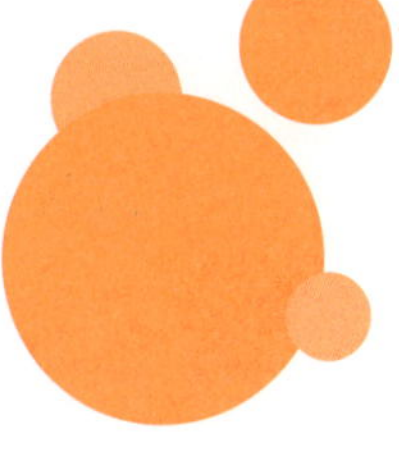

Dandruff

Dandruff particles are visible flakes of skin that have been continuously shed from the scalp.

It is normal to shed some dead skin flakes as the skin is constantly renewing itself. The new cells form in the lower layers. They are gradually pushed to the surface as more new cells form beneath them. By the time they reach the surface, the cells have become flat and overlap each other like roof tiles. By then, these cells are dead and are shed from the surface all the time. They are so small that we do not notice this is happening.

With dandruff, this whole process of skin renewal (or skin turnover) speeds up, so a greater number of dead cells are being shed. Also, the cells are shed in clumps, which are big enough to be seen with the naked eye as embarrassing flakes, especially when they land on dark clothing. The scalp may also feel slightly itchy.

Dandruff is very common. According to Proctor and Gamble, it affects more than 50% of the population of the US – so it is more common to have dandruff than not! It can occur at any age, but is most likely in the early 20s.

Cause of dandruff

Surprisingly, dandruff is a bit of an enigma. About 25 years ago, dermatologists started to blame a tiny fungus, the yeast *Pityrosporum ovale*, on the scalp. (This yeast is a *Malassezia* type of yeast, so its other name is *Malassezia furfur*.) Everyone has some of this yeast on their skin, particularly in the greasy areas such as the scalp and upper back. It feeds on the natural grease produced by the skin.

Although the experts are certain that the yeast is involved, they can not decide which comes first: does a reaction to the yeast actually cause the increased turnover and flaking; or does the flaky skin simply provide an ideal environment for the yeast to thrive? It seems very likely that the former is the case, so getting rid of the yeast should improve the dandruff.

Hormones may also be involved, because dandruff usually starts after puberty and is more common in men than women. For unknown reasons, people with some illnesses, such as Parkinson's disease, are more likely to have dandruff.

Common beliefs – true or false?

'Dandruff is due to dryness of the skin'

False. Dandruff is caused by a rapid turnover of cells, so more dead cells are shed from the surface. In fact, dandruff occurs in areas where the grease glands of the skin are most active, and the skin is not usually dry.

'Dandruff is more common in males than in females'

True. Probably because the grease glands are affected by hormones.

'Dandruff is affected by the weather'

Probably true. Sunlight inhibits the growth of the *Pityrosporum ovale* yeast.

'Dandruff results from poor hygiene'

False. Dandruff is caused by rapid turnover of skin cells, probably as a reaction to the *Pityrosporum ovale* yeast. However, dandruff sufferers do not have more of the yeast than other people – they are just more sensitive to it.

'Dandruff is contagious'

False. You can not 'catch' dandruff from someone else, such as by using his or her brush or comb.

'Wearing a hat worsens dandruff'

Possibly true. *Pityrosporum ovale* yeasts thrive best when protected from sunlight. Also, wearing a hat prevents sweat from evaporating, and this may encourage the yeast.

Getting rid of dandruff

- Hair gels and other hair products can irritate the scalp in some people. For a while, try doing without whatever you have been using, or change to a different product.
- Do not scratch your scalp. When you shampoo, massage your scalp without scratching. Scientists have looked at hair from dandruff sufferers who scratch, using an electron microscope that magnifies 400 times. They could see fingernail marks, damaging the hair at its root.
- If your dandruff is mild, try shampooing your hair twice a week using any shampoo labelled 'frequent use, for dry hair' (not an ordinary 'anti-dandruff' shampoo). This will remove the flakes that are being shed, and the moisturizer in the shampoo will protect the scalp.
- Avoid dyeing your hair (unless you absolutely must). We all have bacteria on our scalp, some of which are beneficial. These 'good' bacteria prevent dandruff yeast, and hair dyes reduce their numbers.
- If you want to try a natural remedy, boil four heaped tablespoons of dried thyme in half a litre of water for 10 minutes. Let it cool and strain it through a sieve into a jar. Massage some of the liquid onto your scalp three times a week. Do not rinse it out.
- Look for a shampoo containing tea-tree oil. Research from Australia (published in the *Journal of the American Academy of Dermatology* in 2002) showed that a 5% tea tree oil shampoo improved dandruff by 41%, which means that, although it did not get rid of the dandruff completely, there was a noticeable improvement.
- For severe dandruff, you need to deal with the yeast. This means looking carefully at the small print on the anti-dandruff shampoo in your local pharmacy. You could start by trying a shampoo containing selenium sulfide, which has an anti-yeast effect. Wet your hair, rub the shampoo onto your scalp and rinse off. Repeat, leaving the shampoo for 3–5 minutes before rinsing off. Do not use selenium sulfide within 48 hours of applying a hair colourant or a perm lotion. Some shampoos contain zinc pyrithione, another anti-yeast chemical.

- The most effective treatment is an anti-yeast shampoo containing ketoconazole, which you can buy from a chemist without a doctor's prescription. Wet your hair, rub the shampoo onto your scalp and rinse off. Repeat, leaving the shampoo for 3–5 minutes before rinsing off. Use it twice a week for 2–4 weeks to clear the dandruff, and then once every 2 weeks, using a normal shampoo in between times.
- Anti-dandruff conditioners are also available.

When to see your doctor

You should certainly see your family doctor if your scalp is red and itchy – or if the skin is flaky around the eyebrows, round the nose or behind the ears – because this suggests you have the more severe form called seborrhoeic dermatitis (seborrhoeic eczema). You should also see your doctor if the dandruff is very lumpy or patchy, or if you have scaly skin elsewhere, because it could be a skin disorder, such as psoriasis.

Useful contacts

Health*Insite* is an Australian government initiative aimed to improve the health of Australians by providing easy access to quality information about human health. Follow the link to find information about dandruff and its treatment.
www.healthinsite.gov.au/topics/Dandruff

The Australasian College of Dermatologists website contains basic information about various skin diseases and problems. It has a helpful section on dandruff under 'A–Z of skin'.
www.dermcoll.asn.au
www.dermcoll.asn.au/public/a-z_of_skin-dandruff.asp

Proctor and Gamble, US are the manufacturers of Head and Shoulders shampoo, which contains antifungal chemicals (selenium sulfide and pyrithione zinc). Their website promotes their shampoo heavily, but also has some helpful information in the 'Ask the expert' section.
www.headandshoulders.co.uk/faqs.jsp

Johnson & Johnson, MSD, are the manufacturers of Nizoral shampoo, which contains ketoconazole. Their UK website promotes their shampoo, but also has useful information in the sections on 'All about dandruff' and 'Common questions and myths'.
www.nizoral.co.uk

The American Nizoral website also has a page on African-American hair.
www.nizoral.com/africanamerican/index.jhtml?id=nizoral/africanamerican/experttips.inc

National Eczema Society website has a factsheet on seborrhoeic eczema.
www.eczema.org/sebadult.pdf

Ears that stick out

Ears are one of the first parts of the body to reach full size. This is why ears that stick out are particularly noticeable in children.

By the age of 5 or 6 years, our ears are about the size they will be when we are adults

What can be done in tiny babies

In about two-thirds of cases, sticking-out ears are evident at birth, so can be dealt with straightaway. The gristle (cartilage) of a newborn baby is soft, so the ears can be corrected by placing a special small splint of cushioned wire in the hollow of the rim of the ear and taping it back for several weeks. This can be done only if the baby is younger than 6 months, and the earlier the better. Parents can buy a kit containing splints with instructions (see Useful contacts below).

What can be done in older children and adults

An operation (otoplasty) to correct sticking-out ears is often done when the child is over 5 or 6 years old. However, there is no reason why it cannot be done at any age. The operation does not affect hearing.

Children need a general anaesthetic, but adults can have the operation with just a local anaesthetic. There are several different techniques. In the most common operation, the surgeon cuts away skin and tissue from behind each ear, and stitches it into its new position. The ears are bandaged for about 10 days after the operation, and after that the stitches are removed. You will have to wear a headband at night for the next 2 weeks so that you do not accidentally bend the ears forward during sleep.

As with any plastic surgery operation, it is important to find a plastic surgeon who is skilled at this particular operation. If it is clumsily done, you may end up with a plastered-down look, or with ears that do not look the same. For general advice on cosmetic surgery see page 339.

Older people have bigger ears. The reason could be that as we get older our ears grow by 0.22 mm a year. Or it could be that people with big ears live longer (for some unknown reason)

Useful contacts

Australian Society of Plastic Surgeons (ASPS) website offers useful information on surgical procedures for ear correction. You can also contact the society for advice and ask for a list of State and Territory members. Society members are all fully qualified in both

reconstructive and cosmetic surgery. All members are Fellows of the Royal Australasian College of Surgeons (FRACS). Each has a record of accomplishment in their field and a commitment to high ethical standards.
www.plasticsurgery.org.au

British Association of Aesthetic and Plastic Surgeons (BAAPS) have available on their website a fact sheet on 'Setting back prominent ears', as well as a list of their members.
www.baaps.org.uk

American Academy of Facial, Plastic and Reconstructive Surgery has a leaflet on 'Understanding otoplasty – surgery of the ear' in the procedures section of its website.
www.aafprs.org/patient/procedures/otoplasty.html

In 1998, a retired company director handed out thousands of large cardboard ears to commuters as they crossed London Bridge into the business area of the City. He filmed the business people wearing the ears, and submitted the film for the contemporary art Turner Prize

Ear Buddies are splints to correct sticking-out ears in babies under 6 months of age. They were invented by a plastic surgeon. The website explains how they work, how to fit them and where to buy them. A share of the proceeds is donated to Mount Vernon Hospital for research into plastic surgery techniques.
www.earbuddies.co.uk

Ejaculation

NOT ENOUGH SEMEN

Sperm are made in the testicles. To reach the penis, they travel along the narrow tube of the epididymis (which lies just outside the testicles) and then along larger tubes (one from each testicle). These tubes join together and go through the prostate gland to the penis. The journey distance is about 6 metres (because the epididymis tube is very tiny and tightly coiled), and can take up to 3 weeks. Nourishing fluids from the seminal vesicle and prostate gland increase the volume, so sperm make up only about 5% of semen (also known as seminal fluid or ejaculate).

During sex, the semen gathers inside the base of the penis. At orgasm (climax), the muscles behind the base of the penis contract, shooting the semen out.

The sensation of orgasm is a relief of tension beginning just before the semen starts to spurt out, and ending with the final spurt – so if there is not much semen the orgasm will be short. Most men ejaculate more fluid at some times than at others – the amount can vary from a few drops to two teaspoonfuls.

Ageing is one of the most common reasons for a decrease in the amount of fluid produced when you ejaculate.

- Men aged 20–30 years typically ejaculate 4.0 mL.
- Men aged 30–50 years typically ejaculate 3.5 mL.
- Men aged 60–70 years typically ejaculate 2 mL.
- Men older than 70 years typically ejaculate just over 1 mL.

These figures come from a survey published in *Human Reproduction* (2003;18:447–54) and they are averages, so some men in each age group will produce a lot more and some a lot less.

Smoking. If you want to increase the volume of semen you produce, stop smoking. The survey found that, on average, non-smokers ejaculated 3.2 mL of semen, but smokers ejaculated only 1.9 mL.

Frequency of sex. The survey also found that abstaining from sex increased the volume of semen produced. Men who had not had sex within the previous 5 days ejaculated a larger volume of semen.

Dry orgasm (no semen) means that although you have an orgasm, no fluid is produced. One possibility is that your semen is going backwards into your bladder (see page 109). This can occur after surgery to the prostate, or with diabetes or some drugs. If you suddenly develop dry orgasm for no apparent reason, you should see your doctor. You will need tests to see if there is a blockage in the tubes.

Each millilitre of semen normally contains at least 20 million sperm and can contain up to 100 million

PREMATURE EJACULATION

Ejaculation is the peak of male orgasm, when the semen squirts out.

How to know if you have premature ejaculation

In premature ejaculation, the point of no return arrives too soon. In the 1950s, a man was said to be a premature ejaculator if he lasted less than a certain time (say 2 minutes) or a certain number of strokes (say 100) before ejaculating.

These arbitrary definitions are rubbish; they were based on ignorance of how long most men actually take to climax. The so-called 'experts' were surprised by the following information.

- Dr Alfred Kinsey reported that 75% of men ejaculate within 2 minutes of vaginal penetration.
- In Shere Hite's survey of 11 239 men, 21% reported that they ejaculated within 1 minute of penetration, and 62% within 5 minutes.
- The Hite survey also showed that there is great variation between men; for example, 7% said they did not ejaculate before 15 minutes.

The best definition of premature ejaculation is climaxing before you or your partner wish you to. This common-sense definition means that climaxing speedily after penetration is not necessarily a problem (for example, if a man pleasures his partner for a long time beforehand until she reaches orgasm).

Some men climax even before they enter their partner. If this is the case, you have the most severe type of premature ejaculation.

Premature ejaculation is common

Many men and their partners wish intercourse could last longer than it does.

- In the Hite survey, about 70% of men said 'yes' to the question, 'Do you ever orgasm too soon after penetration – in other words, are you unable to continue intercourse for as long as you would like?'
- In a survey of 5000 readers of a UK tabloid newspaper, 10.8% responded 'yes' to the question 'Do you always come too quickly?' (*Update* 2005;71(5):39–43).
- A UK study of 5000 men aged 16–44 found that 11.7% had experienced premature ejaculation for at least a month in the past year. The problem lasted for more than 6 months in only 2.7%, suggesting that it probably affects many men some of the time (*British Medical Journal* 2003;327:426–7).

Premature ejaculation is common in young men, but the problem solves itself with time.

Causes of premature ejaculation

Is it a physical problem? It used to be thought that premature ejaculation was the result of a physical problem, such as irritation or inflammation of the urethra (the tube in the penis for urine and semen) or prostate gland, and there were nasty treatments such as squirting silver nitrate into the opening. There is no evidence that premature ejaculation is caused by such conditions. In almost every case, the man is physically normal; very rarely, it can be the result of a neurological condition such as multiple sclerosis.

Is the penis hypersensitive? There is also no evidence that it happens because the penis is hypersensitive. Researchers tested the sensitivity of the skin of the penis in men who considered themselves premature ejaculators and men who were not, and found no difference. It also seems to be a myth that circumcision makes a difference; the American sex researchers Masters and Johnson tested the sensitivity of the glans (head) of the penis in circumcised and non-circumcised men and found them to be the same.

Is it hyperarousal? Premature ejaculation is more likely when the level of sexual excitement and arousal is high. This why it is more likely with a new partner, and why it is common in young men during their first sexual relationships.

Is it just a habit? It is most likely that the time of ejaculation is simply a habit, starting early when a youth learns to masturbate or have sex as quickly as possible for fear of being caught. It is certainly more common in younger men. Like all habits, it can be unlearnt.

Talk about it with your partner

It is very important to discuss the problem with your partner. Otherwise, your partner may wonder what is happening, or think it is their fault. The techniques for 'unlearning' premature ejaculation need your partner's help – another reason for talking about it.

Common-sense measures for dealing with premature ejaculation

- A simple method worth trying is to take a deep breath as you get close to climax. This briefly shuts down the ejaculatory reflex.
- Have sex more often – you are more likely to ejaculate prematurely after a long gap
- For the same reason, masturbating before intercourse may help.
- Stop for a break during sexual activity. Think about something boring. This will allow your level of arousal to fall temporarily.
- Use a condom to decrease sensation. Use a thicker condom labelled 'ultrastrong' or 'superstrong'.
- Have sex with the woman on top – men are less aroused in this position than when they are on top ('missionary position').
- Learn to control your anal muscles. Contract your buttocks around the anus as if you were trying to prevent a bowel movement. Start by doing this 10 times in a row, and increase to 50 times twice a day. Some men find either contracting or relaxing these muscles when ejaculation is near helps them to last longer.
- When your penis is first inside your partner's vagina, try to make shorter thrusts or a circular motion – this can delay ejaculation and you can then progress to the usual in-and-out technique when you and your partner are ready.

Unlearning' premature ejaculation

The main methods are the so-called squeeze technique and stop–go technique. They involve stimulating the penis almost to the point of ejaculation and then stopping. The idea is to train the man to remain in a state of high arousal without actually ejaculating. They require patience. About 90% of men are 'cured' by these techniques, but it usually takes about 14 weeks of practising 3–5 times a week. Unfortunately about 60% of men find that the problem comes back after about a year, and the 'unlearning' has to be gone through again.

Squeeze technique

- The squeeze technique is best done by the couple, but the man can do it alone by masturbation if there is no partner or she is not willing to participate.
- The couple start by being as relaxed as they can, and free from distractions.
- The couple kiss and caress until the man is aroused, and then she takes his penis in her hand and begins stroking it.
- The man concentrates on his feelings of arousal, to increase his sexual awareness (he does not try to think of other things in an attempt to distract himself from ejaculation)
- When he feels he is about to ejaculate, he signals to his partner.
- She immediately stops stimulating him and applies firm but gentle pressure around the penis where the glans (head) meets the shaft. She applies this pressure for 10–20 seconds.
- She then lets go, and they wait without doing anything for about 30 seconds.
- The procedure is repeated several times before ejaculation is allowed to occur.

Stop–go technique

- The stop–go technique is essentially the same as the squeeze technique, but the squeeze is omitted.
- As soon as the man is about to ejaculate, he signals to his partner and she stops stroking his penis for about 30–60 seconds.
- Repeat the 'stop–go' steps four or five times before allowing ejaculation to occur. It is simpler than the squeeze technique, and seems to work just as well.

These techniques are not as easy as they sound. The usual problems are that you go too far and ejaculate, or you lose your erection and can not regain it. If these occur, do not worry – just try again another day. It may take several weeks to master the techniques.

The next step is to do exactly the same, but using a lubricant (such as KY jelly) to increase sensation and more closely resemble the situation of being in the vagina.

When you find that you are beginning to be able to delay ejaculation, you can start to have intercourse with the woman on top. She lowers herself backwards and downwards onto the erect penis and makes gentle coital movements. You signal to her when ejaculation is about to happen. She then remains perfectly still, or lifts herself off and either does nothing or applies the squeeze, before resuming intercourse in the same position.

Drugs

Dapoxetine is a new medication for premature ejaculation. On average, it increases the time before ejaculation by 3–4 times, that is from less than 1 minute to about 3 minutes (*The Lancet* 2006;368:929–37). In the research studies, the men using it and their partners said that sex was more satisfying. It is taken 1–3 hours before sex whenever you need to; it does not have to be taken every day. Some men noticed nausea, diarrhoea, headache or dizziness, especially with the higher strength tablets. Dapoxetine is from the same family as SSRI antidepressants (selective serotonin reuptake inhibitors), but is weaker and shorter-acting, and has been specially tailored for premature ejaculation.

Antidepressants, such as clomipramine (Anafranil), sertraline (Lustral) and paroxetine (Seroxat), delay ejaculation as a side effect, and some doctors used to prescribe them for this purpose (although they are not officially licensed for this use). However, dapoxetine now seems a better option.

Premjact is a local anaesthetic spray, which has been approved by the drug regulatory authorities in the US and UK (see Useful contacts on page 110). It is available from pharmacies; you do not need a doctor's prescription. You spray it onto the glans (head) and shaft of the penis up to 10 minutes before intercourse. It is not totally effective on its own, but is useful if you have successfully 'retrained' with the squeeze or stop–go techniques, but feel that you are in danger of slipping back. A problem is that some of the local anaesthetic may rub off onto the female partner, causing her genital area to lose some feeling temporarily. To prevent this, use a condom after applying the spray.

Semen is made up of 5% sperm from the testicles, 35% fluid from the prostate gland and 60% fluid from the seminal vesicle glands

DELAYED EJACULATION

Delayed ejaculation means that even though your sexual desire (libido) and erections are normal, you have difficulty reaching a climax (i.e. the point at which semen spurts out) when you are inside your partner. In a UK study of men aged 16–44, 5.3% said they had experienced difficulty in reaching orgasm for at least a month in the past year. The problem continues for more than 6 months in only 2.9%, so, like premature ejaculation, it can be a temporary problem (*British Medical Journal* 2003;327:426–7).

For many couples it is a source of pleasure, not a problem, because it allows prolonged lovemaking, but the woman may (mistakenly) assume that it means she is unattractive to her partner.

The UK Sexual Dysfunction Association receives many queries about it and has prepared a special fact sheet (see Useful contacts on page 110). The association says that two categories of men commonly have the problem of delayed ejaculation: sex starters who are paralyzed with guilt or other strong emotions; and older men who have grown psychologically mistrustful of release or who have a need for greater physical stimulation now that age has made lovemaking less spontaneous and orgasm less compliant. Also, some prostate operations and some drugs, such as SSRI-type antidepressants (selective serotonin reuptake inhibitors), can delay ejaculation. Therefore, if you are taking medication and delayed ejaculation is a new problem you should ask your doctor if the medication might be responsible. Alcohol can also have this effect.

How to help a partner with delayed ejaculation

The following advice is provided by the UK Sexual Dysfunction Association.

- There is nothing biologically wrong with most men experiencing ejaculation difficulties. However, men who cannot orgasm inside a woman may have a combination of technique and attitude problems. For instance, many men learn how to perform sex by masturbating. When they bring themselves to orgasm, they may agitate with their hands far more quickly than two people can ever have sex. Thus, when they start making love, the sensations seem under-stimulating. The answer to this part of the problem is to increase the eroticism of foreplay and make your partner wait until he is practically on the edge of climax before allowing him to insert his penis.
- If that does not help, anxiety is probably preventing him from triggering his ejaculatory reflex. Tell him there is a remedy, which you can jointly try over a period of weeks.
- When the time is right, and you are feeling intimate and relaxed, ask him to show you how he masturbates all the way to orgasm. Be light-hearted and make it fun. Next time, ask him to masturbate with a little assistance from you. Next time, see if he can do it just inside your vulva, again with assistance from your hand if he enjoys it. At this point, if the process has proved successful, draw his attention to the fact that you are virtually having normal sexual intercourse and that he *has* managed to ejaculate where you both want him to.
- On the next occasion, he could insert himself fully and try coming deep inside you – and so on. The important point to remember is that, if at any stage he meets with a reverse, you do not fret but simply return to the previous stage and get comfortable with that again.

BLOOD IN THE SEMEN

It is scary to notice blood in your semen (ejaculate). It is likely that you will immediately think that you have a serious disease, such as cancer. Not so; most of the causes of blood in the semen are not serious. There have been several scientific studies of this problem and they all came to more-or-less the same conclusion, which is that the likelihood of finding a reason for the bleeding depends on your age (*Update* 2004;68:6–7, *International Journal of STD and AIDS* 2002;13:517–21).

In people under 40 years old, no cause can be found in about one-third and the problem usually goes away in about a month. Trauma, such as a kick in the groin, may be the reason in some of these men. In the remaining two-thirds, the cause is an infection (such as chlamydia, gonorrhoea or trichomoniasis – see page 126 for more information about these infections). Over 500 people with blood in the semen were involved in the scientific studies, and cancer was not a cause in anyone under 40 years of age, which means it is very unlikely, but not impossible.

In people over the age of 40, a cause can usually be found. It might be an infection or a prostate problem, or some other cause. Prostate cancer has to be considered, especially in older people, but is not a common cause of blood in the semen.

Could the blood have come from your partner, and not from you? This is particularly likely if she is at the beginning or end of her period and the bleeding is not noticeable to her. If she is not menstruating, but you think the blood is from her, she may need a check-up. Use a condom the next few times you have sex. This will enable you to examine the semen and be sure the bleeding is from you.

The male reproductive system has a lot of tubing and the source of bleeding could be anywhere in the system. If the blood is red or pink, it most probably comes from the urethra (the tube inside the penis). If it is dark, it may come from further back (such as the prostate or an area called the seminal vesicles). Because one of the most common causes is inflammation in the urethra or prostate gland, sometimes caused by an infection, it would be sensible to have a check-up at your local sexual health clinic. Otherwise, see your doctor.

EJACULATION BACKWARDS (RETROGRADE)

If your semen goes backwards into your bladder at orgasm, instead of shooting out of the hole at the end of the penis, you have 'retrograde ejaculation'. Men with retrograde ejaculation have orgasm and feel the sensation of having ejaculated, but little or no fluid emerges from the penis. If they urinate after having sex, the urine is often cloudy because it contains semen.

Normally, the muscle around the exit hole of the bladder closes tightly at orgasm to prevent this happening. If the muscle or its nerves are damaged, retrograde ejaculation may occur.

Retrograde ejaculation often occurs after prostate surgery or surgery of the bladder itself. A few people are born with a weakness of the muscle that closes the bladder. Retrograde ejaculation can also occur in people who have had diabetes for many years. Sometimes medications can be responsible, such as prazosin (for blood pressure) and terazosin (for blood pressure or enlarged prostate).

Retrograde ejaculation after a prostate operation is to be expected, and your surgeon will have mentioned the possibility to you beforehand. If this is not the reason in your case, you need to see a urologist to find out the cause. In some cases medications such as ephedrine may help.

To father a child, a man with retrograde ejaculation will probably need help from a fertility clinic. The clinic will be able to remove sperm from urine passed after ejaculating.

Useful contacts

Health*Insite* is an Australian government initiative aimed to improve the health of Australians by providing easy access to quality information about human health. By following the link, you will find information on issues about sex and growing older.
www.healthinsite.gov.au/topics/Sex_in_Later_Years

Impotence Australia is a non-profit organization that was set up to decrease the suffering of men with impotence and their partners by providing quality telephone counseling and information fact sheets on many sexual issues. Some useful information is given on premature and delayed ejaculation under 'Get the facts' section of the website.
www.impotenceaustralia.com.au

British Association for Sexual and Relationship Therapy has a list of psychosexual clinics and qualified sex therapists throughout the UK.
www.basrt.org.uk

Sexual Dysfunction Association has free fact sheets on premature ejaculation and delayed ejaculation. These can also be found on the website.
www.sda.uk.net

Relate (National Marriage Guidance) offer counselling for couples in all relationships. Their website has a facility for locating your nearest Relate centre.
www.relate.org.uk

Brook provides free, confidential sex advice (and free condoms) for young people under the age of 25. Look at the 'Go to Brook' section on their website.
www.brook.org.uk

Premjact (also known as Stud 100). Online order available.
www.premjact.com

How to overcome premature ejaculation by Helen Kaplan is a clear and helpful book. Published by Brunner/Mazel. ISBN 0-87-630542-7.

Erection problems

Common beliefs

'Erection problems are uncommon'

This is untrue – most men simply do not talk about it. A survey sponsored by the pharmaceutical company Pharmacia & Upjohn found that more than 1 in 4 of the UK male population over the age of 16 have experienced erectile disorder to some degree. Of these, over half experienced the problem as one-off incidents and a quarter suffer erectile disorder most or all of the time. There are probably 20 million men with erection problems in the US, and 2–3 million in the UK.

'Erection problems are usually psychological'

This is an old-fashioned view; impotence is most commonly due to a physical cause.

'Testosterone injections/patches are a good cure for erection problems'

Testosterone is of use only in the uncommon situation the man has a proven shortage of testosterone.

'Viagra-type drugs work for everyone'

These drugs are successful in only 50–80% of cases.

Erectile failure (also called impotence or erectile dysfunction) means that you cannot achieve or maintain an erection of the penis sufficient for sexual intercourse. Sex drive is often normal. Impotence can occur at any age, but becomes more common with increasing age. Because the average age of the population is getting older, experts predict that by the year 2010 almost half the men in the UK will have erection problems. But impotence is not inevitable with ageing – 40% of 90-year-olds are able to have a normal erection.

What happens during an erection

The penis contains three long cylinders of erectile tissue. Two of the cylinders lie side by side, while the third lies beneath them. The urethra, which is the urine and sperm channel, runs through this lower cylinder. Sexual excitement causes the cylinders to fill with about 100–140 mL of blood and, as they swell, so the penis becomes erect. And as the erectile tissue swells, it squeezes the veins in the penis. These veins normally drain blood away from the penis, so the squeezing action prevents blood flowing away and keeps the penis erect. (Imagine a bathtub filling with the tap on and a plug in the drain.) After orgasm and ejaculation these events go into reverse, and the penis becomes limp again.

*In men under 60, the greater the time spent watching television, the greater the likelihood of impotence (*Annals of Internal Medicine *2003;139:161–8)*

How the system fails (impotence)

A few years ago it was assumed that most cases of impotence had psychological causes. Now more is known about the blood supply to the penis, and it is recognized that physical problems are often responsible. For example, nerves to the spongy tissue can be damaged by diabetes, blood flow can be impaired by atherosclerosis (clogged arteries) and many medications interfere with erections.

Medications and drugs can interfere with erections. Here are some of the most common culprits:

- cimetidine (for duodenal ulcer)
- some drugs for high blood pressure (e.g. thiazide diuretics especially in high doses, methyldopa, most beta-blockers); erection problems affect about 1 in 5 men taking beta-blockers (*Journal of the American Medical Association* 2002;288:351–7)
- finasteride (for prostate enlargement or baldness)
- phenothiazines (for some psychiatric conditions)
- alcohol and marijuana (cannabis)
- drugs used for prostate cancer (e.g. some GnRH analogues and anti-androgens)
- antidepressants
- cholesterol-lowering drugs (probably)
- non-steroidal anti-inflammatory drugs, also known as NSAIDs (possibly).

Medical conditions. Many medical conditions can cause difficulty with erections by damaging the blood vessels and nerves. Of course, if you have one of these conditions, it does not mean that you will necessarily be impotent. Some of the most important medical conditions that cause impotence are:

- diabetes
- hypertension (high blood pressure)
- vascular disease (clogged arteries) – linked with smoking
- severe liver disease
- thyroid disease
- neurological conditions (spinal injury, multiple sclerosis)
- Peyronie's disease (see page 204)
- tight foreskin (see page 210)
- renal failure.

As cardiovascular disease is one of the most common causes of erection failure, erection problems can be a warning that your arteries are unhealthy. So it is not surprising that men with impotence have an increased risk of angina, heart attacks and stroke (*Journal of the American Medical Association* 2005;294:2996–3002).

Some prostate operations (especially radical prostatectomy) can also cause impotence.

Ageing. The likelihood of erection problems increases with age. The US Massachusetts Male Aging Study reported erection problems in:

- 25% of 65-year-olds
- 55% of 75-year-olds
- 65% of 80-year-olds.

This is because the older you are, the more likely that you have one of the medical conditions that damage blood vessels and nerves causing impotence (see also the section on sex and ageing on page 231).

Smoking. Smokers are much more likely to develop impotence than non-smokers. This is because if you are a smoker your arteries are likely to become clogged (atherosclerosis). During an erection the penis swells because it fills with blood. If your arteries are clogged, the blood cannot flow in efficiently and your erection will not be as good.

A study of 4462 Vietnam War veterans, aged between 31 and 49, showed that smokers had a 50–80% increase in the risk of impotence compared with non-smokers. Another study has shown that for every year you smoke 20 a day, you increase your risk of impotence by 2–3%.

According to a British Medical Association report, about 120 000 men in the UK in their 30s and 40s are impotent as a result of smoking.

Unhealthy lifestyle. A sluggish lifestyle, in which you spend a lot of time watching TV and are too fat, makes impotence more likely. This was shown in a US study of 43 000 men (*Annals of Internal Medicine* 2003;139:161–8). Those who took regular exercise were less likely to have erection problems. And according to Harvard *Men's Health Watch*, a man with a 42-inch waist is 50% more likely to be impotent than a man with a 32-inch waist.

Distance cycling and motorcycling. If you decide to take more exercise, distance cycling may not be the best choice. About 1 in 5 distance cyclists notices some numbness of the genital area after a ride, and 13% experience problems with erections for the following week or longer. The cause is pressure of the saddle on nerves and arteries. For the same reasons, motorcycling may also increase the risk of erectile dysfunction. Choose a wide saddle with plenty of padding that makes you sit back firmly, and dismount if you start to experience numbness.

Psychological factors can, of course, cause impotence. These include:

- guilt
- depression
- losing interest in your partner
- a partner who finds intercourse painful
- low self-esteem
- fear of not performing well.

Often both physical and psychological factors are involved. A physical problem impairs erections, and you then become so preoccupied with the question 'Can I maintain my erection this time?' that sexual arousal becomes impossible. Anxiety actually has the physical effect of contracting the muscles of the erectile tissue, preventing blood entering the penis and allowing the blood to drain away.

Questions to ask yourself

Is it really an erection problem? Or is the actual problem premature ejaculation (see page 104) or a lack of sexual desire (see page 226)?

Can you achieve an erection by masturbation but not with your partner, and do you still sometimes wake with an erection? If the answers are 'yes', a psychological reason, such as stress or depression, is likely.

Did loss of erections come on suddenly, or have erections gradually been failing over a long period of time? Erectile failure which comes on suddenly is usually psychological; physical causes usually have a more gradual onset.

Have you been under extra stress lately? If so, is there any way you can reduce the stress in your life?

Are you taking any drugs (see above) that might be responsible? If so, ask your doctor for alternatives.

Are you drinking too much? Blood alcohol concentrations of up to about 25 mg/100 mL improve erections slightly, but when the level reaches about 40 mg/100 mL erection is inhibited. In some people, only one or two drinks is enough to raise the blood alcohol to this level. Heavy drinking over a long period can cause erectile failure because of nerve damage.

Have you noticed anything else wrong? For example: Peyronie's disease, where the penis develops a lump and often kinks (see page 204), can cause impotence; tightness of the foreskin (see page 210) can prevent full erections; and enlargement of the breasts or loss of body hair might mean a hormonal problem.

Who is really bothered by the problem – you or your partner? Talk to your partner about what each of you wants from sex. As sex counsellor Susie Hayman says, 'It's amazing how many people just lie there wishing their partner was a mind reader.'

Are you a smoker? If so, can you stop? Stopping smoking will not reverse the problem, but may stop it getting worse. Also, impotence is often a sign that your arteries are unhealthy, so stopping smoking is important to reduce the risk of a heart attack.

Have you had your blood pressure checked recently and been tested for diabetes? Many men with impotence have unhealthy arteries and high blood pressure, so a check of your blood pressure and blood lipids (e.g. cholesterol) are necessary. Impotence can also be a symptom of diabetes.

How to approach your doctor

According to *Men's Health* magazine, 'on the Richter scale of embarrassment, impotence comes near the top'. The Viagra publicity has loosened the taboo to some extent, but this is still the problem men least like discussing with their family doctor. A survey by the Sexual Dysfunction Association found that almost half of impotence sufferers took 2 years to summon the courage to seek treatment. So you are not alone in your embarrassment.

But of course impotence is the one problem that the family doctor will not be able to guess that you have, unless you mention it. When you do manage to discuss it, you will probably find that your family doctor is surprisingly matter-of-fact about it. Impotence is a standard medical problem that doctors are now trained to deal with. It is also possible that there is a local specialist hospital clinic in your area.

If you keep avoiding the issue with your family doctor, there are two other possible approaches. Your partner could have a preliminary discussion with the doctor to pave the way. Or you could write to your doctor, marking the envelope 'Confidential' and explaining that you have been too embarrassed to mention the problem, but would like an appointment to discuss it, if possible at the end of a surgery when the doctor would have more time.

Even if you convince yourself that the problem is due to stress, see your doctor. You may be wrong, and even if you are right your doctor should be able to help.

What your doctor can do

Your family doctor will consider whether impotence is the result of some medical condition or any drugs that you are taking. Impotence can also result from depression and from relationship problems, so be prepared for some talk along these lines. However, most doctors believe that there is no point in deep psychoanalytical-type discussions; they prefer to do a few simple investigations and then deal with the problem in a practical way.

Your doctor will also take your blood pressure, and will discuss smoking and weight loss. This is because impotence can be a signal that your arteries are unhealthy, which could lead to a heart attack in the future.

Tests. The following tests are usually carried out.

- Blood or urine are tested for glucose, to check for diabetes.
- A blood test for cholesterol and other lipids (fats) is done, because erection problems can mean your arteries are unhealthy.
- The blood testosterone (male hormone) level can be measured. However, it is unusual for impotence to be caused by a low testosterone level, so the result is usually normal. The exception is when there has been a reduced sex drive for some time before any problem with erections; in this situation a testosterone test is worthwhile.
- Blood prolactin level is sometimes measured if erectile failure was preceded by a reduced sex drive; a high level of this hormone is extremely rare, but may be associated with impotence, and can be an indicator of other diseases.

If a prescribed drug might be the cause, your family doctor will probably be able to change to another pill. For example, if you have high blood pressure, your family doctor might change to a calcium-channel blocker, an ACE inhibitor or an angiotensin-receptor blocker; these are less likely to cause impotence. If the drug was responsible, you can expect to see an improvement in 2–3 weeks. Unfortunately, changing the drug seldom helps, because the real problem is usually the condition for which the drug you need the drug. (For example, high blood pressure causes damage to arteries, which results in impotence. So changing the blood pressure drug will not improve matters if the damage has been done.) Alternatively, you may have developed a psychological block – 'fear of failure' – which may take time and counselling to overcome.

If stress, depression or a relationship problem seems to be a factor, counselling and/or antidepressant medication may be the answer. If you require an antidepressant do not worry that you will be hooked for life; these drugs are given for a limited period to kick-start you out of your depression. However, they may take several weeks to work, and some antidepressants can themselves impair erections.

Your family doctor will then advise you about specific treatments.

Getting treatment

On 1 July 1999, the UK government introduced restrictions on impotence treatments under the NHS. (It was worried that the NHS in the UK would be bankrupted by demand for these medications, perhaps with some reason – for the year 2000, the Viagra bill topped £19 million and, in total, the NHS spent over £73 million on treating impotence.) Only men with certain conditions (prostate cancer, spinal cord injury, kidney failure, diabetes, multiple sclerosis, spina bifida, polio, Parkinson's disease, 'single-gene neurological disease', severe pelvic injury) can receive any kind of NHS impotence treatment. The restrictions apply to all types of impotence treatments, not just tablets. The only exceptions are men who were already receiving impotence treatment on 14 September 1998, the date Viagra was licensed. If your erectile dysfunction is causing 'severe mental distress', you may be able to obtain NHS impotence treatment, but not from your family doctor – it has to be prescribed by a specialist hospital consultant. Doctors have been advised not to prescribe more than one treatment a week.

In the UK, if you are not eligible for impotence treatment under the NHS, your family doctor can give you a 'private' prescription. You will not be charged for the actual prescription if it is written by your NHS family doctor, but you will have to pay the pharmacist for the medication.

Many family doctors are very knowledgeable about impotence. Otherwise, your family doctor may decide to refer you to a hospital specialist called a urologist. The urologist can provide the full range of treatments, and will discuss these with you to see which would suit you best.

Avoid the private clinics you see advertised in the press. *Health Which?* magazine found that some private clinics employed slick salesmen and charged over £1000 for a small supply of anti-impotence drugs.

And do not buy impotence treatments from internet sites. Some of the 'treatments' on offer do not work at all. Medications for impotence (such as Viagra and similar drugs) can be bought from internet sites that first make you fill in a health questionnaire supposedly to ensure that the medication would not be dangerous for you. *Health Which?* investigated some of these sites and found that some were dangerous. The US Food and Drug Administration (FDA) is cracking down on these sites and, in the UK, the Medicines Control Agency is also looking into them. There is also a risk that, unknowingly, you may buy fake medication.

TYPES OF TREATMENT

There are many different treatments for impotence. They include tablets that you take by mouth (oral medication) and other treatments, such as injections and vacuum devices. Your doctor will help you to select the treatment that is best for you.

In the UK, there are three main oral medications (tablets) – Cialis, Levitra and Viagra, which are basically similar. They prevent the breakdown of some of the chemicals in the penis that are involved in erections, so they help the normal erectile mechanism. Therefore the man becomes erect only when he is sexually aroused – unlike some other treatments, which produce an erection automatically, whether or not the man feels sexually stimulated. So these medications seem to produce a more natural erection than other methods.

ORAL MEDICATION

will not take effect unless the man is sexually stimulated

PDE5 Inhibitors

Help to relax the blood vessels in the penis, which enhances blood flow to the penis, causing an erection

	Cialis	Levitra	Viagra
Onset of action	20–60 minutes	20–60 minutes	20–60 minutes
Length of action	24–36 hours	5 hours	4–6 hours
Efficacy	70–80%	70–80%	70–80%
Points to consider	Meals do not affect absorption	A fatty meal may affect absorption	Recent and heavy meals may slow absorption

How Cialis, Levitra and Viagra work

- Man starts to become sexually aroused.
- Nerves send messages to the penis.
- Nerve endings in the penis release nitric oxide.
- Nitric oxide encourages production of a chemical (cGMP) that relaxes muscle in the walls of arteries in the penis, so blood flows in and the penis swells up.
- Without Cialis, Levitra or Viagra, cGMP is rapidly destroyed by an enzyme, PDE5. These drugs knock out PDE5, allowing the erection to maximize.

What happens if you take Cialis, Levitra or Viagra although you do not have impotence?

These medications are not aphrodisiacs, which means that they do not increase sexual desire. They do not improve a normal erection, and they do not give you a better orgasm. If you take it even though you do not have any problem with your erections you could be in for a nasty shock – you might find your erection will not go down and is painful. This is called priapism and it means that blood is flowing into the penis with no flow out. If the erection lasts more than 2 or 3 hours, the blood vessels in the penis become damaged and you will have to rush to your nearest hospital for treatment – probably removal of some of the blood. This is very unlikely to occur in people with previous erection problems, but has occurred in young men with normal erections who were hoping to make them even better with the help of medication.

What you need to know about Cialis (tadalafil)

- Cialis is a tablet treatment for impotence that became available in the UK in February 2003. It works in a similar way to Levitra and Viagra.
- If you take Cialis, you will have an erection only if you are sexually aroused.
- Never take more than one Cialis tablet in a day.
- The effect of Cialis lasts about 24 hours, so you can have sex whenever you choose for about 24 hours after taking it (whereas Levitra and Viagra are taken about an hour before sex).
- Unlike Viagra, Cialis does not have to be taken on an empty stomach.
- Of the men taking Cialis, 1 in 7 experiences a headache and 1 in 8 experiences dyspepsia (indigestion).
- There have been rare cases of sudden loss of sight in men taking Cialis, caused by disruption of the blood supply to the main nerve of the eye (the optic nerve). It is not known whether this is due to the drug or just a coincidence. It is most likely in men who have had a heart attack in the past.
- Unlike Viagra, Cialis does not cause abnormal colour vision.
- Do not take Cialis if you are taking nitrate medication for angina or alpha-blocking drugs.
- Do not drink grapefruit juice if you take Cialis. It could make side effects (such as headache and dyspepsia) more likely.

What you need to know about Levitra (vardenafil)

- Levitra is a tablet treatment for impotence that became available in the UK in 2003. It works in a similar way to Cialis and Viagra.
- If you take Levitra, you will have an erection only if you are sexually aroused.
- Levitra does not have to be taken on an empty stomach, but its effect may be delayed after a high fat meal. It is not affected by alcohol.
- Its effect wears off after 5–12 hours, which is sooner than Cialis.
- Like Cialis and Viagra, you should not take Levitra if you take nitrate medication (an anti-angina medication) or alpha-blocking drugs.
- Do not drink grapefruit juice if you take Levitra. It could make side effects more likely.
- The most common side effects with Levitra are flushing and headache.
- There has been one case of loss of vision in a man taking Levitra, as a result of damage to the blood supply to the main nerve of the eye (the optic nerve). It is not known if this was caused by the drug.
- Levitra can sometimes work for people who do not respond to Viagra.

What you need to know about Viagra (sildenafil)

- Studies originally showed that 88% of men taking it had improved erections, but doctors now think the true success rate may be lower (perhaps about 50%). On average, with Viagra the quality, rigidity and frequency of erections will be about 30% above what you could achieve previously. (This is true only if you previously had erection problems – you will not get a 30% improvement if your erections were previously normal.)
- It is slightly less effective in men whose impotence is caused by diabetes, and may not work if impotence followed a prostate operation (depending on the type of operation).
- Side effects can include headache, flushing, diarrhoea, stuffy nose, nosebleeds and abnormal vision (temporary changes in blue/green colours, increased sensitivity to light).
- There have been rare cases of sudden loss of sight in men taking Viagra, caused by disruption of the blood supply to the main nerve of the eye (the optic nerve). It is not known whether this is due to the drug or just a coincidence. It is most likely in men who have had a heart attack in the past.
- There have been reports of strokes and of deaths from heart attacks in men using the drug. It is unclear whether this was because of an interaction between heart medication and Viagra, or if the Viagra caused clumping of the blood, leading to blockage of a blood vessel, or if unaccustomed sexual exertion was the reason. Viagra is inappropriate if you have had a recent stroke or heart attack.
- Viagra should not be used if you have taken nitrates (for angina) or amyl nitrite (poppers) within the previous 24 hours, under-the-tongue nitrate tablets within the previous 5 days or alpha-blocking drugs. (Viagra with poppers is a potentially lethal combination that has caused a number of deaths.)
- Viagra should not be taken more than once a day.
- If you are taking certain other drugs (such as cimetidine for stomach problems, or erythromycin antibiotic), you will need a lower dose of Viagra.
- A study reported in the *Journal of Urology* in 2001 suggests that after using Viagra for 1 or 2 years, you may find that it becomes less effective.

What if Viagra, Cialis or Levitra do not work?

There are several reasons why Viagra, Cialis or Levitra might not be effective.

- Like all medications, they are not effective for everyone; they do not work in about 1 in 5 people.
- You need sexual stimulation to have an erection with these medications – you will not get an erection automatically.
- Maybe you are not using the medication correctly, or are expecting it to work too quickly. Re-read the information leaflet that is in the pack.
- Maybe you have not tried it for long enough. Most men have a response the first or second time they use the medication, but in some men the response improves after they have used it six or eight times.

- Maybe the dose is too low – this is something to discuss with your doctor.
- Maybe you are a smoker, drink too much alcohol, have poorly controlled diabetes or have a sedentary lifestyle. Research shows that if you deal with these problems, medications for impotence will have a better effect (*Urology* 2002;60:28–38).
- Viagra, Cialis and Levitra seem to have approximately the same effectiveness, but if one does not work for you it might be worth trying another. Your doctor might also suggest taking a low dose of Cialis (which is long-acting) every day; this can improve the effect significantly (*British Medical Journal* 2006;332:589–92). If your testosterone level is low, testosterone gel may help the medications to work. Recent preliminary research suggests that a statin medication (which is normally given to people with high blood lipids such as cholesterol) may improve the response to impotence drugs, but more research is needed.

Other types of treatment

Penile rings (e.g. Rapport RLS) are helpful for people who can get an erection but find that it does not last.

Injecting alprostadil into the penis is probably the most effective method of obtaining an erection. Alprostadil (as in e.g. Caverject and Viridal Duo) is a synthetic version of prostaglandin E1. This chemical relaxes the tiny muscles of the erectile tissue while increasing the blood supply. It is injected 10–30 minutes before intercourse. The doctor will inject the first dose and assess your erection to find the correct dose for you, and will show you how to inject yourself. You will probably be surprised how easy it is to do the injection. It should produce an erection lasting about half an hour. Occasionally a prolonged response develops (priapism). If you have a needle phobia or cannot easily see the penis, an automatic system is available (Autoject 2.25). Some pain in the penis (usually mild) is experienced by 1 in 6 men following the injection, and there might also be some bruising.

MUSE (alprostadil) stands for 'medicated urethral system for erection'. A small pellet of alprostadil, no bigger than a grain of rice, is inserted about 3 cm up the urethra, using a tiny plastic plunger. Although it is not an injection, some men find it painful, but this discomfort can be minimized by urinating beforehand. Another disadvantage is that it makes some men feel slightly dizzy. MUSE takes 5–10 minutes to work, and the erection lasts 30–60 minutes. It does not cause abnormally prolonged erections (priapism). It is not a suitable method to use if your partner is trying to become pregnant and, if she is already pregnant, you should use a condom.

Vacuum devices consist of a plastic cylinder with a pump, which may be hand- or battery-operated. A special ring is placed around the cylinder, and the cylinder is then placed over the penis. The pump is activated to produce a vacuum inside the cylinder, sucking blood into the penis, which becomes erect. When the erection is sufficient, the ring is slipped off the cylinder on to the base of the penis, to maintain the erection. The erection lasts until the ring is removed; you must remove it within 30 minutes. Vacuum devices produce a useful erection in about 75% of men, but they are cumbersome and some people find them off-putting because the penis, while erect, is often blue or mottled, and cold. They are supplied with an instruction video. In the UK, vacuum devices are now available on NHS prescription. Side effects such as bruising are uncommon.

Yohimbine tablets. Yohimbine comes from the bark of the *Pausinystalin yohimbe* tree, which for over a century has been thought to possess aphrodisiac qualities. Various trials have shown success rates somewhat better than the success rates from placebo (dummy) tablets, but mainly in men whose erection problems were not severe. Side effects are usually mild, but may include agitation, anxiety, headache, a slight increase in blood pressure, increased urination and stomach upsets. Also, it is not government regulated, so you cannot be certain of quality.

Surgery to improve blood supply to the penis or to stop blood leaking from it back into the body is possible in certain cases. The results are often disappointing.

Surgical implants to stiffen the penis can be inserted if all else fails, and are helpful if you have Peyronie's disease (see page 204). There are several new types, which are much superior to those used just a few years ago. Some are inflatable, and these are much more natural when inflated, and more easily concealed when deflated, than in the past.

- These inflatables use a reservoir that is inserted beneath the abdominal muscle during a small operation. The reservoir is filled with salty water (saline). When you want an erection, you trigger a pump placed in the scrotum next to the testicle. This signal shifts fluid from the reservoir into the cylinders that have been inserted into the penis.
- An alternative to the inflatables is the 'malleable' (bendy) type, which maintains a constant erection using flexible rods that can be manipulated into a concealed position afterwards.

Both inflatable and bendy implants are expensive and require surgery, but are effective, and most men who have implants are usually pleased with them (especially because the erection is immediately available). The penis is usually shorter after an implant has been inserted, because of scar tissue, and there may be some change in sensation. Implants do not affect ejaculation. The inflatables and the malleable types seem to be equally successful, though one survey showed that female partners tend to prefer the inflatable type. The main problem with the inflatable type is fluid leakage (which occurs in about 3% of men over 3 years, and will need a further operation to correct the problem) and infection (which occurs in about 3–5% of cases and usually means that the implant has to be removed).

Useful contacts

Impotence Australia is a non-profit organization that was set up to decrease the suffering of men with impotence and their partners by providing quality telephone counselling and information fact sheets on many sexual issues. On the 'Get the facts' section of the website there is a number of topics on impotence-related treatments.
www.impotenceaustralia.com.au

Andrology Australia provides access to quality and authenticated information to improve understanding and knowledge of the range, causes and treatment options of male

reproductive health disorders. Specialist clinical opinions have been provided by key medical authorities to ensure information is accurate. Click onto 'Your health' to access information on erectile dysfunction.
www.andrologyaustralia.org

Health*Insite* is an Australian government initiative aimed to improve the health of Australians by providing easy access to quality information about human health. By following the link here, you will find information on issues about sex and growing older, as well as impotence and erectile dysfunction.
www.healthinsite.gov.au/topics/Sex_in_Later_Years
www.healthinsite.gov.au/topics/Sexual_Problems_in_Men

The Sexual Dysfunction Association is a UK non-profit organization. It has a helpline for men suffering from erection problems and an informative website. It also maintains an index of consultants and others who are competent at impotence management; this information can be accessed by your family doctor. The website has excellent information in its section on 'male sexual dysfunction'.
www.sda.uk.net

The National Kidney and Urologic Diseases Information Clearinghouse is a US government organization and has a good website on erection problems.
www.kidney.niddk.nih.gov/kudiseases/pubs/impotence/index.htm

Men's Health Forum is a UK non-profit organization working to improve male health. Its lively website has information about many male problems, including impotence.
www.malehealth.co.uk

The US Food and Drug Administration has a web page providing basic unbiased information about Viagra.
www.fda.gov/cder/drug/infosheets/patient/sildenafilPIS.htm

Diabetes UK (previously known as the British Diabetic Association) has a booklet *Sex and Diabetes – a Guide to Erection Problems.* To obtain a copy, use the order form on their website. Email: info@diabetes.org.uk.
www.diabetes.org.uk

American Diabetes Association is the leading US non-profit health organization providing diabetes research, information and advocacy.
www.diabetes.org

ErectionAdvice.co.uk is a website from Pfizer, the manufacturers of Viagra. The site has lots of good information about erection problems, and a 'Visit the Doctor' role play to help you overcome shyness about your problem.
www.erectionadvice.co.uk

Faecal incontinence (soiling)

It is difficult to know how common this problem is, but various research studies suggest that 2–15% of adults soil their underwear regularly (*Gastroenterology* 2005;129:6).

Causes of faecal incontinence

Diet is the first thing to check. Anything that makes the consistency of the faeces more runny, such as a heavy intake of beer, will make it more difficult for you to hold them in.

In the US, the 'non-fat fat', called olestra (Olean), used in some 'slimming' foods has gained unwelcome publicity for this reason. It is an artificial mixture of fats, none of which can be digested or absorbed. Instead, it goes straight along the gut and is passed out at the other end. This means that the faeces are runny and slippery with fat, and soiled underwear can result. Some snack foods (e.g. some crisps) contain olestra, but the amount in the snacks is too small to cause a problem.

Anything which makes you pass more wind (see page 330) makes leakage more likely. This is because the anus has to relax to let the wind out, and some faecal material may be propelled out at the same time.

Irritable bowel syndrome is the other common cause. In irritable bowel syndrome (also known as IBS), the bowel muscle squeezes strongly, so that it may be difficult to hold the faeces in. If you have abdominal pain as well as leakage of faeces, then IBS is a strong possibility. The pain of IBS can occur anywhere in the abdomen, but is usually felt low down on the right or left side. Passing wind or opening the bowels often relieves it. People with IBS often have to rush to the toilet, and some leakage is common. There is also often a 'morning rush' – the bowels have to be opened urgently several times on rising and after breakfast.

Childbirth. After having a baby, more than 1 in 10 women finds that she has difficulty in controlling wind or faecal leakage. It is most likely if you were an older mother (over 35 years of age) or had a large baby. The reason may be that the anal muscle is damaged by a tear, or by the episiotomy cut made during childbirth. Damage to the pudendal nerve can also occur during childbirth, and result in incontinence. The problem is likely to improve somewhat, but if you first noticed faecal incontinence after having a baby, do see your doctor – a surgical operation to repair the damage often gives good results even if you have had the problem for years.

It is quite common to have both faecal leakage and leakage of urine (see page 283). A study of women with incontinence of urine found that almost 1 in 4 also had some leakage of faeces (*Obstetrics and Gynecology* 2002;100:719–23). The connection is that both are related to childbirth, especially if the baby was large.

Ageing. Faecal leakage is also quite common in older people, because the anal muscle becomes weaker with age. This is something that you should definitely discuss with your doctor, because a lot can be done to help. The real reason may be constipation (see page 79) – if you have hard faeces in the lower bowel, some watery faeces can leak round them and be difficult to control. Doctors are very familiar with this problem (called 'overflow incontinence') and should know how to deal with it.

Medications. Some medications make the faeces looser and therefore more difficult to hold in. Check that you are not taking a laxative from habit. If you are taking an indigestion remedy, check that it does not contain magnesium trisilicate, because this can cause diarrhoea. Misoprostol (a medication for stomach and duodenal ulcers that is sometimes prescribed for elderly people) is another possible culprit.

Orlistat (Xenical) is a diet pill that works by blocking the enzymes that digest fat. This means that the fat cannot be absorbed from the gut. With the correct dose, a third of the fat that you eat is blocked, and is excreted in the faeces instead of ending up as part of your spare tyre. By the time it reaches the lower part of the gut, this extra fat has the consistency of light machine oil. As a result, it can cause oily anal leakage, and the problem gets worse with the more fat that you eat. To stop it happening, you have to eat less than 70 g of fat a day.

What your doctor can do

Your doctor will try to work out what the cause is. Before seeing the doctor, you may wish to keep a bowel diary for a week (look at the Bowel Control website listed under Useful contacts below). In difficult cases, an ultrasound scan can tell if the anal muscles have been damaged (e.g. by childbirth). Medications such as loperamide can be used to prevent the bowel muscle squeezing too strongly and to make the faeces more solid.

Recently, a form of treatment called 'behavioural treatment' has proved to be helpful. This teaches you how to resist the urgent need to rush to the toilet. Look at bowel retraining in the self-help section of the Bowel Control website.

If the anal muscles are weak, injections of 'bulking agents' into the wall of the anus may help, but these have to be done by a specialist doctor and it is uncertain how effective the treatment is (*British Journal of Surgery* 2005; 92: 521–7). For major incontinence, a surgical operation is a last resort and may not be successful.

Useful contacts

Colorectal Surgical Society of Australasia has some very useful information on faecal incontinence under 'Patient info' on its website. Brochures are available through online order.
www.cssa.org.au

Health*Insite* is an Australian government initiative aimed to improve the health of Australians by providing easy access to quality information about human health. Follow the link to find information about faecal incontinence.
www.healthinsite.gov.au/topics/Faecal_Incontinence

Bowel Control. This website is provided by St Mark's Hospital, UK, which is a hospital specializing in bowel problems. The site covers faecal leakage, constipation and wind. It is a first-rate site that is very practical and informative.
www.bowelcontrol.org.uk

American Academy of Family Physicians have two detailed articles on 'Common Anorectal Conditions' on their website. The articles are intended for doctors. They explain how doctors examine the anus. They discuss itching, pain, bleeding, lumps, constipation and incontinence of faeces.
www.aafp.org/afp/20010615/2391.html
www.aafp.org/afp/20010701/77.html

Digestive Disorders Foundation is a UK non-profit organization that provides reliable information about all gut problems. They supply a range of leaflets, which are available on the 'Patients info leaflets' section of the website.
www.digestivedisorders.org.uk

National Digestive Diseases Information Clearinghouse is a US government organization. Its website has information about many gut problems.
http://digestive.niddk.nih.gov/ddiseases/a-z.asp

The Irritable Bowel Syndrome (IBS) Self-Help Group is a Canadian-based organization with an excellent website.
www.ibsgroup.org

InContact (Action on Incontinence) provides information and support for people with bladder and bowel problems through its publications and local groups.
www.incontact.org

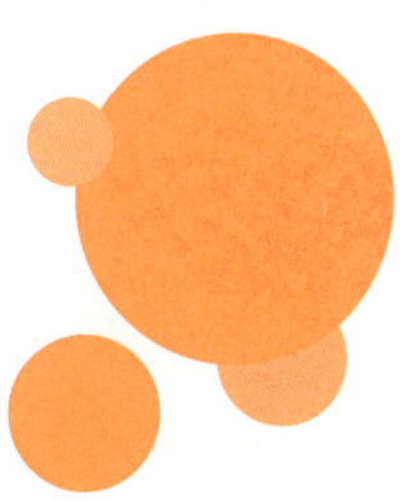

Genital infections

If you are worried because you have noticed a genital symptom, you need to see your doctor or go to a sexual health clinic. This section provides information about some of the most common genital infections and sexually transmitted infections (STIs) for people who have had an infection confirmed by their doctor or by a clinic, or who have a partner with a STI and who want more information.

BACTERIAL VAGINOSIS

Bacterial vaginosis is a very common condition in women. In fact, it is much more common than thrush. If your genital area smells fishy, this is almost certainly the cause. It is an imbalance of the bacteria in the vagina. Its former name was 'anaerobic vaginosis', and some medical textbooks still use this term.

What is bacterial vaginosis?

Every woman has harmless bacteria in her vagina. In bacterial vaginosis, some of the bacteria multiply too much, so that more are present than is normal (especially *Gardnerella* and *Mobiluncus* bacteria). Also the numbers of other friendly bacteria, especially the 'lactobacilli' type, are decreased. In other words, bacterial vaginosis is not an infection caught from your partner – it is due to bacteria that are normally present in the vagina.

Symptoms of bacterial vaginosis

- The main symptom is a fishy smell in the genital area. You may notice that the smell is worse after sex and during your period.
- There is usually a discharge, which is watery and greyish-white in colour.
- Bacterial vaginosis does not cause soreness or irritation.
- If untreated, bacterial vaginosis may possibly increase the risk of pelvic inflammatory disease (infection of the Fallopian tubes that lead from the ovaries to the uterus).

Why women get bacterial vaginosis

Putting antiseptic in your bath water, or using bubble baths, can make a bacterial imbalance more likely. Another cause is douching (squirting antiseptic or soapy liquid into the vagina). Some women douche the vagina because they think it is hygienic, but the opposite is true. The vagina cleans itself very effectively and douching makes infections more likely.

What you should do

If you think you have bacterial vaginosis, you need to see your doctor because the treatment, an antibiotic called metronidazole, is available only with a doctor's prescription. Metronidazole cures the problem in 90% of women, but causes an unpleasant metallic taste in the mouth, though this disappears after the treatment is finished. It can also cause a slightly nauseous feeling. You should not drink alcohol while you are taking it.

If it comes back. Unfortunately, the cure may not be permanent. The symptoms return in about half of women. In this situation, there are three possible courses of action.

- See your doctor again for a repeat of the metronidazole treatment, or to try another antibiotic.
- Try acetic acid vaginal jelly (Aci-Jel), which you can buy from a pharmacy without a prescription. The pack contains a special applicator for inserting the jelly into the vagina – use one applicatorful, twice a day. It restores the natural acidity of the vagina, which may encourage a return to the natural balance of bacteria. It is not known whether or not Aci-Jel damages condoms and contraceptive diaphragms.
- Try yoghurt. Make sure the container says 'live yoghurt', so it contains live lactobacilli bacteria. It is the friendly lactobacilli bacteria that are reduced in numbers in bacterial vaginosis. Gently smear a small amount of yoghurt over the vulva (the area around the opening of the vagina), and also put some inside the vagina. The easiest way to do this is to use a tampon with its applicator. Push the tampon back inside the applicator so you have a space for about a teaspoonful of yoghurt. Then insert the tampon in the usual way, which will push the yoghurt into the top of the vagina. Remove the tampon an hour later. Do this twice a day for a week. According to the medical journal *Bandolier*, which looks at the scientific evidence for treatments, some research has shown that women using yoghurt treatment felt their symptoms were improved (www.jr2.ox.ac.uk/bandolier/band60/b60-3.html).
- If you have an intrauterine contraceptive device ('coil') and bacterial vaginosis is very troublesome, consider having the device removed. Bacterial vaginosis is more common in women using this type of contraception.

If you have a partner. Your partner does not need to be treated, even if you keep getting bacterial vaginosis. There is no scientific evidence to suggest that treating your partner makes a difference.

If you are planning pregnancy. In the past, bacterial vaginosis was thought to be just a nuisance, but not harmful in any way. There is now evidence that it doubles the likelihood of a premature birth. So if you are intending to become pregnant, you should have bacterial vaginosis treated beforehand. If you have had premature labour in the past, your doctor will probably test you for bacterial vaginosis during your pregnancy and treat you with antibiotics if necessary.

CHLAMYDIA

Chlamydia (pronounced *clam-id-ee-a*) is a sexually transmitted infection. Officially, it is a bacterium, but it is more like a virus in being very small and unable to multiply outside living cells. Chlamydia is not life-threatening, but it can do serious damage to a woman's Fallopian tubes. If this happens, the woman could become infertile (unable to become pregnant). The results of chlamydia infection cost the NHS in the UK about £50 million a year.

Is chlamydia common?

In the UK and US, chlamydia is the most common sexually transmitted infection.

- In 2003, 89 431 new cases were seen at sexual health clinics in England, Scotland and Northern Ireland. This is an 8% rise compared with 2002.
- Of those affected, 55% of the men and 73% of the women were in the 16–24-year age group.
- Chlamydia is not just a disease of young people. Among 45–64-year-old women, chlamydia infections increased by 177% between 1995 and 2003.

The true figure must be even higher than the clinic figures suggest, because chlamydia is often a 'silent' infection – not causing any symptoms – especially in women. There must be hundreds of thousands of people with the infection who are unaware they have it, and therefore do not go to a clinic. When doctors in the UK, tested urine samples from sexually active women under the age of 25 (who were visiting their family doctor for any reason), they found about 1 in 10 had chlamydia. In men, the figures were even higher; 1 in 8 tested positive (UK Health Protection Agency, 2004).

How you get chlamydia

Chlamydia is passed on during sex, but using a condom gives good protection if you use it properly (see page 72). You can also catch chlamydia during oral sex, because it can be carried in the back of the mouth. Because most people with chlamydia do not know that they have it, they can pass it on to someone else unknowingly. It is not caught from toilet seats or swimming pools.

How do you know if you have chlamydia?

- About 50% of men with chlamydia have no symptoms, and do not know that they have the infection. In the other 50%, chlamydia irritates the urethra (the tube inside the penis), causing a discharge and making it painful to pass urine. Occasionally (in about 2% of cases), chlamydia spreads to the testicle (usually only on one side), where it causes pain and inflammation; some doctors think that if this happens, the man's fertility could be affected.
- In women, chlamydia infection is usually completely silent, so they are unaware that they have it – 80% of women with chlamydia have no symptoms at all. Some women notice a slightly increased discharge, or slight bleeding after sex. If it has reached the Fallopian tubes (see below), it can cause pain in the lower part of the abdomen (tummy).
- Some men (and a few women) develop 'Reiter's syndrome'. This is a reaction to the chlamydia bacterium, and consists of painful joints (usually knees or ankles) and sore eyes (conjunctivitis). It normally clears up within 6 months, but may keep recurring over several years, even if you never get chlamydia again. Whether or not you develop Reiter's syndrome depends more on your genes than on the severity of your chlamydial infection.

Tests for chlamydia

The best way of knowing if you have chlamydia is to be tested. This can be done at a sexual health clinic or by your family doctor. There are several types of test.

- In women, the cervix (neck of the womb) is wiped with a cotton wool bud, which is then sent to the laboratory for testing. To do this test, the doctor or nurse will insert a speculum into the vagina, like having a smear test. In men, the cotton-wool bud is inserted into the end of the urethra (pee hole) to obtain the sample.
- A urine sample can be tested. However, this test is not available everywhere and, for women, it is not as reliable as taking a sample from the cervix. For this test you must hold your urine for at least an hour beforehand.
- A sample from the vagina in women can be tested using a new, more accurate test (NNAT). This means that women could take their own samples.

In Sweden, they have had a screening programme for chlamydia for 25 years. At present, in the UK, you can be screened for chlamydia at a sexual health clinic and at some other places (such as colleges), otherwise see your family doctor. Free screening in pharmacies is to be tried out in London and Cornwall for 16–24-year-olds. If this works well, it will be extended to the rest of the UK.

When to have a chlamydia test

Several situations in which it would be sensible to have a chlamydia test are:

- if you have symptoms, such as discharge or lower abdominal pain (women), pain on passing urine (men) or pain in the testicles (men)
- if your partner has symptoms
- if you had sex with a new partner without a condom in the past year
- if your partner has had a chlamydia infection and you are not sure if he or she was properly treated
- if you had treatment for a chlamydia infection, but your partner did not have treatment
- if you and your partner had treatment for a chlamydia infection, but had sex before the treatment was completed
- if you have another sexually transmitted infection (such as genital warts, see page 134)
- if you are about to have a termination of pregnancy (abortion).

What happens if chlamydia infection is not treated?

If you have a chlamydia infection, it may or may not give you symptoms. If you have symptoms, such as a discharge, the symptom may disappear in a few days. This does not mean that your body has cured the infection. You are probably still carrying the chlamydia bacterium and can pass it on to other people. Also, if you are a woman, it can start to travel towards your Fallopian tubes. So go for a test, even if the symptoms have gone.

Pelvic inflammatory disease. In most women who have it, chlamydia travels no further than the cervix (neck of the womb at the top if the vagina). But in about 1 in 10, it travels further upwards through the uterus (womb) into the Fallopian tubes. In the Fallopian tubes it can cause inflammation known as 'pelvic inflammatory disease' or PID. Other types of bacteria may then move in making the inflammation worse. PID may be painful, but can occur without any pain at all. If the infection is treated at this stage, the tube may recover completely, or some scarring and other damage may remain.

In Sweden, where young women are screened for chlamydia, the number of women with PID has halved.

Infertility. The Fallopian tube is where the sperm meets the egg, and where fertilization occurs. So if a woman's tubes have been damaged by PID in the past, the egg and sperm will not be able to travel along it easily, and she may not be able to conceive. If she does conceive, there is a possibility that the fertilized egg could get stuck in the tube, and the baby would start to develop in the tube instead of in the uterus. This is called 'ectopic pregnancy' and is a bad situation, because the developing baby almost always dies in early pregnancy, and there will be dangerous internal bleeding.

However, while it is true that chlamydia can cause infertility, this happens in only a small number of women who have it. The risk is not precisely known, but a Swedish study in the early 1990s suggests the following figures.

- If 100 women get a chlamydia infection, 20 will develop PID.
- Of these 20 who develop PID, 2 will have difficulty conceiving and 1 will have an ectopic pregnancy.
- The more times a woman has PID, the greater the damage to the tubes and the greater the chance of later problems. So if those 20 women had another attack of PID, 4 would become infertile and 2 would have ectopic pregnancies.
- If those same 20 women had three or more attacks of PID, 8 or 9 would become infertile and 4 would have ectopic pregnancies.

Treatment for chlamydia and talking to your partner

The good news is that chlamydia is easily treated, usually with doxycycline antibiotic. This treatment is over 95% effective if you take the full course (usually twice a day for 7 days) exactly as instructed by your doctor. Other antibiotics (azithromycin, erythromycin) are sometimes used instead; if you are pregnant or breastfeeding your doctor will probably give you erythromycin.

It is essential that your partner is treated as well. If your partner is not treated at the same time as you, you can catch it again from him or her. This is particularly not good for women, because the more times a woman has a chlamydia infection, the greater her risk of later infertility. So do not have sex (even with a condom) until both of you have completed your treatment.

You may feel anxious about telling your partner about the infection. Sometimes partners do not believe they could have it themselves, because they probably have no symptoms. So explain that most people with chlamydia do not know that they have it. If you think that telling your partner would be problematic, talk to a health advisor at your local sexual health clinic.

GENITAL HERPES

Genital herpes is an infection with the herpesvirus, called herpes simplex. Herpes simplex virus is also responsible for 'cold sores' that occur on the face (see page 68).

How you catch genital herpes

You catch genital herpes during sex, by contact with someone who has the infection on their skin. You are most likely to catch it if your partner has herpes blisters or moist herpes sores.

You can also catch herpes from someone who has no visible herpes sores. About 3% of people carry the virus on their skin without knowing that they have it (because it has never given them any symptoms), but they can pass it on to other people. This is one of the reasons it is important to use a condom with a new partner. Condoms give significant protection against genital herpes (*Journal of the American Medical Association* 2001;285:3100–6).

Because cold sores (see page 68) are also caused by herpes simplex virus, you can catch herpes if your partner gives you oral sex when they have a cold sore.

The herpes virus cannot survive for long outside the body, so it is unlikely (but not impossible) that you will catch it from towels.

How do I know if I have herpes?

With herpes, you do not usually have symptoms all the time. The symptoms usually come and go in 'attacks' (also called 'episodes').

- The first attack is the worst, and starts between 2 and 12 days after you caught the infection (usually about 4 days).
- Later attacks ('recurrences') are less severe.
- Some people never get recurrences, some people get them occasionally and a few people get them regularly.
- The severity of the attacks varies a lot between individuals. At one end of the spectrum, some people have really troublesome attacks. At the other end of the spectrum, the attack may be so mild that the person does not notice any symptoms, which is how people end up carrying the herpes virus unknowingly.

In the UK in 2003, more than 18 000 people visited a clinic for a first attack of genital herpes

First herpes attack

Women. The first time you get herpes can be very unpleasant. First of all, you may feel as if you have flu – muscle aches, feverishness, tiredness and headache. Then small blisters appear on the labia (the 'lips' that surround the opening of the vagina). After 3 or 4 days, they burst to leave small, painful sores. Passing urine may be very painful indeed, and you will probably feel completely miserable and tearful. You may notice that the glands in your groin are swollen and tender.

After 6 or 7 days, the sores start to scab over and slowly heal. So it can be 3 weeks from when you first started to feel unwell to complete healing.

Men. In men, a first attack of herpes is usually less severe than in women. The blisters and sores may be on the glans (head) of the penis, the foreskin, the scrotum, the thighs, the buttocks or near the anus. Passing urine may be uncomfortable, and there may be discomfort or pain around the anus (back passage). You may feel feverish and generally unwell. The ulcers on the glans or the foreskin heal softly, but those on the shaft or scrotum form scabs as they heal.

Later attacks (recurrences)

Do not assume that you will get more attacks of herpes – some people do not. The number and severity of recurrent attacks varies enormously between individuals, but the average number is about five a year in men and four a year in women. Although this sounds bad, recurrent attacks are often very mild. Many people find that recurrences become less frequent and even milder with time.

You will probably not have the flu-like feeling, nor the swollen glands in the groin, that you may have had with the first attack. An uncomfortable tingling feeling in the genital area and buttocks often warns that an attack is about to occur. Some people experience shooting pains in the buttocks, legs or hips. The stage with painful sores will usually last about 4 days, and it will all be over in about 10 days.

Why recurrences occur

After the first attack, herpe svirus often remains because the body has difficulty in getting rid of it completely. The virus travels away from the genitals using the nerves in the pelvic area as a pathway. When it reaches the clusters of cells at the end of the nerves (called ganglia), it stops travelling. The herpesvirus DNA then remains quietly in the ganglia. Fortunately, it does not damage the nerves or interfere with their function.

In some people, from time to time, the herpes virus travels back the way it came, along the nerves towards the genitals. This is called activation. When it arrives in the skin, it causes blisters and sores.

After the sores heal, the virus goes back up the nerve to the ganglion again, where it lies low again. But it can become activated again at any time, and travel down the nerves to the skin to cause another sore. The virus always travels up and down the same or nearby nerve pathways, which explains why herpes sores always recur in roughly the same place.

How recurrences of herpes virus happen

- First genital infection with herpes simplex virus causes sores.
- Herpes virus travels up nerves to the nerve ganglion where it lies low.
- At a later date, herpesvirus may travel down nerves to the genital skin, causing a 'recurrent attack' of herpes.
- Recurrent attack heals, and herpesvirus retreats to the ganglion again.

- At a later date, herpes virus may travel down to the genital skin again, causing another recurrent attack. This may happen several times.

No one really understands why the virus in the ganglia suddenly wakes up from time to time, and decides to go to the skin and cause a recurrent attack. But in some people, there are some definite triggers that make this happen, such as:

- emotional stress
- physical stress (e.g. having another illness)
- damage to the genital skin
- menstruation.

There are two types of herpes simplex virus; recurrences are more likely if you have type 2 than type 1. Recurrences are slightly more likely in men than in women.

In the UK, genital herpes has increased by 19% in men and 9% in women since 1996

What to do if you have an attack of herpes

- If you are female, look at the section on painful vulva (see page 303).
- If this is your first attack, go at once to your nearest sexual health clinic to check that you really do have herpes. There are many other causes of rash or discomfort in the genital area. For example, people sometimes mistake herpes for jock itch (see page 187) or conditions causing anal pain (see page 30). You do not need a doctor's letter to go to the clinic. If you are anxious about going to the clinic, look at the section on visiting the clinic on page 335. The advantage of the clinic is that they will test you for other genital infections, they may also be able to give you some treatment to take away with you and they have health advisors who can talk to you about the whole subject. However, if you prefer, you could see your family doctor instead.
- There is no cure for herpes, but if this is your first attack your doctor will probably prescribe medication to reduce symptoms and speed healing (such as aciclovir, famciclovir or valaciclovir).
- If this is your first attack, recognize that you will be feeling excessively miserable (which is part of the viral illness). Do not force yourself to go to work – stay home until the worst has passed and pamper yourself as much as possible.
- Do not share your towel or wash cloth with anyone – there is no strong evidence that herpes is transmitted this way, but better to be on the safe side.
- Put two handfuls of ordinary salt into a bath of warm water and sit in it for a while.
- If passing urine is painful, do it into the warm bath. Take plenty of drinks.
- Drying the genital area with a hairdryer on the cool setting may help to ease discomfort.
- According to the UK Herpes Virus Association (see Useful contacts on page 145), applying a cold, wet teabag helps. They say that Earl Grey is best!

- Paracetamol (acetaminophen) will help to relieve pain.
- If appropriate (for example, you are home alone), leave the sores exposed to the air to prevent irritation from panties or underpants.
- You could try a herbal cream, such as aloe vera, melissa (a type of mint) or propolis (made by bees from the resin of Canadian poplar trees). These remedies are available from health food stores. But remember that there is very little scientific evidence to back the use of these remedies, their quality is not always controlled and some people may react badly to herbal creams.
- Do not have sex until the sores have completely healed – if this is your first attack, this could be about 3 weeks. One reason is that you are most likely to pass the infection on when you have the sores. Another reason is to protect yourself – open sores give other infections (such as HIV) easy access to your bloodstream.
- After the sores have healed and you start having sex again, use plenty of lubrication to protect your skin from too much friction. Look at the section on vaginal dryness for advice on lubricants (see page 311).

What to do if you keep getting recurrences

It is common to get four or five recurrences a year, but these are usually not very troublesome. You just wait for them to go and avoid sex until the sores have healed. But a few unlucky people have lots of recurrences, which can make their life a misery. Here is some advice for this situation.

- Talk to your doctor about some anti-herpes drug therapy. This medication is most effective if you take it as soon as the attack starts, so your doctor may give you some to keep at home in readiness. For a really severe problem, your doctor might suggest that you take the anti-herpes medication continuously, and will discuss the pros and cons with you.
- Look after your genital skin between recurrences. For sex, use plenty of lubrication to protect your skin from too much friction; look at the section on vaginal dryness for advice on lubricants (see page 311). Try to avoid over-vigorous sex or over-vigorous masturbation. There is general advice for women about vaginal and vulval problems on page 302.
- Keep your immune system in good shape by eating plenty of fresh fruit and vegetables, taking plenty of rest and not smoking.
- Try to keep the problem in proportion. The UK Herpes Association (see Useful contacts on page 145) has a very helpful booklet called *Herpes simplex: a guide*, which will help you feel better about yourself.

In the US, an estimated 1% of sexually active people have genital warts

GENITAL WARTS

Genital warts are caused by a virus – HPV (human papillomavirus). HPV is caught during sexual contact with someone who is already infected with it. If you develop genital warts, try not to feel too upset – remember they are very common and lots of people have them, they are not dangerous and there are many effective ways of treating them.

You may feel angry with the person you think you caught them from. But in fact that person may not know that he or she had HPV for the following two reasons.

- Some people carry HPV, but do not have any warts. In fact 15–40% of people under 40 are carriers of HPV, though it is less common in older people. In most people who carry HPV, it goes away in a year or two.
- A man may not know that he has a wart, because it can be hidden inside the urethral opening (pee hole). Similarly, a woman can have a wart on the cervix (that is, deep inside the vagina) that she does not know about.

In the UK, warts are the most common reason for attending a sexual health clinic. In 2002, more than 70 000 people attended with a first attack of genital warts

Preventing warts

Although you can catch the virus from sexual contact with someone who carries it but has no warts, infection is more likely from someone who has warts. This is because the surface of a wart is teeming with the virus. After infection, warts can develop 3 weeks to a year later (3 months is the average), so do not assume that you caught them from a recent sexual contact.

Recent research among university students in the US shows that condoms halve the risk of becoming infected with HPV (*New England Journal of Medicine* 2006;354:2645–54).

Where genital warts occur

In women, genital warts usually occur around the opening of the vagina (vulva), but they may occur in the folds of skin alongside the vaginal opening, or between the vagina and the anus, and around the anal opening. The figures (*Archives of Dermatology* 1984;120:472) are as follows:

- around the opening of the vagina (vulva) – 66%
- in the vagina – 37%
- between the vagina and anus – 29%
- around the anus – 23%
- on the cervix (neck of womb) – 8%
- at the opening of the urethra (where the urine comes out) – 4%.

In men, genital warts often occur just under the foreskin, but can be anywhere on the penis, on the scrotum, in the groin or around the anus. The figures (*Archives of Dermatology* 1984; 120:472) are as follows:

- on the shaft of the penis – 51%
- around the anus – 34%
- on the glans (head of the penis) – 10%

- inside the opening of the urethra (pee hole) – 10%
- under the foreskin – 8%
- between the anus and scrotum – 3%
- on the scrotum – 1%.

Genital warts are becoming more common. In the UK, the 2003 figures were 2% higher than in the previous year

What warts look like

In women, genital warts begin as small, gritty-feeling growths, which then enlarge and become more frond-like. They can join together so they resemble miniature cauliflowers. Occasionally they are flat, like warts on the fingers. They are not painful, but can feel itchy or vaguely uncomfortable.

In men, warts on the scrotum or shaft of the penis usually resemble the ordinary warts that occur on the hands. Under the foreskin and round the anus, they are usually a shiny pinkish-white. A lone wart may also occur inside the opening of the urethra (pee hole); here it will be a pinkish colour and may look speckled. An individual may have dozens of warts, or just one or two.

What to do

- If you think you have genital warts, the only positive thing you can do yourself is stop smoking, because warts probably persist longer in smokers.
- Do not try to treat genital warts with any of the wart lotions you can buy from pharmacists; these are for use on the hands only.
- You need to see a doctor, either your family doctor or a doctor at a sexual health clinic, whichever you feel most comfortable with. The advantage of going to a sexual health clinic is that you will have tests for other infections; 1 in 5 people with genital warts has another infection that they are probably unaware of. Also, the staff are very used to diagnosing and treating warts. You do not need a referral from your doctor and you simply phone the clinic yourself (see Useful contacts on page 145).

There are several treatments for genital warts. The usual treatments – because they are simple and effective – are podophyllotoxin or imiquimod. Other treatments (such as freezing, burning with acid or laser treatment) are sometimes used, depending on the type and size of wart.

Annoyingly, whatever the treatment, there is a 30% chance that the warts will come back – usually after a few weeks or months. This is because the treatments destroy the wart itself, but cannot get rid of the HPV in the skin beneath the wart.

Podophyllotoxin is a plant extract that comes as a liquid or cream. The clinic will show you how to use it and may give you a supply to take home. You usually have to apply it twice a day for 3 days, followed by a break of 4 days. You then repeat this process until the wart disappears (maximum of 4–5 weeks' treatment). The cream is easier to use than the liquid for warts in awkward places (such as around the anus). It should not be used if you are pregnant or trying to get pregnant.

Imiquimod is a cream that the clinic may suggest if podophyllotoxin does not work. It is applied 3 times a week before you go to sleep, so it can remain on the skin for about 8 hours. It seems to work by stimulating the body's own immune system to destroy the warts. On average, women need 8 weeks of treatment and men need 12 weeks, but it can be used for up to 16 weeks. The disadvantage is that itching, redness and soreness often occur. Its effect is slow and it may be several weeks before you notice any improvement.

There is a particularly noticeable increase in genital warts among teenagers. In women, about 60% of genital warts are in the 16–24-year-old age group and, in men, about 45%

Genital warts and cervical cancer

There are about 120 different types of HPV. Each type has been given a number to identify it. Visible genital warts are usually caused by HPV types 6 and 11.

There is a strong link between HPV types 16 and 18 and cervical cancer. These types of HPV seem to agitate the cells of the cervix (neck of the womb) and encourage pre-cancerous changes. But HPV 16 and 18 do not usually cause visible warts. Therefore if you have genital warts, you are not at a particularly increased risk of cervical cancer.

This also means that people with only the more high-risk type of HPV (types 16 or 18) do not know that they have it, because they probably will not have warts. At present, you cannot be tested under the NHS in the UK to see if you are a carrier of types 16 or 18, but this may be possible in the future. The Department of Health is trying out a screening programme by testing several thousand women for the high-risk strains.

Genital warts in pregnant women

Pregnancy seems to encourage genital warts – they often become bigger or more numerous. Unfortunately, podophyllotoxin may harm the baby, and it is not known whether imiquimod is safe in pregnancy. If very troublesome, they can be treated by freezing (cryotherapy). The good news is that, after the baby is born, genital warts often become smaller or disappear.

The future – a vaccine?

Scientists have developed a vaccine against HPV 16 and 18, and two other types, 6 and 11. It has been trialled in a study involving more than 1000 women, and seems to be very effective (*British Medical Journal* 2005;331:916–8). However, it will be several years before it becomes generally available.

The vaccine would not prevent visible warts. It is directed against the types of HPV that cause cervical cancer and not those that cause visible warts.

GONORRHOEA

Gonorrhoea is a sexually transmitted infection, caused by a bacterium *Neisseria gonorrhoeae*. This infection is often called 'the clap' (from a French word, *clapoir*, meaning 'sexual sore').

Like other sexually transmitted infections, it is especially common in young people. In the UK, 69% of women and 40% of men with gonorrhoea are in the 16–24-year-old age group. In 2003, 24 309 people caught gonorrhoea in the UK.

How gonorrhoea is transmitted

You catch a genital gonorrhoea infection by having sex with someone who has the infection. Therefore it is very important to use condoms with a new partner. Also, you can catch a gonorrhoea throat infection from oral sex.

How do I know if I have gonorrhoea?

Men with gonorrhoea usually develop a discharge from the urethra (pee hole) and pain when passing urine. These symptoms start about 3–10 days after catching the infection. However, some men may have no symptoms so they do not know they have the infection.

In 7 out of 10 women, gonorrhoea causes no symptoms at all. Some women develop vague symptoms, such as an increase in vaginal discharge.

What to do if you think you might have gonorrhoea

If you have a symptom, such as a discharge, or if think you might be at risk of having an infection, you need a check-up at a sexual health clinic or see your family doctor.

Treatment for gonorrhoea

If the clinic or your doctor finds that you have gonorrhoea, you will be prescribed a special antibiotic. In many countries gonorrhoea does not respond to common antibiotics. (This is called 'resistance'.) Therefore the clinic will send your samples to the laboratory to ensure that the antibiotic you are given is the correct one. You will need check-ups afterwards to make sure the infection has gone. You must not have sex with anyone (not even with a condom) until the clinic gives you the all-clear, and your partner(s) will also need to be tested.

Is gonorrhoea dangerous?

If it is not treated, gonorrhoea can spread to other parts of the body. In women, it can travel upwards to the Fallopian tubes. These are the tubes that transport eggs from the ovary to the uterus. If the Fallopian tubes are damaged by an infection such as gonorrhoea, the woman may have difficulty conceiving a baby. Infection in the Fallopian tubes can cause pain in the lower abdomen (especially during sex), or may not cause any symptoms. In men, gonorrhoea can spread to the tubing around the testicle. Gonorrhoea can also spread through the bloodstream to the joints, causing a painful arthritis.

MOLLUSCUM

Molluscum (correct name molluscum contagiosum) is a skin infection caused by a virus. It is transmitted by skin-to-skin contact, so it is commonly caught during sexual contact.

What molluscum looks like

Molluscum shows as white or pink bumps on the skin. They are small (usually 1–5 mm across) and round in shape. If you look very carefully (ideally with a magnifying glass), you will usually see a small dimple in the centre of each one. There are usually several. They are often in the lower abdomen among the pubic hair, or on the upper thighs. In men they may be on the penis, and in women on the lips of the vagina. Sometimes they can be difficult to distinguish from genital warts (see page 134).

How molluscum is treated

In time, molluscum usually goes away on its own. Strangely, molluscum usually goes away faster if the lumps become damaged. Therefore a doctor or nurse will treat them by piercing each one with a sharp sterile needle and digging out some of the material inside. Large molluscums can be treated by freezing (cryotherapy).

Is molluscum dangerous?

Molluscum is not dangerous. If you scratch the lumps, they could become infected, leaving a scar after healing.

THRUSH IN WOMEN

Thrush is caused by the yeast *Candida albicans*. About 2 in 5 women have Candida in the vagina, without it causing any symptoms. Hormones in the vaginal secretions and the friendly vaginal bacteria keep it at bay. Problems arise when this natural balance is upset, and Candida multiplies. This can happen:

- during pregnancy (but thrush is less likely during breastfeeding)
- when you take antibiotics (because these get rid of the friendly bacteria)
- if you have diabetes, especially if your blood sugar levels are consistently too high
- if you wear tight, non-porous underwear, such as nylon panties and tights (because Candida thrives in warm, moist conditions)
- if the vulva or vagina is sore for any other reason, particularly if you scratch (because damaged tissue is more susceptible to Candida)
- if you are ill for any reason
- if you are taking any drugs, such as steroids, which lower the body's resistance to infection.

Attacks of thrush are very common. Most women have had at least one attack by their mid-20s. Thrush is not a dangerous infection, but it can cause a lot of distress if it keeps coming back. It is very uncomfortable and can wreck your sex life.

Common beliefs – true or false?

'The contraceptive pill causes thrush'

Probably false. Doctors are still arguing about this, but there is very little evidence for it.

'Thrush is a sexually transmitted disease'

False. Women who are not sexually active can suffer from thrush. The Candida yeasts are already in the vagina, and they cause thrush when the body's natural balance that keeps it under control is upset.

'Thrush always causes a discharge'

False. Itching is the usual symptom of thrush and there is often no discharge at all, or just a slight discharge.

'Thrush is very smelly'

False. If there is an odour, it is minimal and not unpleasant.

'Thrush can be prevented by douching the vagina'

Very definitely false. Douching is squirting a soapy or antiseptic solution into the vagina to 'cleanse' it. There is no need to do this, because the vagina cleans itself very efficiently. In fact, douching has the opposite effect; it destroys the friendly bacteria, gets rid of the healthy acidity and damages the lining, allowing thrush and other infections to take hold easily.

How do you know if you have thrush?

There are three main symptoms of thrush.

- The most common symptom of thrush is itching and/or soreness around the entrance of the vagina (vulva). The soreness means that you have a stinging sensation when you pass urine and that sex is uncomfortable.
- There may also be a thick, whitish discharge (like cottage cheese), or a watery discharge. The discharge does not smell unpleasant.
- The vulval area looks red, there may be cracks in the skin and the vaginal lips (labia) are often swollen.

It is very difficult to know if thrush is the cause of your problem without having a test, because these symptoms can also occur in other types of infection. For example, an infection in the bladder (cystitis) will also cause stinging when you pass urine, various infections can cause vaginal discharge or vulval soreness, and some skin diseases (which are not infections) can cause vaginal itching.

Researchers in the US tested women who felt sure they had thrush, and were buying thrush medication from a grocery store or pharmacy (*Obstetrics and Gynecology* 2002;99:419–25). They found that only 33% had thrush as their only problem. Another 20% had thrush as well as a different infection that needed a different treatment, such as bacterial vaginosis or trichomoniasis.

This means that if you think you have thrush you have two possible courses of action.

- You could see your doctor or to go to a sexual health clinic to check the diagnosis. If you have never had these symptoms before this is sensible.
- You could buy thrush medication from a pharmacy. According to the American research, there would be a less than 50:50 chance that this would be the right treatment. So if the symptoms persist after the course of treatment, see a doctor for a proper check-up and don't just buy more thrush medication.

Treatment

Creams and pessaries. If you have thrush, the Candida will be on the skin of the vulva, and also in the vagina. Therefore you need:

- an anti-thrush cream to deal with the Candida on the skin
- an anti-thrush pessary to deal with the Candida in the vagina; a pessary is a specially shaped lump of anti-thrush medication for insertion into the vagina.

There are various types of anti-thrush creams and pessaries. Most contain '-azole' drugs, such as clotrimazole, econazole, fenticonazole or miconazole. These drugs are very similar and are all more or less equally effective. Nystatin is another type of anti *Candida* pessary; it may stain your clothes yellow.

Some of these treatments can be bought from pharmacies without a doctor's prescription, in packs containing both cream and pessaries. Read the directions carefully, because some types of pessary (such as nystatin) have to be inserted every night for 2 weeks, but others need to be used for fewer days.

In about 15% of people, these treatments may cause a burning feeling or irritation soon after applying the cream.

Many anti-thrush creams and pessaries can damage condoms and contraceptive diaphragms.

Oral tablets and pills. Some special anti-thrush tablets and pills are now available, such as fluconazole and itraconazole, which can be used instead of creams and pessaries. These oral treatments have to be prescribed by a doctor; do not try swallowing a pessary that is meant to be inserted in the vagina. Although oral treatments are simpler than creams and pessaries, they can have side effects, so most doctors prescribe them only for very troublesome thrush that keeps coming back.

Why do some people keep getting thrush?

A common scenario is that you develop thrush, you treat it with an anti-thrush cream or vaginal pessary, the symptoms disappear, and then a few weeks later they come back again. This is called 'recurrent' thrush. Doctors do not fully understand why some people suffer from recurrent thrush. There are three different theories.

- The 'gut theory' says that Candida yeasts lurk in the lower part of the gut (rectum). When you use an anti-thrush cream, you get rid of thrush from the vulva (the area around the opening of the vagina). According to this theory, you later get a reinfection from your own gut. This theory was very popular in the 1970s, but most doctors no longer believe it, because clearing Candida from the gut (with a long course of tablets) does not prevent recurrent thrush.

- The 'sexual theory' says that your partner reinfects you, even though he does not have any symptoms himself. It is true that about 20% of the partners of women with recurrent thrush have the same type of yeast in their mouth or on their fingers or genital area, but most do not have any. And scientific studies mainly show that treating her partner has no effect on the likelihood of a woman having recurrences.
- The 'vaginal relapse theory' is the one believed by most doctors. It seems that treatment does not eliminate the Candida totally. Tiny numbers of the yeast remain. If the situation is right for them – for instance, the skin is moist and warm – they slowly multiply until there are enough to cause symptoms again.

What to do if you keep getting thrush

Check that you really do have thrush. If it usually goes away with anti-thrush treatment, it probably is thrush, but it is worth making sure. According to research from the University of Leeds (published in the journal *Sexually Transmitted Infections* in 2001), a third of women who attended a clinic because of recurrent thrush did not actually have thrush. There were other reasons for their symptoms.

To check whether or not you have thrush, you should visit your family doctor or local sexual health clinic to have a swab taken. The swab will be sent to a laboratory, which will be able to tell if there is Candida or similar yeasts. Although Candida is the usual cause of thrush, in about 5% of cases symptoms are due to a slightly different type of yeast, for which another treatment might be more effective. With recurrent thrush there is an even greater chance that it is an unusual type.

Look after yourself. It is crucial to make life as difficult as possible for the Candida yeasts, so take a look at our list of common-sense dos and don'ts for anyone with a vaginal or vulval problem on page 314. Avoid anything that might irritate the vulva, such as bubble baths, perfumed soaps, vaginal deodorants and douches. For sex, use a lubricant (see page 311) to lessen the chance of damage to the vulva and vagina.

Keep the vulval area dry. Candida yeasts like warm, moist places so dry carefully after bathing or showering. Avoid tight-fitting or synthetic-fibre panties – choose cotton.

Avoid long courses of antibiotics. The longer a course of antibiotics, the more likely it will lead to thrush. So if you need antibiotics, ask your doctor if a short course would be appropriate.

Natural remedies. If your recurrences are predictable, you could try a natural remedy to ward it off. For example, if your thrush usually comes before a period, on days 21–24 of your cycle, you could try a natural remedy starting on day 18. But remember that you can get a reaction to a natural remedy as easily as to a cream from the chemist, so stop straight away if that happens. Here are some popular natural remedies.

- Gently smear a small amount of bio ('live') yoghurt over the vulva, and also put it inside the vagina. The easiest way to do this is to use a tampon with its applicator. Push the tampon back inside the applicator so you have a space for about a teaspoonful of yoghurt. Then insert the tampon in the usual way, which will push the yogurt into the top of the vagina. Remove the tampon an hour later. However, a scientific study showed that yoghurt did not decrease thrush (*British Medical Journal* 2004;329:548).

- Tea-tree oil is another possibility. Dilute 20 drops of tea-tree oil in half a cup of water, soak a tampon in this liquid and then insert it into the vagina. Change it as frequently as you would a normal tampon.
- Buy some 9% acetic acid gel (Aci-Jel) from a pharmacy. It comes with its own applicator.

Do not bother trying a yeast-free or sugar-free diet. There is no evidence at all that these diets have any effect.

Ask your doctor about oral treatment. A 7-day or 14-day course of an anti-thrush drug taken orally (by mouth) may deal with the Candida yeasts more thoroughly. After that, you could insert pessaries in the vagina once or twice a month to prevent the problem returning.

Oral treatments may have side effects, and are unsuitable if you are pregnant or trying to get pregnant.

Consider long-term medication if you are having many troublesome recurrences. Your doctor can prescribe oral treatment, which is usually taken once a week. After 6 months, you stop the treatment and wait and see if the thrush returns (*New England Journal of Medicine* 2004;351:876–83). However, taking a prescription drug regularly for a condition that is not seriously hazardous to your health is a big decision. It is not suitable if you are pregnant or trying to get pregnant. Discuss all the pros and cons very carefully with your doctor, and go for it only if your symptoms are really distressing.

Consider asking your partner to get treatment. Clinics do not usually advise that your partner is treated (because they do not believe in the 'sexual theory' of thrush). But if you have lots of recurrences, it might be worth asking your partner to be treated as well.

THRUSH IN MEN

Thrush is caused by the yeast *Candida albicans*. It is not just a female problem – men can have it too. In men, Candida can cause itching, redness and soreness of the glans (head of the penis) and the foreskin. In some men, the foreskin swells and becomes cracked; this is probably caused by an allergy to the yeast.

The medical term for redness and soreness of the glans is 'balanitis'. Candida is the usual cause, but there could be other reasons (look at the section on penis problems: red, sore and itchy on page 206). Therefore you need to check with your family doctor or go to a sexual health clinic. Also, thrush in men can be the first sign of diabetes, so your doctor will do a diabetes check.

How do men get thrush?

Thrush is not classed as a sexually transmitted infection, because many people already have small amounts of the Candida fungus on their skin. Whether or not it causes problems depends on the situation. Candida likes warm and moist skin, and skin that is already slightly damaged. It also thrives on the high sugar levels in people with diabetes. So if the skin of your genitals is already irritated by perfumes in soaps or shower gels, or if you are careless about drying yourself after washing, or if you have diabetes that is uncontrolled (perhaps because you are unaware you have diabetes), Candida is more likely to multiply. When it has multiplied, you may begin to notice symptoms.

If you have a regular female partner, it is quite likely that she will also be carrying Candida in her vagina. If she does not have symptoms, she probably does not need treatment. However, if you keep getting thrush, it might be worth her having treatment even if she has no symptoms.

Treatment

Thrush in men is usually cured easily with an antifungal cream. To prevent it coming back, take care over your choice of soaps – avoid perfumed soaps and shower gels, and anything else that could irritate your skin.

TRICHOMONIASIS

Trichomoniasis (pronounced *trick-oh-mon-eye-a-sis*) is infection with *Trichomonas vaginalis*. This is not a type of bacterium; it is a microscopic organism consisting of a single cell, like an amoeba. Under the microscope, it looks a rather attractive creature, because it swims around in a wobbly and rotating fashion, waving its four tiny antennae.

In the UK, trichomoniasis has become less common (whereas most other sexually transmitted infections have increased). No one knows why.

How is trichomoniasis transmitted?

Trichomoniasis is sexually transmitted. It does not always cause symptoms, so people may not know that they are carrying it. In fact, most men and about half of all women with trichomonas have no symptoms themselves, but can unknowingly pass it on to someone else.

Symptoms of trichomoniasis

- Trichomoniasis seems to be most common in young sexually active women, and in women nearing the menopause. In about half the women who have it, trichomonas causes no symptoms. In the other half, it causes a foul-smelling discharge. The vulva (area round the opening of the vagina) is often itchy and sore. Passing urine may be painful.
- Men commonly have no symptoms, or they may notice burning when they pass urine and/or a discharge from the urethra (pee hole).

What you should do

- To relieve the itching and discomfort, put a couple of handfuls of salt in a bath of warm water, and sit in it for a while. If passing urine is painful, it may help to pee into the bath water. The salt bath will help symptoms, but will not get rid of the trichomonas.

- See a doctor for treatment with metronidazole tablets. You should not drink alcohol while you are taking them. It is a good idea to go to a sexual health clinic, because the clinic will be able to test you straightaway, tell you whether or not you have trichomonas, and give you the treatment. The clinic will also be able to check for other infections, which are quite common in people with trichomoniasis.
- Your partner will also need to be checked and treated.

If you are pregnant

Trichomonas infection can cause a premature birth, so doctors are keen to treat it if you are pregnant. However, there have been worries about using metronidazole in pregnancy, so a low dose is used.

Useful contacts

Family Planning NSW has a 'Useful contacts' link on their website to other family planning and sexual health clinics in Australia. The website also provides fact sheets and FAQs under the section 'Sex matters'.
www.fpahealth.org.au/sex-matters

Health*Insite* is an Australian government initiative aimed to improve the health of Australians by providing easy access to quality information about human health. Follow the link to find information on a variety of sexually transmitted infections
www.healthinsite.gov.au/topics/Sexually_Transmitted_Infections

Reach Out! is a web-based service aimed to improve young people's mental health and wellbeing by providing support information and referrals in a format that appeals to young people. The website has a topic section on 'Sex and pregnancy' with related fact sheets about sexually transmitted infections.
www.reachout.com.au

Playing safely is a website funded by the UK government Department of Health. It has information about all types of genital infections. It also has a 'Where to get help' section, where you can locate a genitourinary medicine clinic (sexual health clinic).
www.playingsafely.co.uk

Society for Sexual Health Advisers has a website for health advisers who work in sexual health clinics, informing and counselling patients. The site has information about all types of genital infections, with photographs. But be warned – the pictures are explicit, and not for the squeamish.
www.ssha.info/public/index.asp

Leeds University has pictures of the Candida yeast on its website.
www.bmb.leeds.ac.uk/mbiology/ug/ugteach/icu8/std/candidosis.html

Health Protection Agency is a UK government organization that monitors infection, including sexually transmitted infections. If you are interested in the latest statistics about genital infections, look in the 'Topics A–Z' section of their website.
www.hpa.org.uk

Herpes Virus Association is a UK non-profit organization. It publishes an excellent booklet called *Herpes Simplex – A Guide*. The website has a FAQ section.
www.herpes.org.uk

American Social Health Association provides information about sexually transmitted infections. Its website is very informative and has detailed Q&A sections on each of the main infections, and a section on how to discuss infection with your partner.
www.ashastd.org/stdfaqs/index.html

US Centers for Disease Control and Prevention is a US government organization that has information about sexually transmitted infections on its website. It also sponsors the US National STD Hotline (see website), which gives advice about sexually transmitted infections.
www.cdc.gov

Pharmaceutical companies thrush websites

- The Thrush Advice Bureau website is sponsored by the pharmaceutical company Pfizer. Pfizer makes Diflucan thrush treatment, so the section of the site on 'Treatment' promotes this drug. The other sections of the site have excellent information about thrush and some other genital infections.
  www.thrushadvice.co.uk
- The Canesten websites are sponsored by the pharmaceutical company Bayer. Bayer makes Canesten thrush treatment, so the sites promote this treatment. They also have information about symptoms.
  www.canesten.co.uk
  www.canesten.com

Prodigy is an NHS website that provides information about thrush in one of its patient information leaflets.
www.prodigy.nhs.uk/PILs/index.asp

Hair loss

Hair loss is a big worry to many people, both male and female. If you have a worrying amount of hair in the basin after shampooing, you may think you are on the way to baldness. But this is not usually the case. The 50–100 hairs that everyone loses each day often become tangled with the rest of the hair, but are washed out when we shampoo. So we see what seems like a lot of hair in the basin after shampooing, but in reality these hairs have been shed earlier.

Of course, bald areas are an obvious sign of hair loss, but otherwise it can be difficult to tell whether your hair is getting thinner. To find out, try the 'tug test'. Hold a small bunch of hair – about 15 or 20 hairs – between the thumb and index finger. Pull slowly and firmly. If more than six hairs come out there may be a problem.

We each have about 100 000 hairs on the scalp

How hair grows

The portion of the hair that we can see is called the shaft. Each shaft of hair protrudes from its follicle, which is a tube-like pouch just below the surface of the skin. The hair is attached to the base of the follicle by the hair root, which is where the hair actually grows and where it is nourished by tiny blood vessels.

Like the rest of the body, hairs are made of cells. As new cells form at its root, the hair is gradually pushed further and further out of the follicle. The cells at the base of each hair are close to the blood supply and are living. As they get pushed further away from the base of the follicle, they no longer have any nourishment and so they die. As they die, they are transformed into a hard protein called keratin. So, each hair we see above the skin is dead protein. It is the follicle, which lies deep in the skin, that is the essential growing part of the hair.

The thickness of each hair depends on the size of the follicle from which it is growing. At puberty in boys, hormones increase the size of the follicles on the chin, chest and limbs so that each hair becomes more thick and wiry. In the elderly, the follicles shrink and the hair becomes finer.

Stages of hair growth

Hair growth is not a continuous process. It has several stages.

- The first phase is the growing stage. Hair grows at about 1 cm each month, and this phase lasts for anything between 2 and 5 years.
- This is followed by a resting stage, during which there is no growth. This phase lasts about 5 months, and is called telogen.
- At the end of the resting phase, the hair is shed and the follicle starts to grow a new one.

- At any moment, about 90% of the hair follicles of the scalp are growing hairs in the first phase; only about 10% are in the resting phase.
- If a follicle is destroyed for any reason, no new hair will grow from it.

What happens to cause baldness

Excessive hair loss can occur if any of the stages of hair growth become disrupted. For example, if follicles shut down (meaning that they stay in the resting phase and then shed the hair) instead of growing new hairs, there will be less hair on the head.

Another reason might be interference with the formation of new hair cells at the root during the growing phase; this occurs with some anti-cancer drugs. If follicles have been destroyed (as they might be by, for example, a burn by some skin diseases), there will be baldness in that area.

An individual can also look bald if the hairs are growing but are so fragile that they break just as they emerge from the follicle, or if they are very small and thin.

In 1998, scientists at Columbia University in New York announced the discovery of a gene that appears to be the 'master switch' for hair growth. They found the gene after comparing the genes of hairless mice belonging to a mutant breed, and comparing the genes of 11 members of the same family who had lost all their hair. This discovery is a step towards understanding how the hair follicle works and how baldness happens, and may lead to effective treatments in the future.

It is normal to lose 50–100 hairs from the head each day

Common beliefs – true or false?

'Some hairstyles can cause hair loss'

True. Styles that put tension on the hairs – such as tight ponytails, plaits or cornrows – can cause hair loss. Winding hair tightly onto rollers (particularly heated rollers) can have the same damaging effect.

'Brushing the hair 100 times a day will stimulate the circulation and prevent hair loss'

False. Vigorous brushing is more likely to injure the hairs and make the problem worse.

'Hair needs to breathe, so wigs and toupees worsen loss of hair'

False. Hair does not need to breathe. Only the root of the hair is alive and this gets its oxygen from the blood in the scalp. Wigs and hairpieces will only damage hair if they are too tight.

'Frequent shampooing makes hair fall out'

False. Shampooing simply gets rid of the hairs that have already fallen out.

'Blow-drying and heated brushes can worsen hair loss'

True. The reason is that extreme heat damages the proteins in the hairs, making them fragile and liable to break off. Brushing the hair during blow-drying causes more damage.

Careless use of heated brushes can even burn the scalp, so that the hair follicles are permanently damaged in that area.

'Protein-containing conditioners and shampoos nourish the hair and help it to grow'

False. Protein-containing conditioners only temporarily fill in defects on the surface of the hair shaft, making it smoother and thicker.

'Hair dyes, perms and hairsprays worsen hair loss'

False. Hair dyes, perms and hairsprays do not affect thinning hair. Perms and hairsprays can help to disguise the problem.

'If your father has a full head of hair, you will not go bald'

False. A tendency to baldness is inherited and probably involves a combination of genes. So you are not automatically in the clear even if your father has a full head of hair. It is not true, as sometimes claimed, that only genes from the mother's side are involved.

'Baldness means that you are more likely to have a heart attack'

Partly true. In 1999, doctors at Harvard Medical School found that men who had lost hair at the crown of the head had a 32% increased chance of coronary heart disease. Hair loss at the front of the head (a receding hairline) hardly increased the risk at all. So if you have baldness at the top of your head, you should stop smoking, eat healthily, have your blood pressure checked and do some exercise.

'Low levels of zinc in the body are a reason for hair loss'

Probably false. There is no evidence that low zinc levels cause hair loss in people taking a balanced diet or that zinc supplements improve hair loss.

'Stress can cause hair loss'

True. Scientists have now identified some chemicals that are produced in the body during periods of stress, which can affect hair growth (*Journal of Investigative Dermatology* 2004;123:455–7).

'It is normal to lose hair from our early 30s'

True. A person aged 20–30 years typically has 615 hair follicles per square centimetre. The number falls to 485 by 50 years of age and to 435 at 80–90 years of age. Also each hair is thinner. So, with ageing, hair becomes both finer and sparser.

'MALE PATTERN' HAIR LOSS

Most men eventually lose hair at the sides of the forehead. This mainly occurs at or after middle age, but it can start at any time after puberty. In fact, most balding men say that they first noticed the problem when they were in their mid-20s. Some men also lose hair from the top of their head, then eventually only the sides and back of the head have hair, forming a horseshoe shape. This is known as common baldness, androgenic alopecia or male pattern baldness.

If you were able to look at the bald area under a microscope you would see that there are the same number of hair follicles as before, but each is shrunken, the hairs being produced are fine and short and pale, and more of the follicles than usual are in the 'resting phase'.

It is impossible to predict how quickly anyone will lose hair. One study found an average rate of hair loss of about 5% per year. Once they have started to notice hair loss, most men take 15–25 years to lose most of their hair, but a few are completely bald after 5 years. The rate of hair loss usually varies; a lot of hair may be lost over a 3–6-month period, and then no more for 6–18 months. This makes it very difficult to tell whether 'treatments' are having an effect.

Each hair on the head grows for about 5 years before being shed

Causes of male pattern hair loss

Male hormones. 'Maleness' was recognized by Aristotle as a cause of baldness. He wrote that 'no boy, woman or castrated male ever becomes bald' and he thought that baldness was a sign of virility (he was bald himself!). To a large degree, science has proved him right. Baldness is the result of hair follicles reacting to male hormones. However, men with male pattern baldness do not have more male hormone than other men. It is simply that their hair follicles are more responsive to the hormones.

The main male hormone is testosterone. Both men and women have testosterone in the blood, but men have more. The skin of the scalp converts testosterone to another substance called dihydrotestosterone (DHT for short). Hair follicles in areas that are destined to become bald are especially sensitive to DHT – it makes them shrink. Follicles on the sides and back of the head are not affected by DHT.

Confusingly, DHT helps growth of the beard and hair on the chest. This explains why bald men can have bushy beards and hairy chests. Nobody knows how DHT produces opposite effects on hair growth on different parts of the body.

Heredity (genetics). If you have relatives with thin hair or who are bald, you may well develop the same problem. This tendency can be inherited from either the mother's or the father's side of the family (but the mother herself would usually be unaffected, or her hair might start thinning after the menopause). Inheritance probably makes the follicles extra-sensitive to DHT.

Ageing. Baldness is more likely with increasing age: 40% of men have noticeable hair loss by age 35; and 65% by age 60. Most elderly people have thin, fine hair even if they are not noticeably bald.

What you can do

Go bald gracefully: cut your losses. If you do go bald, is it really a disaster? Before embarking on expensive and possibly disappointing treatments, consider the alternative. Bald men look clean and elegant (as long as they keep their remaining hair close-cropped and avoid the notorious 'comb-over' of 25 strands of hair across the bald patch!).

Baldness shows the world that you don't wish to spend your time fussing with lotions, pills or hair transplants. It also demonstrates that your male hormone system is fully functioning. If anyone comments, remind them of the traditional belief that bald men are so vibrant and fiery that their passion burns out the roots of their hair. Think Pablo Picasso, Michael Jordan, André Agassi, Sean Connery, Captain Jean-Luc Picard of *Star Trek* and the Italian referee Pierluigi Collina. Zinedine Zidane said after his team's demolition of favoured Brazil in the World Cup, 'My baldness gives me strength!'

Most surveys show that women do not care if men are balding, but can not bear the scrape-over. So cut your losses – keep your hair really short and go bald gracefully.

Wash your hair regularly. Wash your hair once or twice a week with a mild shampoo; dirty hair lies flatter and looks more sparse.

Look after your hair and scalp. Avoid anything that could make the hairs liable to break. For example, after washing do not rub your hair vigorously or use a hot hairdryer. Instead, pat it dry with a soft towel or use a low setting on the dryer or, even better, let it dry naturally. Use a brush with soft bristles. Undo any tangles with your fingers, rather than pulling with a comb.

Protect bald areas from sun damage. ScalpBloc has been specially prepared for this purpose, and is available from pharmacies. It is non-scented and non-greasy.

Consider Regaine (minoxidil) lotion. If you are really bothered by your hair loss, you could consider using Regaine. It can be bought from pharmacies without a prescription; in fact, it is not obtainable on an NHS prescription in the UK.

Regaine stimulates hair growth in balding areas. It works by keeping hair follicles in the growth phase for longer, so hairs grow bigger and the rate of further thinning slows down. The lotion is applied to the scalp and spread lightly with a finger – it does not need to be massaged in. With the 2% lotion, no effect is seen for the first 3 or 4 months. The 5% lotion (Regaine Extra Strength) may be slightly more effective.

To decide whether Regaine is likely to help, you need to examine your scalp closely, preferably with a magnifying glass. It is tricky to look at the top of your own head, so next time you visit the barber take a magnifying glass with you. Ask the barber to tell you whether the 'bald' areas actually have plenty of fine, short hairs. Or ask a friend to look.

You are a good candidate for Regaine if:

- you have been bald for less than 5 years
- your bald area is less than 10 cm across and/or your main problem is general thinning
- hair loss is mainly at the top of the head
- your bald area has lots of tiny, fine hairs.

Regaine is not likely to help if:

- you are completely bald
- your main problem is receding hair (frontal loss)
- the bald scalp has very few tiny, fine hairs.

In the US and UK, there has not been a bald President or Prime Minister since the television age began

What you should know about Regaine

- It is not successful for everyone – only about 35% of men have noticeable regrowth of hair, and this is often fine and downy – and the manufacturers advise users to give up if there has been no regrowth after using it for 1 year.
- It has to be applied twice a day, 7 days a week and does not produce a permanent cure. If the treatment is stopped, the follicles go back to how they would have been without Regaine. About 10–12 weeks after starting Regaine you may notice some extra hair loss. Take no notice; these are simply the old short downy hairs at the end of their life.
- It is important to read the manufacturer's leaflet, as Regaine is probably not suitable for some people. For example, it should probably not be used by people taking drugs for blood pressure, or who have angina. The solution contains alcohol, and can cause irritation in some people.
- It is an expensive treatment – around £25 for a 1-month supply. This means that you have to spend £100 before seeing any benefit. If you continue for a year and then give up because it has not had any effect, you will have spent £300 for nothing. Regaine 5% lotion is probably more effective, works faster and is also cheaper (about £70 for a 3-month pack).

What your doctor can do

Your doctor can discuss two other treatments with you: the drug finasteride; and 'hair transplantation' or 'scalp reduction' surgery.

Finasteride (Propecia) is a drug that prevents testosterone from being converted into DHT. In the UK, it is now available from family doctors on a private prescription. This means that you have to pay the full cost of the drug (about £167 for a 3-month supply), but the doctor will not charge you for writing the prescription or for the consultation. (The same drug, in a larger dose, is used to treat prostate problems.)

Because finasteride is a once-daily tablet rather than a lotion, it is more convenient than Regaine, and it seems to be at least as effective as Regaine. It seems to be more effective for baldness at the top of the head than at the front. Like Regaine, it works best if the 'bald' areas have lots of fine, thin hairs. It has to be taken indefinitely if hair growth is to continue. If you stop taking it, about 6 months later you will notice a change, and by 9–12 months you will be back to where you started. Studies of men who have taken it for 2 years suggest that the longer it is taken, the thicker and longer the hairs become. Men have continued to take it for 5 years with good results (*European Journal of Dermatology* 2002;12:38–49).

How effective is finasteride? In a 1998 study, 945 men with male pattern baldness took 1 mg finasteride and 600 similar men were given dummy tablets to act as a comparison group. The results of the study (*Journal of the American Academy of Dermatology* 1998;39:578–89) were as follows.

- Some hair growth occurred in 66% of men who received finasteride.
- On average, a bald patch 2.5 cm in diameter grew 107 extra hairs.
- Not much improvement occurred before 3 months.

Does finasteride cause any problems? The 1998 study showed that finasteride causes sexual problems in a few people.

- Decreased sexual desire was reported by 1.8% of men (but also by 1.3% given the dummy tablets).
- Difficulty in achieving an erection was reported by 1.3% of men (but also by 0.7% given the dummy tablets).
- A decrease in the amount of semen was reported by 0.8% (but also by 0.4% given the dummy tablets).

However, these sexual problems gradually lessened with long-term finasteride use and they were not permanent (they disappeared when treatment was stopped).

The most worrying problem with finasteride is that, in a pregnant woman, it might possibly interfere with development of the baby's genitals if the baby in her womb is male. This means that a woman who is pregnant or who could become pregnant should not handle crushed or broken finasteride tablets. And when a man is taking finasteride, there will be a tiny amount in his semen; during intercourse this will be transferred to the woman. Therefore some doctors believe that a couple should not try to conceive if the man is taking the drug.

Future treatments

Unfortunately, we are stuck with the number of hair follicles that we are born with – no new follicles ever develop naturally. Treatments such as Regaine (minoxidil) and finasteride do not grow new follicles; they work only if there are living follicles left, and encourage these badly-performing follicles to produce hair. Researchers are now concentrating on the possibility of actually growing new follicles.

One of the most interesting discoveries was made by researchers at the University of Pennsylvania, US. For years, scientists have suspected that hair follicles contain 'stem cells' that have the potential to develop into new follicles, but no one could separate these cells from the other cells in the follicle. At the University of Pennsylvania, they have now managed to separate these cells in mice, and transplanted the cells into other mice. The transplanted cells produced new hair follicles (*Nature Biotechnology* 2004;22:411–17).

Other scientists in the US have discovered the natural signals that instruct stem cells in the skin to form hair follicles. These signals depend on protein molecules called 'noggin' and 'Wnt'. The molecules activate genetic instructions that tell cells to make a pit in the skin from which hair will eventually grow (*Nature* 2003;422:317–22).

Hair transplants and surgery

Hair transplantation is a surgical procedure, based on the fact that hair follicles from the sides and back of the head will continue to grow, even when transplanted to bald areas.

In the past, small plugs of skin less than half a centimetre across and containing about 100 hair follicles, were transplanted. These 'plug grafts' were not very successful, because they gave an unnatural 'tufted' appearance, like doll's hair, but are still sometimes used to give coverage in the middle of large areas.

The hairs on the scalp are not spaced evenly. If you look at someone's scalp with a magnifying glass, you will see that the hairs are in groups with 2–4 hairs in each group, with single hairs scattered between. Nowadays, surgeons are able to transplant tiny groups of hairs, so the result looks much more like the natural pattern.

- Minigrafts (3–4 hairs/graft) are commonly used for men who are thinning over a large area, to fill in gaps around plug grafts.
- Micrografts (1–2 hairs/graft) are often used along hairlines, especially if the hairline has receded only slightly.
- Unigrafts (1 hair/graft) look very natural and so are used along the frontal hairline, or for areas that are thinning but not yet bald. They are also suitable for men who have a large bald area and would be satisfied with light, but natural-looking, thin coverage.
- Some surgeons use a mixture of unigrafts, micrografts and minigrafts. This technique (vari-grafting) helps to give a natural appearance with good coverage.

What is involved? After a local anaesthetic injection, a small piece of skin is removed from an area where there is still plenty of hair and where it will not show, such as the back of the head, just above the neck (the 'donor site'). The surgeon cuts out the tiny grafts from this piece of skin (the most skilful part of the procedure), and then places them into tiny incisions in the bald area. The hole to receive each graft is made with a needle, a scalpel or a laser. The grafts do not need any stitches; they are held in place by the clotting action of the blood. The donor site and the grafts heal very quickly, because the scalp has a very good blood supply.

Usually, an individual will need 300–700 grafts, but of course this depends on the size of the bald area. About 100 are done at each session, which takes about 3 hours. The hair can usually be washed the next day. After a few months it is often difficult to distinguish between the grafts and the areas of normal hair.

Issues to think about. Hair transplantation is a cosmetic surgery operation, so you need to think about it carefully to ensure that it is done properly, that you will not be overcharged, and that you have an accurate idea of what the result will be. Look at the section on choosing a cosmetic surgeon on page 339 and discuss the operation with your family doctor.

The main disadvantage of hair transplantation is that the procedure is drawn out and costly. Also, many men are dissatisfied with the result. This may be partly because expectations are too high. It also depends on the skill of the surgeon. Choose a reputable clinic and have a detailed preliminary discussion so that you know what the result will be. Find out how many sessions you will need, what coverage you will achieve and precisely what the total cost will be.

You should also ask what possible problems might occur. For example:

- as with any surgical procedure, there is a risk of infection of the skin
- the new grafts may not grow properly (and if this happens, nothing can be done)

- the transplanted hair may be a slightly different colour from the surrounding hair, but this can be disguised by a colorant if necessary
- scarring or a lumpy appearance known as 'cobblestoning' may occur, but are unlikely with the modern small grafts.

If you have tight curly negroid hair, you need a particularly detailed discussion with the surgeon, because hair transplantation could be problematic. Firstly, the hair follicles are curled, so it is more difficult for the surgeon to prepare the tiny grafts; they may be damaged and not grow well. Secondly, each graft may develop an unsightly lumpy scar, so the surgeon should do an initial test by transplanting just two or three to an inconspicuous area.

Implantation of artificial hair. Some clinics also offer implantation of artificial hair, which has the same strength, thickness and colour as your hair. Each 'hair' is inserted individually by an injection technique. This is also not to be recommended, because the scalp never gets used to the 'foreign' material, and there is always a risk of infection and rejection with inflammation. Although the result may look good to start with, in time the hairs will break.

Scalp reduction (scalp excision) is a surgical operation in which the hairless portion of the scalp is pulled up tightly and the excess removed surgically, so that the area that has no hair is reduced. It is best for older men whose scalps are looser. There will be a scar from the incision, but this will fade in time. The result can sometimes look odd, because the remaining hair may be pulled up to an unnatural position. The advantage is that it is usually a 'one-off' procedure, unlike hair transplantation.

What not to bother with

Some treatments certainly do not work. The most popular medical book of our great-grandparents' day, *The Household Physician*, advised that baldness could be prevented by 'quickening the circulation in the scalp, such as by washing the head every morning in cold water, then drying with a rough towel by vigorous rubbing, and brushing with a hard brush until the scalp becomes red'.

Others recommended smearing the area with fresh cowpat or rubbing in onion juice, curry paste or Marmite with a stiff brush to irritate the scalp.

In fact, lack of circulation is not the problem in baldness and these measures would make the problem worse by damaging the hairs. Similarly, hanging upside down to improve the circulation in the scalp will not produce any improvement.

It used to be thought that excess grease on the scalp caused hair loss, and male pattern baldness was called seborrhoeic (greasy) baldness. In fact, bald areas appear greasy only because there is no hair to take up the grease; the actual amount of grease being produced is normal. Some baldness 'cures' claim to act by reducing grease; they make no difference. Removing grease makes hair look more fluffy, but does not actually increase the amount of hair.

Some treatments probably do not work. Thousands of products for baldness are advertised in the classifieds and on the internet. They claim to make hair regrow, or simply to stop further loss. Almost all are a complete waste of money.

Most have not been assessed by proper research studies, and aim to persuade by one or two 'true life' success stories. Because hair loss is often noticeable for a month or two and then stops for a few months, it is easy to imagine that a product is having an effect. Without proper research studies, treating hundreds of people with the product and an equal number of similar people with a dummy version of the treatment (a randomized, placebo-controlled trial) it is impossible to know one way or the other about effectiveness and safety. So before trying a private treatment, ask the company for a copy of published evidence about the treatment and ask your family doctor to check it.

- Fenugreek is a herb with a chemical structure similar to the drug minoxidil (see page 151). It is claimed that it may delay hair loss when applied to the scalp. (It is also claimed to help baldness by dilating blood vessels, but this is nonsense.) It can be taken as a tea or as tablets.
- Saw palmetto extract comes from a palm tree. Its chemical structure is similar to finasteride (see page 152), but its action is very weak and so it is unlikely to make any difference to baldness. Proper scientific studies to investigate whether it is effective have not been done.

BALD PATCHES

Baldness in patches, which is not in the typical male pattern, is usually alopecia areata. However, braiding and other tight hairstyles, hair pulling and fungal infection also cause bald patches.

Alopecia areata occurs in about 3% of people and affects men and women equally. It can occur at any age, but in most people it occurs between the ages of 5 and 40 years. The cause is not known. Most experts think it is an 'auto-immune' condition, in which the body's immune system attacks the hair follicles by mistake. It is slightly more common in people with thyroid disease. There may be a link with stressful life events. About 1 in 5 people with alopecia areata says that other family members have the same problem, so genes are important.

The hair is lost completely from the patch, leaving a smooth, shiny scalp. A magnifying glass shows that the openings of the hair follicles are still present, but there are no hairs protruding from them. There may be short, distorted hairs at the edge of the bald patch. There may be only one patch, or there may be several. Sometimes there is a more diffuse 'moth-eaten' appearance, rather than distinct patches.

Alopecia areata can be very distressing, but the good news is that the hair follicles are not permanently damaged so regrowth of hair usually occurs. Regrowth is unpredictable, but usually occurs in 6–9 months. At first the new hair may be white, but after 12–18 months the colour returns to normal. In some people the problem recurs after a few years.

In about 1 in 20 people with alopecia areata, the hair loss continues, so there will be total hair loss (see page 157).

- In a few people, regrowth can be temporarily encouraged with Regaine solution, but the effect lasts only while the lotion is being used. Some doctors inject steroids into the scalp or prescribe steroid creams, but these only occasionally result in some regrowth.

- Dithranol is a cream or paste made from tar, and is used mainly to treat the skin disease psoriasis. In some people it produces some regrowth of hair. It is rubbed into the scalp and washed off after a few hours. Dithranol is messy, and stains clothing.
- Essential oils may help, according to research at Aberdeen Royal Infirmary, Scotland (published in the *Archives of Dermatology* in 1999). Patients massaged a combination of thyme, rosemary, lavender and cedar wood oils into their scalps at night, and then wrapped a warm towel around the head to encourage the oils to soak in. After a few months, 44% had growth of hair (compared with 15% of those using dummy oils).

Hot-combing with pomades. Some women apply a pomade to the hair and then use a hot-comb to straighten or style the hair. This can cause problems. The hot-comb melts the pomade, which drips down the hair to the root and into the hair follicle, where it can cause inflammation. The inflammation can damage the hair follicles and cause a bald patch, which can be permanent in severe cases. Hot-combing or using pomades alone is all right – it is using them together that causes the trouble.

Braiding and other tight hairstyles. Some hairstyles, such as braiding and cornrows, pull the hair very tightly. This can result in a bald area, usually at the hairline around the forehead. If you give up this kind of hairstyle, the scalp usually recovers and the hair will grow normally, but the area can remain permanently bald.

Hair pulling. Children quite commonly develop a habit of pulling the hair; there will be a patch of hair loss with stubbly regrowth. Adults (particularly women) can develop a similar habit, which becomes a psychological compulsion and is hard to stop.

Fungal infection. In children, a bald patch is probably caused by a fungal infection. The bald area usually looks red and scaly. After the fungal infection is treated, the hair will grow again.

Other diseases. Some other diseases, such as systemic lupus erythematosus (SLE) and sarcoid, can cause bald patches, so it is worth discussing the problem with your doctor.

Eyebrow hairs grow for only 10 weeks

TOTAL HAIR LOSS

Hair loss is a side effect of some chemotherapy treatments for cancer. Although this is very distressing, at least the sufferer is prepared for it and knows the hair will regrow after the chemotherapy is over. A lot of research is being carried out into ways of preventing hair loss during chemotherapy, so we can hope that this problem will be solved soon.

Suddenly losing all your scalp hair out of the blue, for no apparent reason, is a frightening and distressing experience. It can happen to both men and women. Elizabeth Steel, who has written a book about her experience, says, 'When you suddenly lose all your hair as an adult, you feel immediately humiliated. It destroys your confidence in yourself in every aspect of your life. When your hair goes and self-esteem with it, your self-image is shattered.' This condition is called alopecia totalis. If it affects the body hair as well as the scalp hair (eyelashes, pubic hair), it is known as alopecia universalis. However, the fact that it has a name does not mean that it is understood. Doctors at St John's Institute of Dermatology in London have found a gene that is involved in some hereditary cases. In most cases it is a mystery, but the follicles are not destroyed so regrowth is always a possibility. It may start as a small bald patch of alopecia areata that extends over a few months until there is no hair left, or all the hair may fall out over just a day or two. Regrowth can occur, but is not as likely as in the smaller patches of alopecia areata.

Scalp hair grows at a rate of about 1 cm a month

What your doctor can do

Your doctor should refer you to a dermatologist, who may try some of the following treatments. Unfortunately, the results of the treatments are very unpredictable.

Regaine may produce regrowth of hair but, as in male pattern baldness, it may take several months before any effect is seen and the new hair will start to fall out after the treatment is stopped (also see the section on Regaine on page 151).

Injecting steroids into the scalp is not suitable for the large area of total baldness, but steroid creams produce slight regrowth in some cases.

Dithranol. As in patchy alopecia, dithranol sometimes produces some regrowth, but it is often scanty.

PUVA therapy is long-wave ultraviolet light. It is painless. It produces regrowth in up to 50% of people, and often works for people who have not responded to any other treatments. However, when the treatment is stopped, only a few are cured. This means that the treatment has to be continued, which has two disadvantages. Firstly, it is time-consuming because between two and five sessions per week are needed. Secondly, like sunlight, it causes ageing of the skin and the risk of skin cancers.

Immunotherapy is based on the idea that, in alopecia, the hair follicles are attacked by the body's own immune system. The treatment involves making the scalp sensitive to a chemical and then repeatedly applying the chemical. Some doctors believe this works by turning the immune system away from attacking the hair follicle, by making it attack the chemical instead. The chemicals used most often are dinitrochlorbenzene, squaric acid dibutyl ester and diphencyprone. This technique results in hair growth in 30–40% of people, but the treatment has to be given weekly for many months. The result may not be permanent, but usually lasts for at least 6 months.

What you can do

The main task of anyone with alopecia totalis or alopecia universalis is a psychological one, and it is not easy. It involves working out a way of living with the condition and for this, Hairline International, the patients' society founded by Elizabeth Steel (see Useful contacts on page 163), is a great help. It is important to remember that the hair follicles are not destroyed, so hair growth can occur at any time, even after many years. Steel herself now has a full head of hair.

THINNING OF THE HAIR

If you think your hair is thinning, although you do not have any real baldness, it is important to check that this is actually the case. Try the tug test, and remember that it is normal to lose 50–100 hairs a day. Sometimes, thinning of the hair can be entirely in the mind, as a symptom of depression.

Thinning of hair all over the scalp (rather than patchy baldness) can be due to various causes. In the case of mental or physical stress, it often occurs 2–3 months after the event. This is because at the time of the stress many follicles enter telogen (the resting phase) prematurely, and are then shed together at the end of telogen a few months later. In this situation, the hair loss usually recovers completely.

If you believe your hair is thinning, do not assume it is due to stress. See your family doctor, who will be able to rule out the common causes (such as thyroid deficiency and iron deficiency). Many drugs – not just those listed below – can cause hair loss, and your doctor will be able to check if this is a possibility.

Some skin disorders, such as eczema or psoriasis of the scalp, can cause thinning of the hair. Usually the hair grows again once the skin problem is treated.

Some drugs that may cause hair thinning

- Anti-cancer drugs
- ACE inhibitors for blood pressure or heart failure (captopril, enalapril, lisinopril)
- Blood-thinning drugs (warfarin)
- Drugs for gout (allopurinol)
- Anti-malarials (chloroquine)
- Drugs for epilepsy (valproate sodium, vigabatrin)
- Drugs for Parkinson's disease (e.g. pramipexole, bromocriptine)
- Anti-thyroid drugs (carbimazole, propylthiouracil)
- Lipid-lowering drugs (clofibrate, bezafibrate)
- Anti-acne drugs (isotretinoin)

Often no cause can be found. In some of these cases the hair will recover in time, but in others it remains thin.

It is important to keep thinning hair as healthy as possible (see page 161 for general recommendations). If there is no curable cause and the thinning is distressing, it may be worth trying Regaine. Bear in mind that Regaine will take several months to show any effect, and works in only a proportion of cases.

A survey has shown that about 7.9 million men and 1.6 million women in the UK have hair loss problems

HAIR LOSS IN WOMEN

In the words of Elizabeth Steel, hair loss is 'miserable enough for a man: a downright catastrophe for a woman.' A survey by Hairline International, the baldness support group, found that 78% of its female members no longer felt like women, 40% said their marriage had suffered and 63% had considered suicide.

Women who lose their hair often worry that they are going bald like a man, and that their hormones are becoming masculinized. In fact, patchy baldness (alopecia areata) and total baldness (alopecia totalis and alopecia universalis) are unrelated to hormones and occur equally commonly in men and women.

Thinning hair after the menopause

Like men, most women develop widening partings and thinning of the hair all over the scalp with age; this is normal. It actually starts in the teens or early 20s, and by the age of 50 over half of all women have thinning hair. After the menopause, thinning of the hair is more pronounced. Hair can also become thin at the front, similar to the male pattern. This is because the hair follicles are responding in exactly the same way as in balding men to the testosterone in the blood. All women have testosterone; this is perfectly normal. The balding does not mean that the woman has more testosterone; it simply means that the hair follicles on her scalp are oversensitive, which is probably inherited. The hair will eventually not become any worse. There is no need to worry that you will become completely bald.

Hair loss and other symptoms

A few women develop male pattern baldness with other problems such as growth of hair on the face, lumpy acne, deepening of the voice and irregular periods. In rare cases, this can mean that too much testosterone is being produced by a tumour, so it is important to see your family doctor so that appropriate tests can be done.

Causes of thinning hair in women

Thinning hair may be caused by:

- age (most old people have thinner hair than when they were young)
- heredity (some people are programmed to have thin hair, particularly as they get older)
- a hormone disorder (particularly an underactive thyroid gland)
- drugs
- iron deficiency (most likely in women who are vegetarians)
- severe mental stress (such as bereavement), 2–3 months previously
- severe physical illness of any sort, 2–3 months previously (particularly a high fever or severe infection – the hair grows again when the body has fully recovered)
- childbirth (it is common to shed a lot of hair for 1–6 months after childbirth, but it usually grows again afterwards)
- Systemic lupus erythematosus (SLE, a disease affecting the connective tissue)

- damage from bleaches and relaxers, which can make the hair become 'soapy' in texture and break off (Afro-Caribbean hair is especially vulnerable).

Treatments for thinning hair in women

Looking after your hair. Just because your hair is thinning there is no need to avoid hairsprays, careful perming or hair dyes. These will not worsen the problem. In fact, perms and hairsprays lift the hair and disguise thinning. However, you should avoid bleaches and hair relaxers. Short, bouncy hairstyles give lift and body. It is also all right to use hair colorants on thinning hair, but darker shades may make thinning more obvious.

Diet. Low stores of iron in the body can sometimes cause hair loss so, particularly if you are vegetarian, ask your doctor for a blood test. Iron-rich foods include lean red meat, game, offal, egg yolks, dark green leafy vegetables and pulses. Vitamin C helps your body to absorb iron. Although hair follicles need plenty of the essential amino acids – the building blocks of proteins – it is doubtful whether increasing your intake of protein or taking amino acid supplements will really help.

Regaine (minoxidil) produces some improvement in about 50% of women with thinning hair. Only the 2% strength is suitable for women. A few women (about 1 in 20) using Regaine notice hairiness of the face, even though the lotion is only applied to the scalp. Hairiness occurs on the cheeks, above the eyebrows and sometimes on the upper lip and chin. The reason for this is not known; perhaps the Regaine is carried in the blood from the scalp to the face, or maybe it is rubbed off onto a pillow that is in contact with the face while sleeping. If Regaine is continued, facial hairiness usually lessens over a year; if the drug is stopped, it goes away within 1–6 months.

Oestrogens used to be prescribed for women with hair loss, but no proper research has been done to find out whether or not they worked at all. They are seldom prescribed now because Regaine is more effective.

HRT, depending on the type, can affect the hair. If you are taking HRT containing progestogen, ask your doctor for a 'third-generation' type of progestogen HRT, which is less similar to male hormones and may be better for women with hair loss.

Drug treatment. If you have male pattern baldness (receding at the front and balding on the crown), you need to see your family doctor for some tests. Male pattern baldness is treated with Regaine or cyproterone acetate (as in polycystic ovary syndrome, see page 168). Another drug, spironolactone, is promising, but needs more research (*British Journal of Dermatology* 2005;152:466–73). The drug finasteride (used for male baldness) is not used for women, because it does not work in women. Also, it could affect the developing baby if a woman became pregnant while taking it.

Hair transplantation. If you are very distressed by thinning hair, and Regaine has not helped, you might consider hair transplantation (see page 153), which can be done for women as well as men.

WIGS AND HAIRPIECES

Most people with extensive hair loss – usually caused by alopecia totalis or cancer chemotherapy – prefer to wear a wig. In recent years, wigs have improved greatly and it is no longer painfully obvious that someone is wearing one.

Wigs

In the UK, the NHS will supply a wig if a consultant (e.g. your dermatologist) considers it necessary. These are free of charge for hospital inpatients, for under 16s, for 16–18 year olds in full-time education and for those receiving income support or family credit. People on low incomes may get some help towards the prescription cost. Otherwise, the cost is about £50 for each wig. (See Useful contacts below for details of a useful leaflet.)

Acrylic wigs are lightweight and look extremely natural, although they may feel hot to wear. They can be washed (but do not use a hairdryer – the heat can make them frizzle or melt). It does not matter if an acrylic wig is worn in the rain.

Because they are in stock sizes, acrylic wigs can be obtained quickly. They need to be replaced every 6–9 months. Most people have two: one to wear and one to wash. For totally bald heads, special adhesive pads are available to stop the wig slipping, and some women also use them for extra security.

Real-hair wigs. Some people still prefer a real-hair wig, but when obtained through the NHS in the UK even these cost almost £200 each . However, they last for 3–4 years. They are made to measure and this takes 6–8 weeks. They cannot be washed, and must be protected from rain. They are also more trouble than an acrylic wig, because they have to be styled and set like real hair, and you will have to buy a wig block for styling it. (See Useful contacts below for information on wigs and VAT.)

Buying and living with a wig. In her useful book, *The Hair Loss Cure*, Elizabeth Steel makes the following points about wigs.

- If you decide to buy your wig privately from a department store, explain your predicament and ask for a private fitting room.
- You will probably feel you look very odd in the first few wigs you try on – partly because you have not seen yourself with hair for a while. Persevere until you find one you like.
- Each time, make sure you put the wig on properly – it is quite easy to put a wig on backwards. (The tapes to adjust the size will be at the back.)
- At home, do not leave your wigs lying around.
- If you feel happier going to bed in your wig, do so.
- Remember that at a party you will not be the only one wearing something false. What about false nails, bosoms and teeth?

Hairpieces

For male pattern baldness, some men like to wear a hairpiece. Like wigs, these have improved in recent years and some now look very natural if carefully matched to the existing hair. Some clinics suggest implanting clips into the scalp to hold the hairpiece more firmly in place, but this is not to be recommended because it can result in inflammation and infection of the scalp. Modern hairpieces are glued to the scalp and remaining hair, so there is no danger of them coming off. However, they usually need to be adjusted every 6–8 weeks as your own hair grows.

Each year, American men spend about $900 million on efforts to regrow hair

Useful contacts

The Australasian College of Dermatologists website contains basic information about various skin diseases and problems. It has a helpful section on hair loss and baldness under 'A–Z of skin'.
www.dermcoll.asn.au
www.dermcoll.asn.au/public/a-z_of_skin-hair_loss_baldness.asp

Alopecia Support Group Sydney offers a supportive environment for all Alopecia sufferers through the exchange of information and the development of personal skills.
www.alopecia-sydney.com

Alopecia Areata Support Association is a voluntary group established to provide information and support for people with alopecia (areata, totalis or universalis), and their family and friends. The association holds quarterly meetings which are open to all members of the public free of charge, and an annual open day.
home.vicnet.net.au/~aasa/

Health*Insite* is an Australian government initiative aimed to improve the health of Australians by providing easy access to quality information about human health. Follow the link to find resources relating to hair disorders.
www.healthinsite.gov.au/topics/Hair_Disorders

Cancer BACUP, the UK national charity that provides information, counselling and support for anyone affected by cancer, publishes a free booklet called *Coping with Hair Loss*. The information is also available on their website.
www.cancerbacup.org.uk/Resourcessupport/Controllingsymptoms/Hairloss

Hairline International is a self-help society for people with alopecia, founded by Elizabeth Steel.
www.hairlineinternational.com

The Hair Loss Cure: How to Treat Alopecia and Thinning Hair by Elizabeth Steel is a practical guide to coping with different types of hair loss. It is published by Thorsons and is available through bookshops or from Hairline International.

Wigs. In the UK, the Department of Health's leaflet HC11 *Help with Health Costs/35002* has full details of who can get a wig free.
Email: dh@prolog.uk.com.
Alternatively, order online (use the search facility).
www.dh.gov.uk
If you buy your wig privately in the UK, you may be able to get it free of VAT, because it is being supplied to someone with a medical condition. You can do this only if the wig supplier

has made a special agreement with Customs and Excise, so check before buying. You will have to sign a special form, which the shop will give you at the time of purchase (you cannot claim at a later date).

Bald is Beautiful. This site includes reasons to be pleased about being bald, a baldness hall of fame, miscellaneous information (bald animals, bald places, bald quotes, bald literature), details of bald pride organizations and more.
www-personal.umich.edu/~pfa/bald.html

Bald-headed Men of America was founded in 1974 and strives to cultivate a sense of pride for all bald-headed men.
www.members.aol.com/baldusa

The National Alopecia Areata Foundation is an American organization that supports research and funding to find a cure for alopocia areata. It has a helpful website tthat provides details of various support networks available.
www.alopeciaareata.com

Regaine. Pharmacia & Upjohn, the manufacturer of Regaine, has a website for consumers that promotes their product, but also has useful information.
www.regaine.co.uk

Bald stories are folk tales about bald men.
www.pitt.edu/~dash/bald.html

Strange facts about hair. Some interesting facts about hair can be found on the following website.
www.keratin.com/didyouknow.shtml

European Hair Research Society is an organization for scientists and doctors, but its website has useful links for anyone seeking detailed information.
www.ehrs.org

Hairloss Talk is a website packed full of information about baldness and its treatment.
www.hairlosstalk.com

ScalpBloc is a thin, non-greasy SPF 20 sunscreen for use on bald scalps. It is not oily, and it forms an invisible film over the skin. It is available from pharmacies.

Hairiness

Each person has about 2 million hairs and only about 100 000 of these are on the scalp. We have hairs over our entire body, except the lips, soles of the feet and palms of the hands. In the UK, £25 million is spent every year on hair-removing products.

HAIRINESS IN WOMEN

Excess hair (hirsutism) in women often appears in the places where men have body hair, such as the upper lip and chin, the chest (including around the nipples), the tops of the shoulders and the lower abdomen. The excess hair is usually coarse and dark (different from the fine hair that some women have on their upper lip, chin, breasts and stomach). The hairs also grow longer than normal so, for example, hairs on the upper lip may grow to 1 cm long instead of remaining short, fine and fair.

25% of normal middle-aged women have unwanted facial hair

Reasons for excess hair

Extra-responsiveness to hormones. Women often worry that hairiness means that they have male hormones and are not fully female. In fact, all women have a small amount of the 'male' hormone, testosterone, circulating in their bodies. It is produced mainly by the adrenal glands, which are situated over the kidneys. If the skin is extra-responsive to it, testosterone encourages hair growth on the upper lip, chin, chest and lower abdomen. The hormone levels are normal; the problem is that the skin is too responsive to testosterone. Women with this problem gradually develop more body hair from puberty until the menopause, after which the amount of body hair slowly lessens – except for facial hair, which continues to increase.

There are many reasons for this extra-responsiveness to normal amounts of testosterone.

- Often, it is inherited; your mother or aunts may have had the same problem.
- Some drugs can be responsible, particularly phenobarbitone and phenytoin taken to control epilepsy. Long-term steroids (taken for conditions such as arthritis or inflammatory bowel disease) and ciclosporin (taken for psoriasis, dermatitis or arthritis) can also cause extra hair growth.

Polycystic ovary syndrome is the cause of hairiness in some women. This syndrome is usually caused by an imbalance between the pituitary and adrenal glands with cysts on the ovary. As a result, the level of male hormone rises. It often develops in the late teens or early 20s and there are usually other symptoms as well as excess hair. Polycystic ovary syndrome sometimes runs in families. It is diagnosed by blood tests and, usually, an ultrasound scan of the ovaries. It can be treated with medication. Women with polycystic ovary syndrome are often obese, and the hirsutism (hairiness) improves if they lose weight.

Symptoms of polycystic ovary syndrome

- Excess hair
- Scanty or irregular periods, or periods stop altogether (but periods may be normal)
- Acne and greasy hair
- Difficulty in getting pregnant

Tumour. Very occasionally, a tumour of the ovaries or an adrenal gland can be responsible for the excess male hormones, but this is very rare.

After the menopause, the face becomes hairier, while the rest of the body's hair is slowly lost

What you can do

Lose weight if you are overweight. This may greatly improve the problem.

Bleaching is a good way of disguising upper lip hairs unless your skin is dark.

Depilatories (hair-removing creams) do not leave stubble, but can irritate the skin. Test beforehand by applying a small amount to the inside of your wrist. If there is no reaction the next day, it is probably safe to use the cream. Weaker creams for use on the face are available.

Plucking, waxing, sugaring or threading will deal with the problem temporarily. These all work by pulling out the hairs. If you pull out a hair, a new hair immediately starts to grow in that follicle. (If you shave a hair, it may be in its resting phase and will not grow for some time.) So plucking, waxing and sugaring may have to be repeated quite frequently.

Plucking is not a good idea for the face because it can easily cause scarring. In waxing, strips of hot wax are placed over the hairy area and pulled off, taking the hairs with them. This is painful, and difficult to use on the face. Sugaring is similar, but uses a special sugar paste obtainable from pharmacies.

Shaving will need to be done every day. In spite of the old wives' tale, it does not make the hairs grow back more quickly, but they will be stubbly, so they may be noticeable if shaving is not repeated daily.

Laser treatment is quicker and less painful than electrolysis. It works best on dark hair with pale skin, because the dark pigment helps to transmit the laser energy down the hair shaft. The results can be very good, but there are also a few problems.

- In general, it is not suitable for black skin, because the pigment (melanin) in the skin will pick up the laser energy, causing scarring and loss of pigment. People with Mediterranean or pale Asian skin tones might be able to risk the treatment. However, new long-wavelength lasers that can be used on dark skin are becoming available.
- In general, grey or blonde hair is unlikely to respond well. However, some new types of laser are able to treat pale hair.

- It is slightly uncomfortable – like having rubber bands flicked over the skin. Your skin may tingle for several hours afterwards.
- It takes time. Although an area 9 cm in diameter takes only 1 or 2 minutes to treat with the newest fast lasers, most people will need two or three treatments at intervals of a few months. This is because laser treatment works best on hair that is in the growing phase – at any time, only a proportion of hairs are in this phase. Also, at the first visit, the therapist should treat just a small area and wait at least 8 weeks before starting the full treatment.
- Complete and permanent removal of the hair is unlikely. The hair usually disappears for 2–3 months, and then slowly regrows (but the new hair is less dense and less coarse). Six months after the treatment, you would probably have about half the amount of hair you had originally.
- It is still a fairly new treatment, so no one knows if there are any bad long-term effects.
- Almost anyone can get hold of the equipment and set themselves up as a therapist. It may be difficult to be sure that a therapist is properly trained. Find out who will actually be doing the procedure, and their qualifications. They should be a doctor (plastic surgeon or dermatologist). In the UK, check that the doctor is a member of the British Association of Plastic Surgeons or the British Dermatology Association (see page 339 about choosing a cosmetic surgeon).
- It is expensive. Before embarking on it, ask the price of a complete treatment, and how large an area will be treated in each session.

Electrolysis is probably the best method of getting rid of the unwanted hair long term (possibly permanently). Electrolysis is a slow process, because each hair is dealt with separately and it may take months or years of treatment before all the unwanted hairs disappear. A fine needle is inserted into the hair root, which is then destroyed by a chemical reaction and by heat.

- Electrolysis treatment can be uncomfortable. It is important that you use a qualified practitioner, such as those in the UK registered with the Institute of Electrolysis (see Useful contacts on page 170).
- Treatments are given 2 weeks apart (to allow the skin to recover), and the whole process may take 6–9 months.
- Check that the practitioner uses new, disposable (not simply re-sterilized) needles.
- If it is too expensive for you, contact a local college of continuing education – they may have training courses for beauticians where you could be treated by trainees who will be supervised and have good equipment.
- Home kits for electrolysis are not a good idea; the current used is too low to destroy the hair root, so the effect is similar to plucking.
- Electrolysis is unsuitable for anyone with a heart pacemaker.

How your doctor can help

See your doctor if any of the following apply:

- you have any of the symptoms of polycystic ovary syndrome, such as periods becoming irregular or stopping altogether

- you are taking any medications that might be responsible (check the information leaflet in the packet)
- excess hair starts to appear suddenly in adult life
- no one else in your family has excess hair
- if, at the same time, you are losing hair from your scalp, especially at the sides of your forehead
- you are having to spend a lot of money on electrolysis
- you are depressed and worried by your appearance.

10% of 65-year-old women have noticeable chin hair

Polycystic ovary syndrome. If this is a possibility, your doctor will refer you to an endocrinologist (hormone specialist). The endocrinologist will check for other problems, such as diabetes, that can sometimes accompany polycystic ovary syndrome. The medication used to treat polycystic ovary syndrome is effective, especially if you also lose weight; greasy skin and acne clear up in about 6 weeks, but it can take 12–18 months for maximum improvement in the hirsutism (hairiness).

No hormone abnormality. If there is no hormone abnormality, and the hirsutism (hairiness) happens simply because your skin is especially responsive to testosterone, your doctor may prescribe the combined oral contraceptive pill containing the progestogens desogestrel, gestodene or norgestimate. Both the oestrogen and progestogen in the combined pill have an effect, so the progesterone-only pill would not be as effective in reducing hair. About 1 in 10 women will see an improvement, but it may take 12–18 months.

If this does not help, your doctor may decide to try a combination of ethinyloestradiol and cyproterone acetate (Dianette) or drospirenone (Yasmin), which stop testosterone having an effect on the skin. It will take about 3 months before there is any improvement, and 12 months to achieve the full effect. After this, the drug is stopped. Hair may regrow about 6 months later, in which case another course of the drug can be given.

If none of these treatments work, your doctor can refer you to a hospital dermatologist or endocrinologist who could suggest other medication.

Laser treatment and electrolysis. In the UK, some hospital dermatology departments provide laser or electrolysis treatment under the NHS, but this is usually available only for individuals with a great deal of excess hair, or who are particularly distressed by it.

Eflornithine (Vaniqa) is a cream that slows hair growth. It reduces hair growth in about 60% of people who use it (*American Journal of Clinical Dermatology* 2001;2a:197–201). It contains a chemical called eflornithine, which blocks a key enzyme in the hair follicle. Because it does not destroy existing hairs, it may take weeks or months before you see any result. It is probably best used after hair has been removed by another method (such as laser), to slow down the return of unwanted hair (*American Family Physician* 2002;66:1907–11). Eflornithine is not a permanent method of hair removal; when you stop using it, the hair will regrow, usually within about 8 weeks. The cream can cause a burning or stinging sensation and acne.

Research among medical students in the USA found that 45% of male medical students were very hairy, compared with 10% of the general population

HAIRY BACKS

Hairiness is something to be proud of – hairy men are more intelligent. Hairy chests and backs are more likely to be found among the highly educated than in the general population. (However, there are also very intelligent men with little or no body hair. Einstein had hardly any body hair!)

If you want to get rid of the hair on your back or shoulders, you could consider waxing or laser treatment. Electrolysis is also a possibility.

In Kerala, in southern India, research among medical and engineering students and manual labourers found that the students had more body hair than the labourers; the top six in the class of engineering students were far hairier than the bottom eight

Waxing. In 2000 Tesco, the UK supermarket chain, reported that sales of home-waxing kits rose by 41%. Their research showed that men were using them (but were asking women to buy the kits for them). Back waxing for men in beauty salons is also increasing. For best results, the hairs should be at least 0.5 cm long. In a salon, the process takes about 30 minutes. Waxing is not a permanent solution. It works by pulling out the hairs, but a new hair will then start to grow in the hair follicle. Regrowth will start to become obvious in 1–2 months.

Laser hair removal. For general information about laser hair removal, refer back to page 166 and see Useful contacts below]. To deal with your entire back you will need three or four treatments at 6–8 week intervals. Your back will be shaved first, and the treatment will then take about 30 minutes. Laser treatment does not get rid of hair permanently – after a few months, it will start to regrow slowly. However, the hair that regrows is likely to be less dense.

Electrolysis removes hair permanently. Each hair is treated individually, so if you are very hairy over a large area, it might not be practical. Contact the beauty salon first to check that they are willing to treat men.

A study of 117 male members of the brainy society Mensa (you have to have an IQ of over 140 to join) showed that Mensa members had a tendency to thicker body hair – and the most intelligent had hair on their backs as well as on their chests

Useful contacts

Verity is a self-help group for women with polycystic ovary syndrome. Its website has useful links to other sites connected with the condition.
www.verity-pcos.org.uk

Polycystic Ovary Syndrome Association is a US support group for women with polycystic ovary syndrome. The website has useful information, including 'What is PCOS' in the 'Support' section.
www.pcosupport.org

Women's Health is a useful and reliable non-profit organization. Its website has a good section on polycystic ovary syndrome.
www.womenshealthlondon.org.uk

Institute of Electrolysis. The website explains electrolysis very clearly.
www.electrolysis.co.uk

Lasercare is a chain of private laser clinics in the UK, some of which are based in NHS hospitals. Their website has a page about hair removal.
www.lasercare-clinics.co.uk/treatments_hair.htm

Head lice

Lice are small, wingless insects. They have six legs with hook-like claws for grasping onto hairs. They feed on human blood. There are three types of lice.

- Head lice are common in children.
- Body lice are common in vagrants, they live in clothing and only visit the skin to feed.
- Crab or pubic lice are found in the pubic hair area (see page 89).

Although the itching is annoying, and scratching can sometimes result in skin infections, head lice are not really a health problem. Sometimes people scratch so much that they damage the skin and bacterial infections can then occur, but there is no evidence that they carry any serious diseases. Head lice are so common that they are now just a fact of life, and nothing to be embarrassed about. On average, someone with head lice will have about 20.

In the UK, each month 20% of hairdressing salons see head lice in a client's hair

The short life of a head louse

- The louse begins as an egg, with a hard brown shell.
- The egg hatches after 7–10 days, leaving behind the empty egg case, which appears white.
- The baby louse takes 10 days to grow into an adult, shedding its skin 3 times as it grows.
- When the louse reaches adulthood, it is about the size of a sesame seed (about 3 mm long).
- The louse clings to hairs with its claws, and sucks blood from the scalp several times a day. If it is a female, it busies itself laying five eggs each night and attaching them to the base of hairs close to the scalp where they will be kept warm.
- The louse keeps looking for any opportunity to get onto another head, by clambering across a 'bridge' of hair. It cannot jump.
- After 30 days of being an adult, it dies.

How you get head lice

- Lice are genetically programmed to move from one head to another. They want to meet different lice (not their brothers and sisters on the same head) and breed with them. Lice cannot jump, hop, fly or swim, but have several ways of moving onto another person (*The Lancet* 2003;361:99–100).
- The most common method is to grab onto another person's hair during head-to-head contact. They grab the hair with one leg and then climb onto it.

- If they are in danger (if you agitate the hair), they may go to the end of the hair and drop off, hoping to land somewhere better.
- Head lice can live for 3 days away from the head, and eggs can survive for 5 days. Therefore they could be spread by shared hats or helmets, combs, brushes, earphones or bedding. (Experts used to think this was unlikely, but have now changed their minds.)

In the UK, it is estimated that 5% of the population have head lice

Who gets head lice

People of all ages can be infected by head lice. They are most common in children aged 4–11 (especially girls), probably because children have more head-to-head contact than adults. Some people blame modern schooling, where young children are grouped round tables, instead of sitting at separate desks. Other people, such as grandparents, can then become infected. Outbreaks of head lice have occurred in residential care homes for the elderly, probably brought in by a child visitor.

Clean and dirty people are equally affected – head lice do not care. It is untrue that they prefer dirt. It is also untrue that washing gets rid of them. When the hair is washed, they crouch down close to the skin and stay still, to prevent themselves being washed out, so people who wash their hair every day are as likely to have lice as anyone else.

All social classes are affected. In some parts of the UK, head lice are more common in posh private schools than in state schools.

Length of hair does not matter to lice, because they stay near the scalp. Short and long hair are equally likely to be infected. The only advantage of short hair is that it is easier to 'wet-comb' (see below) and very short hair makes it easier to spot the lice.

Type of hair can make a difference. In the UK, head lice are less common in Afro-Caribbean-type hair. The reason is probably that the lice in the UK are not well-adapted to clinging on to this type of hair. On the other hand, if a person of European descent, with straight hair, goes to Africa, he or she is unlikely to be infected by head lice there. The reason is that head lice in Africa are adapted to African hair, and are not good at clinging on to straight hair.

*Head lice have probably been annoying humans for at least 72 000 years (*New Scientist *2003;23 Aug)*

How to tell if you have head lice

Itching. Only 1 in 3 people with head lice experiences itching. It is worse behind the ears and at the back of the neck. Itching is caused by an allergy to the saliva of the louse, and it may be several weeks before it occurs.

Seeing the lice. There are various ways of looking for lice.

- Tip the head down and brush or comb the hair thoroughly from root to tip over a piece of white paper. Inspect the paper and the brush or comb closely for signs of life. You may see the skins that the young lice have cast off – these look like lice.

This method is not very reliable because, in dry hair, lice move away from the area that is being disturbed.

- A better method uses a 'lice comb' (a special comb with narrow-spaced teeth), which you can buy from a pharmacy. Wash the hair, leave it damp and comb out tangles with an ordinary comb. Rub some ordinary conditioner into the hair. Then divide the hair into sections and carefully comb each section with the lice comb, starting at the scalp. Every now and again, wipe the comb on a tissue and look closely for live lice. This works better than the dry hair method, because lice stay very still when hair is wet, so they can be combed out.
- If you have Afro-Caribbean hair, do not bother with a lice comb – it will be too uncomfortable. Instead, use lots of conditioner and an ordinary comb.

Look for nits. The nits are egg cases, attached to the hairs. They are oval in shape. The empty egg cases (left behind after the baby louse has hatched) are white, and easier to spot. As the hair grows, the egg case will move further up its shaft, so the position of the nits on the hair gives you an idea of how long you have had them. Hair grows at about 1 cm a month. Therefore nits 1 cm from the scalp mean 1 month, 2 cm mean 2 months, and so on.

If you have never seen them before, it can be difficult to decide whether a white speck is a nit or not. Globules of hair lacquer and bits of dandruff can be confused with nits. And if you pull out a normal hair, you may notice the whitish thickening at its root, which you may mistake for a nit. A magnifying glass will help.

Look for black specks on the pillow or collar, these are louse faeces.

Look for tiny, inflamed bites on the scalp, or a rash on the back of the neck or behind the ears.

Each year in the UK, the NHS and the general public together spend £29 million on head lice treatments

What to do about head lice

In the UK, you do not have to tell the school if your child has head lice. It makes sense to tell the parents of your child's 'best friends', with whom they might have had head-to-head contact in the last 4–6 weeks. Friends do not necessarily need treatment – they need to be checked for lice, but not treated 'just in case'. Do not use any treatments unless you are sure there are lice, that is, you have actually found at least one live louse.

Talk to your pharmacist, health visitor, school nurse or doctor if your child has eczema or asthma, and you are thinking of using head lice lotion, or if your child is under 4 years old.

How to get rid of head lice

Washing will not get rid of lice. Head lice batten down their hatches to keep water out, and can survive without breathing air for about 24 hours.

Head lice or 'nit' lotion. You can buy this from a pharmacy or get it on prescription from your doctor. Your pharmacist, school nurse, health visitor, family doctor or, in the UK, a NHS walk-in centre (see Useful contacts on page 177) will advise you. You should certainly talk to them if your child has any skin problems such as eczema or asthma, because a water-based (rather than alcohol-based) preparation would be advisable. Special shampoos are available that claim to get rid of lice, but in fact they do not work very well; you need a lotion or mousse. The lotion will not remove the empty egg cases (nits) and you either have to wait for them to grow out, cut the hair they are stuck on, or use a lice comb to remove them.

Lousy, nitwit, nit-picking, nitty-gritty, go through something with a fine-tooth comb – all these phrases come from lice

How to use head lice or 'nit' lotion

- Read the label and follow the instructions exactly.
- You will need to treat the head twice, with 7 days between treatments. This way, you will get rid of lice that have hatched from their eggs since the first treatment.
- Do not use the lotion after you have been swimming, because chlorine can interfere with its action.
- Put the lotion on dry hair, parting the hair into sections and combing the lotion through carefully.
- Most head lice lotions are very flammable, and some horrible burns have occurred when people's hair has caught fire. When you or your child have lotion on your hair, keep well away from fires, candles, gas cookers, pilot lights, matches and cigarette lighters.
- Dry the hair naturally – hot-air hair dryers can deactivate the lotions, and a malfunctioning dryer could set the hair alight.
- Wash the lotion off after 12 hours.
- Repeat the treatment once more 7–10 days later to get rid of any newly hatched lice (because the first treatment will not kill lice eggs).

Are head lice lotions dangerous? This is a very difficult question to answer. Some of the chemicals in head lice lotions have toxic effects, but only in large doses.

- Lindane was used as a head lice treatment in the UK for many years, but has now been withdrawn, partly because lice have become resistant to it worldwide, but also because of worries that it might promote cancers or cause nerve damage.
- Carbaryl (available only on doctor's prescription in the UK) caused cancers when given to rats in large doses throughout their lives. Therefore it should not be used repeatedly.
- Malathion is an organophosphate insecticide. There have been concerns that organophosphates might damage nerves. However, the body breaks down and eliminates malathion very quickly. Official UK Government advice is that 'malathion does not have the potential to cause a specific polyneuropathy because, unlike some other organophosphates, it cannot bind to the relevant target protein' (*Communicable Disease Report,* 1997).

- Permethrin and phenothrin are 'pyrethroid' chemicals that occur in chrysanthemum plants. (It has been known for centuries that chrysanthemum flowers can kill insects.) If these chemicals are absorbed by the body, they are eliminated very quickly and they do not appear to be dangerous.
- In fact, the most likely serious danger from head lice lotions is the risk of fire with alcohol-containing lotions. Also, head lice lotions, especially those containing alcohol, can irritate the scalp, so talk to your doctor if your child has skin problems, such as eczema.
- On present evidence, it is unlikely that applying a head lice lotion on two occasions, a week apart, would cause any dangerous effects. But it would seem sensible to use them as little as possible. And do not use them unless you are certain live lice are present (that is, you have actually seen a live louse).

'Bug busting' (also called 'wet combing with conditioner') is something to try if you are worried about using strong chemicals on the scalp. Wet the hair with ordinary conditioner, and thoroughly comb it all the way from the roots with a plastic (not metal) lice comb. You can wipe the comb on a tissue from time to time to see if you have caught any lice. It removes lice, but not eggs, so you have to repeat the process several times to remove lice that have hatched since the last time that it was done. Do it three times a week for at least 2 weeks. In fact, you should carry on for three further sessions after finding the last louse. In the UK, you can buy a kit containing all the equipment you need (see Useful contacts on page 177).

There are three problems with this method.

- According to research published in *The Lancet* in 2000, bug busting is not as effective as lotions. Its cure rate was only 38%. However, since this research was carried out, the design of the bug-busting combs has been improved.
- It takes a long time to do bug busting properly. Each combing session will take about 30 minutes so do not try it unless you are willing to spend several hours a week on it.
- It is unsuitable for tight, curly hair – it would be difficult to do it properly and would be too uncomfortable. It is easiest on short, straight hair.

In medieval Gothenburg, in Sweden, lice helped to choose the mayor. Candidates sat round the table with their beards on the table. A louse was put in the centre and the owner of the beard it crawled into became the new mayor – a virile man was supposed to attract lice

1.5-volt battery-powered combs are available from some pharmacies. The comb kills the head lice by making them lose their grip. It is unsuitable for children under 3 years of age or for anyone with an electrical device, such as a pacemaker. More research is needed to find out how effective this method is. It does not kill the eggs.

Herbal remedies are another possibility if you wish to avoid ordinary anti-lice lotions. Rosemary, neem tree, tea-tree, bergamot and geranium oils are popular choices. However, some herbal remedies are strong natural chemicals, so you need to watch out for allergies and sensitivities, and stop using them if they seem to be irritating the scalp. Concentrated essential oils are toxic, so they must be diluted. In fact tea-tree oil is more toxic than either permethrin or malathion (*Prescriber* 5 June 2003).

- Add six drops of a selection of these oils (3 or 4) to 30 mL (2 tablespoons) of sunflower oil. Massage it well into the scalp and leave for 6 hours. Then shampoo the hair and, when it is wet, go through it with a lice comb. Repeat every 3 days until you think the lice have gone.
- Alternatively, use a preparation such as Nice 'n Clear (see Useful contacts on page 177).

It is difficult to know how effective herbal remedies really are, because there have not been any good scientific studies of them.

*The average person with head lice has about 20 lice. During their 30-day life, 20 lice will lay 2652 eggs (*The Lancet *2003;361:99–100)*

What to do if treatment is ineffective

No treatments are 100% effective. The cure rate for lotions is just over 90%. There are several reasons a treatment might not seem to work.

- May be it has actually worked. Nits (the empty white eggshells) can remain after the lice are dead. Lotions do not get rid of the eggshells, and even special lice combs may not remove all of them, because the mother louse has fixed them very firmly to the hair. Itching can persist for weeks after the lice have gone, because it is caused by an allergy to louse spit. Remember that if itching is the only symptom, there may be another reason, and repeated use of head lice lotions could further irritate the scalp.
- The most obvious reason is that the treatment has not been carried out properly. Did you make sure the lotion saturated the scalp (where the lice live), not just the hair? Did you leave the lotion on for the correct time? Did you repeat the treatment 7–10 days later to get rid of newly-hatched lice? If you were bug busting, did you do it thoroughly, or were you fed up and half-hearted?
- It is possible that your child has simply caught lice again.
- Some head lice are resistant to one or other head lice lotions. So talk to your pharmacist, school nurse, health visitor or family doctor, and try one that contains a different chemical.
- Bug busting is not 100% effective. If some lice remain, after a few weeks they will multiply. But using this method will certainly keep the numbers down, even if it does not eliminate them entirely.

*After mating, a female head louse keeps spare sperm in a special container in her body (spermatotheca), so that she does not have to bother with mating again, but can use the sperm she has kept (*The Lancet *2003;361:99–100)*

Ways of preventing re-infection

- Tell the parents of 'best friends' that your child has head lice, so they can be checked.
- Check everyone in your family, but treat them only if you find live lice.
- Think about your choice of treatment. Malathion is absorbed into the keratin of the hair and skin surface, and gives protection even after you have washed it off. This effect dwindles away over about 6 weeks. Permethrin and phenothrin (but not carbaryl) also have a protective effect lasting several weeks.
- Get into the habit of brushing and combing your hair thoroughly twice a day. This might kill some lice.
- Wash the hair 3 times a week, apply conditioner and, while it is wet, comb through carefully with a plastic lice comb. This will kill some lice and help prevent reinfection.

Head lice are fairly speedy. They can move at 23 cm per minute
*(*The Lancet *2003;361:99–100)*

Useful contacts

There are lots of head lice websites. It is such a common problem that some dubious sites see it as a money-making opportunity to sell remedies that do not work, accompanied by misinformation. For reliable information, look for government-sponsored sites, non-profit organization sites and sites run by well-known pharmaceutical companies.

Health*Insite* is an Australian government initiative aimed to improve the health of Australians by providing easy access to quality information about human health. Follow the link to find information relating to head lice and their treatment and control.
www.healthinsite.gov.au/topics/Head_Lice

Victorian Government Health Information website offers guidelines for the control of infectious diseases such as pediculosis or head lice.
www.health.vic.gov.au/ideas/bluebook/pediculosis

Harvard School of Public Health provides the best site on the internet about lice. It answers every possible question you might have. It is a US site, and mentions treatments (such as lindane) that might not be available in some other countries. It has some good photographs of lice and nits.
www.hsph.harvard.edu/headlice.html

NHS Direct Online Health Encyclopaedia is a UK government site. It has a reliable section on head lice, with photographs. Use the search facility on the home page.
www.nhsdirect.nhs.uk/en

National Pediculosis Association is a US non-profit organization ('pediculus' is Latin for louse). The website has up-to-date news about lice and a FAQ section.
www.headlice.org

Community Hygiene Concern is a UK non-profit organization that developed the 'bug-busting' method. They give full advice about how to do it, and also supply the Bug Buster Kit containing four special combs of different sizes (for nits, for adult and baby lice, for untangling hair and for small children).
www.chc.org/bugbusting

Lice Advisory Bureau is part of the pharmaceutical company Pfizer. The website has good advice on recognizing lice, and a comprehensive FAQ section. There is a separate section for teachers. You can request a free booklet *Having a Lousy Time*. As would be expected, the treatment section emphasises their product, Lyclear.
www.headliceadvice.net

Herbal treatments

- Boots pharmacies in the UK sell Boots alternatives Children's Head Lice Removal Kit, which contains a fine-toothed comb with a conditioner.
- Nitty Gritty combines a fine-toothed comb with a lotion containing neem oil.
  www.nittygritty.co.uk
- Nice 'n Clear is a head lice treatment containing a mixture of natural ingredients including oils of the Indian neem tree, tea-tree oil, lavender, nettle and thyme. It is available from pharmacists and health food stores.
  www.lice.co.uk

Headache during sex

Headaches during sex sound like a joke, but they are not funny to anyone who experiences them. Mysteriously, the headache may occur on some occasions but not on others, even with the same sexual technique. Sexual intercourse, or just masturbation, may bring on the pain.

Who gets headaches during sex?

- Sexual headaches can occur at all ages, but are most common in the early 20s and between 35–45 years of age (*Neurology* 2003;61:796–800).
- Men are 3 times more likely than women to have sexual headaches.
- Sexual headaches tend to occur during male, but not female, orgasm, and during female, but not male, masturbation.
- Sexual headaches are also more common in people who already suffer from migraine or tension headache.

Why the headache occurs

Sex can cause various sorts of headache.

- At the moment of orgasm there can be a sudden, severe pain. This is probably due to contraction of some of the small blood vessels in the brain, similar to migraine, and in fact half the people with this type of headache are also migraine sufferers. This pain generally lasts less than an hour, but may be gone in 10 minutes or linger for a few hours. It may be throbbing, dull or stabbing.
- Less commonly, as sexual excitement increases, some people experience a dull, cramping, tight feeling at the back of the head. This is probably due to excessive contraction of the muscles of the neck.
- If you suffer from migraine, you may find that sex triggers a migraine attack. This headache will be identical to your 'usual' migraine. It occurs after sex, but not during sex.

Some people have only one of these headaches, but many people have a combination, so they experience a headache that increases with sexual excitement, and culminates in an explosive headache at orgasm.

Often, the headaches occur in bouts lasting a few weeks, and then disappear for a while.

Other causes of headache during sex are pills for the treatment of erection problems, such as Viagra (sildenafil), Cialis (tadalafil) and Levitra (vardenafil). Headache is one of their side effects.

What you can do about it

- If you have severe headache at orgasm, you must see your doctor to check that there is no serious reason for the headache. Your doctor may then be able to prescribe a drug such as propranolol to prevent it.

- If you mainly have the dull headache at the back of the neck, make a deliberate effort to relax your neck muscles. This usually relieves it.
- Try intensifying your sexual excitement more gradually. This works in about 50% of men with sexual headache.
- Most people find they are more prone to these headaches when they are tired or under stress, attempting intercourse for the second or third time in close succession, or when they are using an uncomfortable or strenuous position. Try to avoid these situations!
- Sexual headaches are also more likely if you are in poor physical shape, overweight and with high blood pressure – so if you become fitter they may improve.

Hiccups

Everyone experiences hiccups from time to time, especially after eating too much food or drinking too much alcohol. But some people get hiccups frequently for no apparent reason, and the attacks can last a long time and be distressing.

Charles Osbourne, an American, hiccuped for 69 years and 9 months, from 1922 until his death in 1991

Why hiccups occur

Hiccups (sometimes spelled hiccoughs) are caused by sudden contractions of the diaphragm. This is the large flat muscle that lies across the body, just below the lungs. At the same time, the glottis (a flap at the top of the windpipe) shuts off the windpipe, causing the 'hic' sound.

It used to be thought that the diaphragm itself was the cause. Later, it was believed that the nerves that control the diaphragm (the phrenic nerves) were firing inappropriately. Now it is thought that a 'hiccups reflex centre' in the upper spinal cord is responsible.

An ancient throwback?

Hiccups may be a throwback to 370 million years ago, when our ancient ancestors lived in the ocean and breathed with gills as well as lungs (*New Scientist* 8 February 2003). They needed to shut the glottis to stop water entering the lungs. Researchers think this mechanism remained because it allows babies to close the windpipe when sucking milk, so milk does not enter the lungs.

Triggers for hiccups

Hiccups can be triggered by:

- sudden expansion of the stomach by swallowing air while eating
- sudden expansion of the stomach by excessive eating or drinking
- fizzy drinks
- sudden excitement or emotional stress
- acid reflux from the stomach.

If your hiccups are very persistent there could be a medical cause such as:

- conditions that irritate nerves to the diaphragm (such as an enlarged thyroid)
- some medications (such as methyldopa for blood pressure, some tranquillizers)
- uncommonly, a low level of salt in the blood.

Persistent hiccups usually decrease or disappear during sleep, but resume when the person wakes

Babies in the womb start hiccuping from the age of only 8 weeks

How to stop an attack of hiccups

Everyone has their favourite method for curing hiccups. Next time you have an attack try one of the following.

- Pull your tongue fairly forcefully.
- Use a teaspoon to lift the uvula. This is the fleshy tag that hangs down from the back of the roof of the mouth.
- Use a cotton wool bud to tickle the roof of your mouth, at the point towards the back where the hard roof becomes softer.
- Hold your breath for as long as possible, then swallow when you feel a hiccup is about to come.
- Pant deeply.
- Breathe into a paper bag 10 times, holding the edges of the bag tightly against your face to make a good seal.
- Swallow while holding your nose closed.
- Take a teaspoonful of sugar, swallowed dry.
- Drink a glass of water very quickly, while a friend puts their hands over your ears.
- Gargle with water mixed with vinegar.
- Bend forward and drink water from the wrong side of a glass.
- Chew and swallow some dry bread.
- Pull your knees up or lean forward to squeeze your chest.

Persistent hiccups are more likely in men than women

Frequent, distressing hiccups

See your doctor if you suffer from frequent attacks of hiccups, or the attacks go on for a long time and distress you. Your doctor will give you a general check-up to make sure that there is no lung or stomach problem that is irritating the phrenic nerve, or any other cause. There are various drugs that can be used to treat extreme cases of hiccups. These include chlorpromazine, haloperidol and some anti-epileptic drugs. All these drugs have side effects, and do not work for everyone. In very, very rare cases, surgery to cut the phrenic nerve is needed.

Itching

Itching is a distressing symptom. A survey of people with eczema showed that they minded more about the itching than about the appearance of their skin. There are lots of possible causes of itching but, quite often, no cause can be identified.

3% of people seeing their family doctor do so because of itching

Questions to ask yourself

Is there anything to see? Maybe there is a rash that is red and/or scaly, or maybe there are itchy patches. If so, your doctor should be able to work out the cause.

Is your skin too dry? For an unknown reason, dry skin is itchy skin. This is a particular problem as we get older. Skin produces its own grease to moisturize the skin, but as we get older less grease is produced. Add to this the effects of soaps and central heating, skin can become dry, scaly and itchy. Our legs have the fewest grease glands and so are particularly affected, producing a 'crazy-paving' appearance.

Could it be flea bites? Flea bites are usually raised, red areas up to 1 cm across. They are usually in groups of three or four. They are often on the neck, lower leg or at the waist (under the waistband of your clothing). Cat fleas are the usual culprits. You can get cat flea bites even if you do not have a cat, because they can remain in a dormant state in carpets for up to 1 year. When people arrive nearby, the vibration wakes them up. So if you move into a house where there were cats previously, the house can suddenly 'come alive' with fleas.

Could it be scabies? This is the most overlooked cause of itching. It is a strong possibility if anyone else is itchy. Scabies is caused by infection with scabies mites, which are tiny creatures that live on the skin. The mites burrow into the skin, especially between the fingers. After about a month, an itchy rash occurs, which is actually an allergy to the mite. The rash can be over most of the body, or may be on the finger webs, wrists, elbows, armpits, waist, feet or penis.

Is the itch all over, or just in one part of your body? If you are a woman, and the itch is in your genital area, look at vulval itching on page 305. If your scalp is itchy, look at the section on head lice on page 171. If your bottom is the problem, look at anal itching on page 26. If the itch is in the groin, see jock itch on page 187.

Have you recently had shingles? The area affected by shingles can remain itchy for weeks or months, but it will eventually stop.

Does the itching come and go? If so, you may be able to work out the cause. Intermittent raised, red, itchy patches could be 'urticaria', a condition that is often the result of an allergy.

Is the itching worse at night? Psoriasis is a skin condition that causes scaly patches. It also causes itching that is worse at night and affects the normal-looking skin as well as the scaly areas (*The Lancet* 2003;361:690–94). Eczema is another skin condition that can cause bothersome itching at night.

Could you be sensitive to something? Nickel in jewellery can cause itching in people who are sensitive to it. The itching, and often a rash, occurs where the jewellery has touched the skin. Chemicals from plants or from the workplace can sometimes cause the skin that has been exposed to the chemical to itch.

Do you have an itchy pet? If so, it could be fleas or 'dog scabies' (which can affect humans). In the case of dog scabies, your dog would have scaly, bald areas as well as itching.

What you can do

Break the scratching habit. You know you are doing it, but cannot stop. This is quite a common problem. Often it starts as scratching to relieve itching, but then the scratching makes the itching worse, so you scratch more and then itch more. The scratch–itch cycle is hard to get out of, especially if you are feeling stressed, anxious or depressed. Doctors at Chelsea and Westminster Hospital, London, have developed a programme to break the habit of scratching (*Dermatology in Practice* 2202;10(2):28–30). You could try their method at home.

- The first stage is simply to become aware of how much you are scratching. Obtain a counter (from sports shops) and click it each time you scratch. You will probably be surprised at the high count. Also, note the circumstances in which you are likely to scratch.
- The second stage is to replace the action of scratching by another 'safe' action. For example, you could clench your fists to a count of 30, then if the itch remains (often it will have gone), pinch the skin gently. Continue to log your scratching using the counter.
- As your scratching decreases, concentrate your efforts on the times you scratch most (usually first thing in the morning, getting home after school or work, and last thing at night).

Use a moisturizer (emollient)

- If the urge to scratch is overwhelming, try smoothing on some moisturizing (also called 'emollient') skin cream; this will be less damaging to your skin. A pharmacist will be able to recommend something suitable. For some people, emollient cream (such as aqueous cream) can itself be irritating if left on the skin (but all right for washing); if this happens, change to an ointment (*Dermatology in Practice* 2204;12(3):16–20).
- Take advice from readers of the Dr Le Fanu column in the *Daily Telegraph*. To relieve itching, they recommend gently rubbing the itchy area with the inside of a banana skin.

Keep cool

- Itching is usually worse when people are warm. Also, dry air will dry out your skin and worsen itching. So try to keep cool, do not overdress and turn your heating down, especially for sleep.

Your clothes

- Avoid wool or rough synthetic fabrics against your skin. Cotton is less irritating.
- Check the detergent you use for washing your clothes. Avoid those labelled 'biological' or 'enzyme'. Instead, choose one labelled 'for sensitive skin'. Choose an unperfumed fabric softener or one labelled 'for sensitive skin'.

When you wash

- You do not have to bathe every day to be clean. Bathing strips natural, protective grease from your skin. If you think your skin is dry, bath or shower only twice a week – you can easily wash the smelly parts of your body separately.
- Avoid perfumed or drying soap. Choose an unperfumed 'cream bar' type or use aqueous cream (from pharmacies) instead of soap.
- Do not put any disinfectant in the bath or, worse, directly onto your skin. This can start a dermatitis reaction and make the problem even worse. An unperfumed, 'dermatological' bath oil is a good idea, because it will help to prevent dry skin. You can buy a suitable oils from pharmacies – ask the pharmacist for advice. But remember that bath oils can make the bath or shower very slippery!
- Do not scrub your skin.
- Take warm, not hot, baths or showers.
- Moisturize your skin after bathing, when the skin is still slightly damp, as this seals in the moisture. So after washing, towel-dry your skin gently, then apply a moisturizing cream such as E45.

If your pet is itching

- Treat the pet for fleas. If this does not work, take your animal to a vet. Human itching from dog scabies goes away when the animal is treated.

In Roman times, hot sulphur baths were taken to get rid of scabies

How your doctor can help

If the simple measures given in the previous section do not control the itching, you should see your doctor.

Diagnosing the problem. Your doctor will check your skin for signs of skin disease, such as eczema or folliculitis (an infection that is sometimes picked up from hot tubs), and will also look for scabies. If you think you have urticaria, your doctor can help work out the cause. Itchy skin with nothing to see can sometimes be caused by diseases (such as diabetes, thyroid dysfunction, iron deficiency and liver problems). Therefore your doctor will ask about your general health and do some blood tests.

Possible treatments. Obviously, if your doctor finds a reason for the itching, you will receive the appropriate treatment. Sometimes it can take a while for the itching to go. For example, after scabies is treated, the itch may persist for a few weeks.

If no specific cause can be found, don't be too dismayed. This is a common situation. The good news is that this type of itching often clears up after a few weeks or months. Meanwhile, a moisturizing cream (also called an 'emollient') and an antihistamine drug can help. Some antihistamines can make you feel drowsy and have been responsible for road accidents, so be very careful about driving while taking them. An antihistamine before bedtime can help night itching. If antihistamines do not deal with the problem, various other drugs can be tried.

*A few days after the euro was introduced in Spain, 20 people needed hospital treatment for itching of their hands. Nickel in the euro coins was responsible. A spokesman for the European Central Bank said people were so excited by the new coins that they were handling them excessively (*Independent*)*

Useful contacts

Eczema Association of Australasia (EAA) has an educational website which offers practical information about living with, or caring for, someone with eczema. General information includes eczema, symptoms and potential causes, as well as international eczema-related organizations and support groups and a unique 'skin condition information service'. The site also features information about treatments available from Australasian-based eczema product manufacturers.
www.eczema.org.au

The Australasian College of Dermatologists website contains basic information about various skin diseases and problems. It has a helpful section on eczema under 'A–Z of skin'.
www.dermcoll.asn.au
www.dermcoll.asn.au/public/a-z_of_skin-eczema.asp

Zoological Institute of St Petersburg has a collection of 50 000 dead fleas. Take a look at the website if you want to know more about fleas.
www.zin.ru/Animalia/Siphonaptera/index.htm

National Eczema Society provides information and advice about all aspects of eczema.
www.eczema.org

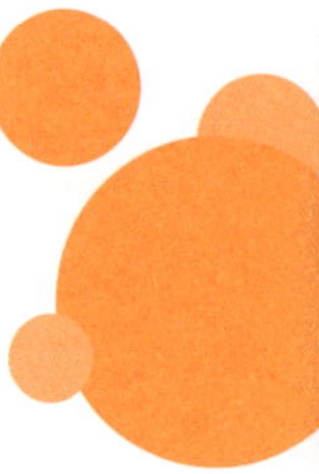

Jock itch

Jock itch with a rash

Jock itch is usually an itchy rash in the fold of skin in the groin. In men, the skin fold beneath the scrotum is often affected as well, but not the penis. Usually the area is red and slightly scaly. It usually has a sharp border, demarcating it clearly from the unaffected skin. If you look closely at the border, you may see small pimples. The rash spreads outwards and, as it does so, the centre may clear. Both sides are usually affected.

This is sometimes known as 'sweat rash', but it is not caused by sweat. The actual cause is a tinea fungus – the same fungus that causes athlete's foot. In fact, jock itch is probably 'caught' from your own feet. Check between your toes for the red, scaly appearance of athlete's foot. Athlete's foot is very common in people who do a lot of sport, because it is easily caught from the floors of communal changing rooms and showers.

What to do

Although sweat does not cause the rash, the fungus does thrive in warm, moist, sweaty conditions, so you can help yourself by:

- not wearing tight underpants
- wearing 100% cotton underpants instead of synthetic fabrics
- drying yourself carefully in the groin and around the testicles after bathing or showering
- losing weight if you have a paunch
- looking after your feet to avoid athlete's foot (look at the section on sweaty feet on page 258).

Fungi also thrive on skin that is slightly damaged. Skin damage is commonly caused by perfumes in soaps, shampoos and shower gels, and enzymes in washing powders. So you can help yourself by:

- washing with an unperfumed soap
- if you wash your hair in the shower, not letting the foam run down your body into the groin creases
- not using 'enzyme' or 'biological' washing powders for your underpants.

These self-help measures will discourage the fungus but probably will not eliminate it, so see your doctor for an antifungal cream.

Jock itch without a rash

Sometimes the groin area can be very itchy but there is no rash to be seen. In this case, a fungal infection is unlikely. Probably your skin is very sensitive to soaps and perfumes, so follow the advice above and look at the section on itching on page 183.

Lumps on the genitals

IN MEN

Sometimes we look at our bodies in a new light, and notice things that we have never seen before, and we think they are not normal. This often happens with the genital area, partly because it is not easy to compare with other people. If you notice any new lumps or bumps, ask your doctor to check, or go to a sexual health clinic. This is because any lumps might actually be warts or other conditions, which should be treated.

Lumps and bumps on the penis that are normal

Pearly penile papules are small lumps, about 1–2 mm across. They look like pimples and are all roughly the same size and shape. They are in a row around the margin of the head of the penis, and can be seen when the foreskin is pulled back. In some men they are hardly visible at all, and in others they are quite noticeable. They usually develop in the teens. People often worry that they are warts or an infection, and pick or squeeze them. In fact they are perfectly normal tiny glands. Leave them alone!

Lymphocele. This is a hard swelling that suddenly appears after sexual intercourse or masturbation. It is usually on the shaft of the penis, near the foreskin. It is caused by temporary blockage of the lymphatic channels at the margin of the head of the penis. It will go away on its own, and there are no after-effects.

Lumps and bumps on the penis that are not normal

Genital warts are very common and are caused by a virus. (See page 134 for more information.)

Molluscum (correct name molluscum contagiosum) are pinkish-white round lumps, each about 1–5 mm in diameter, which are caused by a virus. See page 139 for further information.

Lichen nitidus consists of tiny, shiny, flat-topped, flesh-coloured pimples, which are difficult to distinguish from warts. The pimples are usually seen on the shaft of the penis and their cause is a mystery. They may remain the same for years, or may disappear of their own accord. They do not usually need any treatment.

Sores (ulcers) on the glans may be due to genital herpes, an infection caused by a virus (see page 131), or less commonly the ulcer may be a special form of skin cancer. If an ulcer or ulcers develop, you should consult your doctor without too much delay.

Lumps on the scrotum that are normal

Chicken-skin scrotum. It is normal for the skin of the scrotum to look like the skin of a plucked chicken. This is because the hair follicles on the scrotum are quite far apart and prominent, while the hairs themselves may not be very obvious.

Sebaceous cysts are swollen, blocked grease glands that look like yellowish pimples. They often occur on the skin of the scrotum, and there may be a dozen or more. The skin contains millions of glands that make grease to keep the skin waterproof and in good condition. The openings of these glands easily become blocked, so they become distended with grease. For some reason, the skin of the scrotum seems particularly susceptible to this problem. They are harmless, but if they become infected (red and sore) or you do not like the look of them, a sexual health clinic will be able to treat them.

Angiokeratoma of Fordyce are tiny, bright-red blood-blisters. They usually occur on the scrotum, and there may be lots of them. They are quite common in the late teens, and are normal. Their only problem is that they can be itchy, and may bleed if you scratch them.

Lumps and bumps on the scrotum that are not normal

Genital warts are discussed on page 134.

Varicoceles are the result of swelling of the veins around the testis (see page 272). They often feel like a 'bag of worms' and are more noticeable on standing. About 15% of men have a varicocele, usually on the left side.

Lump in the scrotum. A lump attached to the testicle may sometimes be felt through the skin of the scrotum (see page 271). While many of these are harmless cysts, occasionally a lump may be due to the development of testicular cancer. If you do find a lump in your scrotum you should consult your doctor who will usually refer you to a urologist. Most tumours of the testis are curable (that is, they do not come back), if removed early.

IN WOMEN

Cervix

The main 'lump' in the vagina is the cervix (neck of the womb). This projects into the far end of the vagina and is about 3 cm across. You can usually feel the cervix by inserting the first two fingers into the vagina and pushing upwards. It is easier to feel if you 'bear down' (contract your stomach muscles as if you are trying to open your bowels). The texture of the cervix is similar to the end of your nose, but it has a hole in the middle. In a woman who has not had a child, the hole is about the size of a pencil lead, but it is usually larger in women who have given birth. Menstrual blood passes through this hole from the womb into the vagina.

The cervix usually feels smooth, but sometimes pimples can be felt on it. These are usually small glands called nabothian follicles, and are normal.

However, a pimple on the cervix could be a wart (see page 135), though it would be unusual to have warts on the cervix without having any at the opening of the vagina.

A small, soft lump which seems to be coming out of the hole in the cervix is probably a cervical polyp. This is not cancerous, but can bleed, especially after intercourse, so it is best to have it removed.

Vagina

The inside of the vagina can normally feel crinkly. This is because it is designed to stretch for intercourse and childbirth, so when it is not stretched the walls may have wrinkles.

However, it is not normal to have distinct small lumps in the vagina. If you feel any, see your family doctor or go to a sexual health clinic, because they could be warts (though it is unusual to have vaginal warts without any at the opening of the vagina).

Prolapse

A bulge in the vagina is probably a prolapse. The vagina rests between the bladder and the rectum (back passage); the bladder lies in front of it and the rectum lies behind. The bladder, vagina, cervix and rectum are held in position by muscles that stretch across the pelvis – the pelvic floor muscles. If these muscles are weak, the bladder and/or rectum can lean towards the vagina and press on it, or the womb may sag downwards.

Treatment for prolapse is really surgery, but other measures may be of some benefit.

- Lose weight if you are obese. This will certainly help; excess weight puts pressure on the pelvic floor and makes the problem worse.
- Stop smoking if you have a smoker's cough; coughing puts pressure on the pelvic floor.
- Do pelvic floor exercises (see page 288). They will help leakage of urine due to prolapse.
- Surgery is needed if prolapse is troublesome, particularly if it is causing incontinence of urine. The surgeon cuts away flabby parts of the vagina and strengthens the supporting tissues. It is important to tell the surgeon if you are still sexually active, so that the vagina is not made too narrow, or intercourse may later be uncomfortable.
- A pessary is a special ring placed in the vagina to give support. Pessaries are made of plastic and are changed every 6 months. They are usually used as a stop-gap measure while waiting for an operation, or for women who cannot have surgery for any reason.

Entrance to the vagina

In many women, the entrance to the vagina normally feels lumpy. This lumpiness is the remains of the hymen which stretches across the entrance in young girls. The hymen is a thin piece of tissue with a hole to let menstrual blood flow out. The hole becomes enlarged during sports, by inserting tampons and by sexual intercourse, but the remnants of the hymen can remain as irregular, firm lumpiness.

A woman who has given birth to a child, and who needed stitches afterwards, may be left with a lumpy scar at the vaginal opening.

Genital warts (see page 134) are increasingly common and often occur around the vaginal entrance.

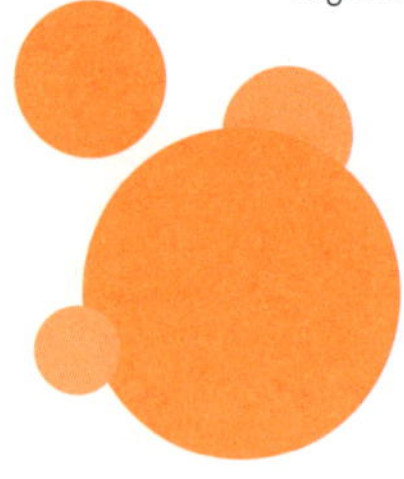

Memory problems

If you notice that your memory is poor, it is natural to think of the worst explanation – Alzheimer's disease. In fact, there is usually another reason and the problem is usually temporary.

Causes of memory problems

Depression is the most common cause of memory problems. With depression, many of the mental processes are slowed, and memory is particularly affected. Unfortunately, worry about memory loss can worsen the depression, producing a vicious circle.

Stress is another common cause of memory problems. Almost any worry or stressful life event can affect our ability to store and recall memories. When the problem is resolved, or time has healed the pain, memory becomes as efficient as it was before.

Stressful life events that can affect memory

- Work-related problems
- Divorce or other relationship problems
- Being charged with an offence
- Being involved in litigation
- Bereavement

Normal ageing. During your mid-40s and 50s, it is quite normal to believe you have become more forgetful. Surveys find that 75% of people over the age of 50 report that they have had some 'memory problem' over the past year. But it may not be as bad as you think – young people forget things and do not bother about it, but older people take more notice of their memory lapses and worry. Do not make the mistake of thinking that everyday memory lapses are Alzheimer's disease – forgetting where you put your keys is not Alzheimer's!

A study of 111 people aged 90–100 years showed that over half had a strikingly good memory (*Neurology* 2003;60:477–80), so memory loss is not automatic as we get old. Other studies have shown that old people are better at judging whether people are honest or intelligent, so some aspects of mental function actually improve with age.

The 'tip-of-the tongue' phenomenon is a very common experience – your mind suddenly freezes when you need a crucial word, such as a name (often of someone you know well). This is more likely to happen if it is a name that you seldom speak aloud, because scientists believe you are simply having trouble retrieving the actual sound of the word from your memory bank of word sounds. It is a nuisance, but does not mean you are on the way to serious memory loss.

Alzheimer's disease. Of course, a failing memory does occur with Alzheimer's disease. Alzheimer's is mainly a disease of the elderly. About 1% of people in their 60s, 20% of those over 85 years and 30% of those over 90 are affected.

Stroke. It is common to have some memory loss after a stroke, but this usually improves over the following 3–6 months.

What you can do

Look for a reason

Could it be stress or depression? Try to work out if you have had an unusual amount of stress recently, or if there is any possibility that you are depressed. For example, has there been any change in your sleep pattern? Sleeping a great deal less or more than in the past, difficulty getting to sleep, or waking early in the morning are all pointers to depression or anxiety. Unless there is an obvious cause that you can deal with for your stress or depression, see your doctor.

Could it be the medications you are taking? Some sedatives, antidepressants and other drugs can affect memory.

Have other people noticed? Ask a close friend or family member whether they have noticed that your memory has deteriorated. As a general rule, if memory loss is due to anxiety or depression, people notice it themselves and worry about it; if it is due to Alzheimer's, other people are much more aware of it than the sufferer.

Keep your mind active. Although it is normal for our memory to be less efficient as we grow older, this can be offset by activities that require thinking and learning. Memory is like a muscle; keep working it so it stays in shape.

- Consider taking up a hobby that uses your brain such as reading, evening classes, card games, crosswords or discussion groups.
- When you are reading a good book or a newspaper article, pause every now and again and imagine you are telling someone about what you have just read.
- Even better, join a book group to discuss your reading with other people.
- In the evening, try to recall the day's events as vividly as possible.
- Pick a topic and think of the opinions opposite to those that you usually hold; for example, if you love pets, think about all the disadvantages of having a pet.

Take exercise. A study of over 71-year-olds in the US has shown that moderate exercise (for example, walking more than 3 km a day) helps to keep the brain, as well as the body, in good shape (*Journal of the American Medical Association* 2004;292:144–61).

Be sociable. People who have lots of social contact with other people are less likely to develop serious memory problems.

Use common sense to help your memory. There are a number of simple things that you can do to really make a difference.

- Pay attention! We best remember things we are most interested in.
- Establish a routine for putting frequently used items (keys, pens and spectacles) in the same place each time.

- When you are introduced to new people, repeat their names once or twice to commit them to memory.
- Write down things that you need to remember – carry a notebook, use lists and keep an appointment diary.
- It is easy to forget whether or not you have done something if you do it on automatic pilot. Instead, pause and register what you are doing; speaking it aloud may help. A common example is wondering whether you have turned the iron off, so when you finish ironing, pay special attention to your act of turning it off and say aloud 'iron off'.
- If you often forget names, go through your address book from time to time, saying the names of your friends and acquaintances out loud. This helps to bring the sounds of their names to the surface of your memory bank. Similarly, before you go to a social gathering, say out loud the names of the people you might meet.

Do not smoke. Do not listen to people who say smoking prevents memory loss. This idea was popular a few years ago, but there is no scientific evidence for it. Nicotine can improve brain function very temporarily, but smoking is likely to damage brain blood vessels and make the problem worse in the long term.

Get enough sleep. When you sleep, your brain processes the information that you have learnt during the day. If you are deprived of sleep, the memories will not stick properly, so students who spend half the night cramming for exams may be wasting their time.

Do not take HRT to help your memory. It is untrue that the menopause causes memory loss (*British Journal of General Practice* 2004;54:434–8, *Neurology* 2003;61:801–6). If this is happening to you, it is more likely that you are depressed or anxious. HRT does not improve brain function and may actually make it worse (*Journal of the American Medical Association* 2004;291:2959–68).

Consider a ginkgo biloba supplement. Extracts of the leaves of the gingko tree (also known as the maidenhair tree or fossil tree) have been used for hundreds of years in Chinese medicine. Over the past few years, gingko supplements have become very popular with people who think their memory is poor, but the scientific evidence to support this is very confusing. Many of the so-called 'scientific' studies have been flawed for several reasons, so their results cannot be trusted.

- For a good scientific study, you need a large number of people. Half of them need to be given the gingko supplement, and the other half a dummy tablet that looks and tastes exactly the same. Then you compare the results in the two groups to see if the supplement is having a real effect. One difficulty is that ginkgo has a very pronounced taste and smell, so most researchers have been unable to make a similar dummy tablet.
- Some of the best studies of gingko have been in patients with Alzheimer's disease. But even if it does help in Alzheimer's, it would not necessarily improve memory in people who do not have Alzheimer's disease.
- Herbal remedies are very big business. So, like standard pharmaceuticals, there are vested interests promoting them.

Contradictory studies on gingko and memory

For

- Several studies have concluded that gingko does have some effect, but many were flawed. In one of the better studies, people with Alzheimer's disease or similar dementia diseases were given 120 mg gingko each day for a year, or a dummy tablet. Those given the gingko did not deteriorate as quickly as those on the dummy tablet (*Archives of Neurology* 1998;55:1409–15, *Journal of American Medical Association* 1997;278:1327–32).

Against

- In a Dutch trial of elderly patients with memory impairment given either gingko or a dummy tablet for 24 weeks, there was no difference between the two groups in a large number of memory tests. This was a good trial, because the researchers used a very convincing dummy tablet with the same taste and smell as real gingko (*Journal of American Geriatric Society* 2000;48:1–12).
- An American study of elderly people found no benefit from ginkgo – each given 40 mg, 3 times daily – on learning, memory and concentration. However, these people did not have any memory problems to start with (*Journal of the American Medical Association* 2002;288:835–40).

Despite the lack of firm evidence, it might be worth trying a gingko supplement. It might take 2–3 months to show any effect. Side effects (allergic reactions, gastrointestinal symptoms, headache) are rare. It would probably be unwise to take it if you are on blood-thinning medication.

What your doctor can do

Depression can creep up so gradually that you may not be aware that you are suffering from it, so your doctor will first assess whether or not you are depressed. If so, antidepressant medication would be the most appropriate treatment and would restore your memory. The improvement might not be immediate, as antidepressant drugs can take several months to have an effect. Your doctor could also help you to identify stresses or problems that may be affecting your memory, and could advise on coping strategies.

If you or your doctor cannot work out the reason for your memory problem, he or she could refer you to a special clinic. In the UK, there are about 20 NHS memory clinics. Memory clinics assess whether or not you have a memory impairment and what the cause might be. They also teach strategies to improve the ability to acquire new information and to memorize it.

Useful contacts

Alzheimer's Australia is the peak body providing support and advocacy for Australians living with dementia. Information on the website supports people from culturally and linguistically diverse backgrounds. The website provides contact details for other State and Territory

organizations, as well as helpline and interpreter services.
www.alzheimers.org.au

Health*Insite* is an Australian government initiative aimed to improve the health of Australians by providing easy access to quality information about human health. You can find information on dementia and about support services for sufferers, their carers and families by clicking on the link below.
www.healthinsite.gov.au/topics/Dementia

myDr is an Australian healthcare website compiled by a team of experienced Australian healthcare writers, with contributions from practising Australian healthcare practitioners and recognized Australian health organizations. The website has an interesting article on the treatment of sweating. Type in 'memory loss' in the Quick search form fill for a list of related articles.
www.mydr.com.au

The Royal College of Psychiatrists has a useful fact sheet on memory problems. It has useful tips on coping with forgetfulness and a list of recommended self-help books on its website.
www.rcpsych.ac.uk/info/help/memory/index.htm

The Alzheimer's Society in the UK has an excellent website with a number of fact sheets and many pages of information about dementia and Alzheimer's disease, and how they differ from normal forgetfulness.
www.alzheimers.org.uk/
www.alzheimers.org.uk/Facts_about_dementia/factsheets.htm

The Alzheimer's Association in the US has an informative website, which includes a page listing the ten warning signs of Alzheimer's disease.
www.alz.org
www.alz.org/AboutAD/Warning.asp

American Academy of Family Physicians has a web page on 'Memory Loss and Ageing: What's Normal, What's Not?'.
www.familydoctor.org/124.xml

Mouth ulcers

We all have mouth ulcers occasionally. The medical term for them is 'aphthous ulcers'. They are round, painful sores inside the mouth, which interfere with eating and teethbrushing, because of the pain. The centre of the sore is white or greyish. Usually, eating spicy or salty foods is especially painful.

An unlucky 1–2% of the population suffer from mouth ulcers repeatedly. Usually the problem starts in childhood or adolescence, and seems to get better in the 40s. Typically, the ulcers come in crops of 1–5 at a time. The mouth is remarkably good at healing, so the ulcers last for only a week or two. Then a few weeks later it may happen again.

Causes of mouth ulcers

Although the cause of most mouth ulcers is unknown, accidental damage is a common reason; for example, biting the tongue or cheek lining by mistake, eating foods that are too hot or wearing badly-fitting dentures can all produce a mouth ulcer.

In 1 in 3 sufferers, it seems to run in the family; this is because of an inherited tendency, not an infection. A few people who constantly get mouth ulcers are anaemic or short of iron, folate or vitamin B12. Zinc deficiency, food hypersensitivity and general psychological stress have all been blamed for mouth ulcers, but specialists now think these are unlikely to be responsible. A few women find that mouth ulcers are more likely before their periods, so hormones might perhaps have an influence. Some people develop mouth ulcers after stopping smoking.

Repeated mouth ulcers can be part of several medical and skin conditions. Though these disorders are unusual, you should see your doctor if you have mouth ulcers often.

Very rarely, a mouth ulcer can be cancerous. A cancerous ulcer does not heal, and is more common in older people, especially long-term smokers and drinkers. So you should see your doctor if you have an ulcer that does not heal within 3 weeks.

What to do about mouth ulcers

Unfortunately, there is no reliable way of preventing ordinary mouth ulcers.

- You could try chlorhexidine gluconate mouth rinse, which in the UK you can buy from a pharmacy without a prescription. Use it twice daily. There is some evidence that this may reduce the frequency and severity of recurrent mouth ulcers, but long-term use can stain the teeth.
- Look for a toothpaste that does not contain sodium lauryl sulphate (SLS). One study showed that switching to an SLS-free toothpaste more than halved the likelihood of recurring mouth ulcers, but another study found no difference (*Oral Disorders* 1999; 5:39–43).

There are various ways of relieving the pain while waiting for the ulcer to heal itself.

- Avoid spicy, salty or sour foods until the ulcer has healed.
- Dissolve a tablet of soluble (dispersible) paracetamol (acetaminophen) in water and swirl it round your mouth before swallowing it.
- Before eating, rinse your mouth with iced water. This may dull the pain, so that eating is more comfortable.
- Buy a mouth ulcer liquid rinse or gel from a pharmacy. These contain an anaesthetic. Many people find the rinse easier to use than a gel, especially if they have several ulcers at the same time, and the rinse forms a protective barrier over the ulcer as well as relieving pain.
- Some people find that warm (not hot) chamomile tea is helpful. Swirl it round the mouth before drinking it.

What your dentist can do

Dentists are experts on all types of mouth problems, so your dentist will be able to give you general advice about mouth ulcers. Another reason to see your dentist is that trauma from a sharp tooth, a brace or ill-fitting dentures are common causes of mouth ulcers.

What your doctor can do

Your doctor can prescribe a corticosteroid paste. This is the best treatment for getting rid of ordinary mouth ulcers (aphthous ulcers), but of course it does not prevent them from occurring again. Apply it as soon as you suspect that an ulcer is forming. Dry the area with a tissue first, so that the paste sticks on.

Although ordinary aphthous ulcers are the most likely, there are other possibilities. Mouth ulcers can be part of several medical and skin conditions, so tell your doctor if you have any other symptoms, or if you have blisters or sores on any other part of your body. Your family doctor may wish to check a blood sample for levels of iron, folate and vitamin B12. Of course, anyone with a mouth ulcer that does not go away in 3 weeks should see their doctor, because a persistent ulcer that refuses to heal could be cancerous.

Nipple problems

Nipple discharge

Nipple discharge is usually harmless and does not signify anything seriously wrong. In fact, most women can squeeze some discharge out of their nipples, especially if they have had children in the past. This may be whitish or may be yellow-green or almost black.

On the other hand, nipple discharge can be a symptom of breast cancer, particularly if it is bloodstained. Therefore, you should definitely discuss any nipple discharge with your doctor. If you are a man, you should see your doctor straightaway, because the usual cause is a tumour and you will need treatment.

What your doctor will do. Your doctor will check your medication, because some drugs can cause (non-bloody) nipple discharge. The most common culprits are:

- cimetidine (for stomach problems)
- oral contraceptives
- some antidepressants and other drugs for psychological problems
- domperidone (for nausea).

Your doctor will ask whether there is any possibility that you could be pregnant. Some women have nipple discharge very early in pregnancy. Your doctor will then examine your whole breast thoroughly (not just the nipple), to make sure you have no lumps.

Even if you have not noticed any blood, your doctor may ask you to try to squeeze a few drops out, and will test it for microscopic blood.

Each nipple has about 15–20 tiny pores on it. These pores are the openings of ducts that connect with the glandular tissue in the breast. You and your doctor should try to work out whether the discharge is coming from just one pore, or from several.

- The cause is very, very unlikely to be breast cancer if the discharge is coming from several pores, it does not contain any blood and you are under 50 years of age.
- If the discharge is bloodstained, or it is emerging from just one pore, your doctor will refer you to a hospital clinic for tests (such as ultrasound, mammography and looking at the discharge under the microscope) to make sure that breast cancer is not responsible.
- If the discharge is milky and coming from both breasts, your doctor can do a blood test to check for an imbalance of the hormone prolactin.

If all the tests are normal, you can stop worrying, but the discharge may still bother you (perhaps soiling your clothes). A possible cause is some inflammation (mastitis) around the ducts. This is linked with smoking, and may improve if you stop smoking and avoid squeezing. A course of antibiotics may help.

It is possible to have an operation to close or remove the ducts that the discharge is coming from. This operation may not be a good idea for anyone who plans to become pregnant afterwards – depending on the number of ducts involved, it might make breastfeeding difficult and the breast might become congested. For more information about the breast, see the section on breast problems on page 54.

Inverted nipples

Most women's nipples protrude (stick out) about 5–10 mm. Usually they become about 10 mm longer and 2–3 mm wider during sexual arousal. Some women have nipples that are flat, but become erect during sexual arousal or when a baby is sucking on the nipple. Nipples that are tucked into the breast, instead of being flat or sticking out, are called inverted nipples. Both nipples may be inverted, or just one.

Nipples that have always been inverted. If your nipples have been inverted for as long as you can remember, it is nothing to worry about. It is just the way you are, and a lot of women are the same. A survey of 3000 women attending an antenatal clinic found that 10% had inverted nipples.

A nipple that suddenly becomes inverted can be a sign of a cancer underneath it, so you should see your doctor straightaway.

Breastfeeding should not be too much of a problem if your nipples become erect in the cold or when you are sexually aroused. It will be harder for the baby to draw the nipple into the back of its mouth, so breastfeeding will require some patience, but eventually the baby's strong sucking will draw the nipple out. You will be able to help by applying an ice cube wrapped in a flannel to the nipple beforehand and by stroking the areola (the pink area round the nipple).

If stimulation does not make the nipple protrude, breastfeeding may be more difficult. During the last 6–8 weeks of pregnancy, you may be able to encourage the nipples to stick out by wearing breast shields under your bra. These are small devices that press gently on the breast around the nipple. They are quite comfortable. They are worn for 1 or 2 hours at first, and the time is gradually increased. Your midwife will be able to advise you.

Ways of making your nipples protrude. Even if you do not intend to breastfeed you may wish to have protruding nipples. Teenagers often have flat nipples and, in some women (especially if their periods did not start until late), they remain flat until the early 20s. So if you are young, there is a possibility that they may gradually start to protrude. Otherwise, you could try stroking the areola with warm hands for a few minutes each day to bring the nipple out. You could also try wearing breast shields. Do not wear them for too long at first, otherwise the breasts may become sore, and do not continue wearing them for more than 6 weeks.

If these measures do not work and your nipples are really distressing you, it is possible to have a small operation to make the nipples protrude. This involves a small incision on each side of the nipple, and the cutting of some ducts and tissue. The drawback is that some women cannot breastfeed after this operation, and the operation is very expensive (and in the UK not available on the NHS).

Hairy nipples

Coarse, dark hairs around the nipple are quite common. You can pull them out with tweezers, but this can cause irritation because the skin round the nipple is very sensitive. It is probably better simply to cut them off close to the skin. This is easier if you hold the end of the hair with tweezers to keep it taut. The hairs will grow again, so you will have to cut them off again from time to time.

Hairs round the nipple are nothing to worry about unless you have excess hairiness on other parts of the body and your periods are irregular. If this is the case, you may have polycystic ovary syndrome (PCOS) and you should see your doctor. PCOS is discussed further on page 168.

Itchy, scaly nipples

If your nipples are itchy, scaly and cracked, you probably have eczema. The itching can make this an embarrassing condition. It occurs mainly in women in their late teens, and usually affects both nipples. It may be only on the nipple, or may affect the flatter area surrounding the nipple (the areola). A steroid cream from your doctor will deal with it. Your doctor will check that it is not scabies (see page 183), which can cause a similar appearance.

'Jogger's nipple' is another possibility. This is caused by friction from clothing, especially during long-distance running. Protect your nipples with petroleum jelly (Vaseline) or surgical tape (Micropore, from pharmacies) before exercising. A silk running vest is less abrasive than synthetic fibres.

Very rarely, eczema of a nipple can signal a cancerous growth beneath. This is uncommon, but it is why you should see your doctor if you have eczema on only one nipple. It occurs mainly in middle-aged or elderly women. It is not usually itchy, but there may be a pricking or burning feeling.

Extra nipples

Most people have only two nipples, but about 1 in 50 people (both males and females) has more. These extra nipples are not as well formed as the main nipples, so you may have them without realizing what they are. Imagine a line drawn between the armpit and the inner thigh; the extra nipples are usually on this line.

Oral sex

Oral sex can take place in various ways.

- The woman can stimulate the man's penis with her mouth and tongue (fellatio, blow job)
- The man can stimulate the woman's vulva with his tongue (cunnilingus)
- One partner can stimulate the area round the other partner's anus (rimming) with his or her tongue.

Are there any risks?

It is possible to catch infections by oral sex but, in general, the chances are probably lower than with penetrative sex. The risks also depend on whether you are the partner performing oral sex, or the partner who is having it done to them.

Risks to the partner performing oral sex

Gonorrhoea. It is quite easy to catch a gonorrhoea throat infection by performing oral sex on a man who has it. He will have some discharge from the urethral opening (pee hole), and this discharge will be teeming with gonorrhoea bacteria. Unfortunately, the discharge is not always noticeable, so neither partner may be aware that he has the infection. Alternatively, he may have noticed a discharge previously, but may have assumed that the problem had cured itself. See page 138 for more information.

Similarly, it might be possible to catch gonorrhoea throat infection by performing oral sex on a woman who has gonorrhoea.

Chlamydia. You can catch chlamydia in your throat by performing oral sex on a man who has it. A man who has a chlamydia infection may have pain passing urine and/or a discharge, or he may have no symptoms. See page 127 for more information.

Warts. It is not a good idea to perform oral sex on a man who has genital warts. The warts may not be obvious – check around the edge of the head of the penis under the foreskin, and just inside the opening of the urethra (pee hole). Although the risk is not great, a woman can develop a wart on the roof of her mouth as a result of oral sex. The wart may take weeks or even months to appear. If you develop one, see your doctor or go to your local sexual health clinic (see page 335).

Similarly, it is possible for a man to develop a wart on his lips from performing oral sex on a woman who has genital warts. Again, if this happens, see your doctor or go to your local sexual health clinic.

HIV. It is possible to catch HIV by oral sex. Although the risk is low, it is not absolutely safe, and oral sex with someone who might be HIV positive cannot be described as 'safe sex'.

The body fluids (including semen and the natural fluids that lubricate the vagina) of a person who has HIV will contain the virus. Therefore HIV can infect the cells that line the mouth of the person performing oral sex, and then enter the bloodstream (*Journal of*

Virology 2003;77:3470–6). The risk is likely to be greater for a woman performing oral sex on a man than the other way round. Withdrawing the penis before the man's orgasm (ejaculation) would lessen the risk; however, when a man is sexually aroused, small amounts of semen leak out before ejaculation so infection could still occur.

Syphilis is uncommon in the UK, but seems to be increasing. An outbreak was reported in the journal *Communicable Disease and Public Health* in 2001. Most of the people infected were homosexual men who had oral sex without using a condom.

Mouth and throat cancer. Oral sex can lead to mouth or throat cancer, but the risk is tiny. The reason is that the genital area can be infected with type 16 human papillomavirus (HPV). This type of papillomavirus can cause mouth and throat cancers (*Journal of the National Cancer Institute* 2003;95:1772–83).

Risks to the partner who is receiving oral sex

Herpes. Apart from being bitten, catching genital herpes from a cold sore on the face is the main risk. Cold sores are also infectious at the tingling stage before the sore has developed. If your partner has recurrent cold sores, he or she will recognize this tingling feeling, and should avoid performing oral sex until the sore has healed completely.

Chlamydia and gonorrhoea. In theory, it is possible to catch gonorrhoea or chlamydia by receiving oral sex from someone who has it in their mouth. Chlamydia and gonorrhoea in the mouth tends to be mainly at the back of the mouth (throat) and does not usually cause a sore throat or any other symptoms.

HIV. Contact between your genitals and the mouth of someone with HIV means that your genitals are in contact with their saliva, which will contain the virus. The amount of virus in the saliva would be very small and there would probably be a very low risk of infection, but it would not be absolutely safe.

Safe oral sex

- Do not perform oral sex on a man who has a discharge, or has recently had one that was not treated.
- Do not perform oral sex on anyone whose genitals look unhealthy or unclean.
- If your partner has a cold sore on the face or lip, do not let him or her perform oral sex on you. Similarly, do not offer oral sex if you have a cold sore or think you might be getting one.
- Some experts say you should avoid mouth-to-genital contact unless you are very sure that your partner is HIV negative.
- Avoid brushing your teeth beforehand, because this could open up cracks in the gum which would make it easier for infection (such as HIV) to enter.
- Consider using condoms for oral sex. If you are concerned about infection during oral sex, but do not like the idea of condoms because of their off-putting rubbery taste, try flavoured ones. Textured, knobbed or ribbed condoms are not suitable for oral sex, because they can make the mouth sore.

- Swallowing semen during oral sex is not harmful. The main risk of infection is in the mouth (see above). Swallowing semen is unlikely to increase the risk of HIV, because the stomach contains acid that destroys HIV.
- 'Rimming' (licking round the anus) is not to be recommended. The lower bowel contains many bacteria and viruses, which could enter the mouth, even if the anal area is washed beforehand.

Useful contacts

Family Planning NSW has a 'Useful contacts' link on their website to other family planning and sexual health clinics in Australia. The website also provides fact sheets and FAQs under the section 'Sex matters'.
www.fpahealth.org.au/sex-matters

Health*Insite* is an Australian government initiative aimed to improve the health of Australians by providing easy access to quality information about human health. Follow the link to find information on a variety of sexually transmitted infections.
www.healthinsite.gov.au/topics/Sexually_Transmitted_Infections

Terence Higgins Trust gives information about all aspects of HIV. Its website has a page on oral sex that gives clear and factual information about the risks of HIV from oral sex. The page is mainly about gay men, but also has information about heterosexual oral sex.
www.tht.org.uk/gaymen/oral_sex/faq02.htm

Health Protection Agency is a UK government source of information about infection. Its website has various reports about oral sex and sexually transmitted infections, which can be found using the search facility.
www.hpa.org.uk

The Guide to Getting It On by Paul Joannides is a straightforward and informative sex guide, with practical information about oral sex. The website contains some extracts from the book and is not for under-16s. Published by Goofy Foot Press. ISBN 1-885535-00-7
www.goofyfootpress.com

Penis problems

BENDING AND TWISTING
What's normal?

An absolutely straight penis is unusual – most have a slight curve when erect. But this should not be more than about 25° from straight, like a banana. If your penis bends more than this, you might have Peyronie's disease. It is also quite normal and harmless for the penis to have a slight twist (usually anticlockwise).

Peyronie's disease

A condition called Peyronie's disease, in which the penis becomes crooked when it is erect, occasionally develops in men. This can make sexual intercourse difficult, if not impossible. The condition is named after Dr François Gigot de la Peyronie (physician to King Louis XV of France) who wrote about it in 1743, but it has probably been around for much longer; sculptures dating from the 6th century BC depict angulated erect penises. It is estimated that about 1 in 100 men has Peyronie's disease.

Peyronie's disease most commonly occurs in men aged 50–60, but it can occur in young men and in old age. The cause is thickening of the fibrous tissue in the penis on one side. This means that, during an erection, one side of the penis cannot lengthen, and the penis will bend. The direction of the bend depends on the position of the thickening (which can often be felt as a lump or lumps when the penis is limp).

- If the thickening is on the top of the penis, the erection tends to curve upwards; this is the most common type.
- If the thickening is on either side, the penis will bend towards the side that is thickened.

You may be able to feel the thickened area; it feels like a hard piece of toffee.

Will it get better? For the first 9–18 months after Peyronie's disease starts, it is often quite painful, especially when the penis is erect. During this period, the thickened area increases in size. After this 'active period', it is unlikely to become worse. In 20% of cases, the penis will go back to normal without any treatment. Those who have had the condition for a long time feel no pain but sometimes have difficulty achieving an erection (perhaps because the lumpiness is obstructing blood flow in the penis).

What causes Peyronie's disease? No one knows why the thickening occurs, but it is not a cancerous condition, nor is it the result of sexually transmitted disease or of any odd previous sexual practices. It is more common in smokers. There seems to be a link with some other conditions. For example, men with Peyronie's disease are quite likely to have Dupuytren's contracture, a thickening of fibrous tissue in the palm of the hand. They are also quite likely to have raised blood pressure; some doctors think that the blood pressure itself might be responsible for the penis problem, while others blame the drugs used to treat blood pressure (particularly beta-blockers).

Treatments. There is no need to feel embarrassed about discussing the problem with your family doctor, because doctors are very familiar with the condition. It may be difficult for your doctor to assess how severe the problem is, because the curvature shows only when the penis is erect. If you have a digital or instant-picture camera, take a photograph of your erect penis and show it to your doctor. (You might wish to tell your doctor that you were advised to do this in a book written by a doctor.) If it is only mild and does not cause any inconvenience, no treatment is necessary.

Cocoa butter cream. Some men with mild Peyronie's disease say that massaging cocoa butter cream (available from pharmacies) into the curved area is helpful.

Steroid injections. In the past, the most common treatment was steroid injection into the thickening, but this is now less popular.

Vitamin E tablets are sometimes recommended, but scientific evidence to show that they help is scanty. Do not take more than 250 mg of vitamin E a day, because higher doses may damage your health.

Tamoxifen is a medication that may reduce the thickened area. This medication is also used for breast cancer, but Peyronie's disease is not related to breast cancer.

Sound waves are a new treatment for Peyronie's disease. Preliminary research has shown that high energy sound waves reduce pain, and also decrease the size of the thickened area somewhat. More research is needed to see how effective this treatment really is.

Verapamil is a medication that is used to treat blood pressure. Injections of verapamil into the thickened area may help, but more research is needed.

Surgery to correct the deformity is the most effective treatment. In the usual operation, the surgeon cuts out some tissue from the opposite side to balance out the thickened area. After the operation the erect penis will be straight and 1–3 cm shorter than before when erect, but many men do not notice any difference. Studies have shown that only 58–88% of men are satisfied with the result of the operation, partly because it straightens the penis but leaves the thickened area in place so it may still be painful. Also, a few men have difficulty achieving an erection after the operation.

In another type of operation, the surgeon cuts a slit in the thickened area and inserts a piece of tissue (usually a piece of vein from the groin or ankle). This makes the area more flexible, and there is no shortening of the penis. However, 10–15% of men have difficulty in obtaining an erection after this operation.

DISCHARGE

The hole at the end of the penis is the opening of the urethra (the tube for urine and semen that is inside the penis). Discharge is usually a sign of infection in the urethra.

Non-specific urethritis (NSU) is a common cause of discharge. 'Urethritis' means inflammation of the tube, and 'non-specific' means that it is difficult to know the exact cause. NSU causes a discharge that is usually clear, and is worse in the mornings. You may find it uncomfortable to pass urine, and you may feel irritation along the urethra inside the penis.

NSU is caught during sex. Several types of bacteria may be responsible; about half of cases are caused by chlamydia (see page 127) and about 40% are caused by other bacteria (such as Ureaplasma and Mycoplasma). These bacteria do not cause a discharge in women, or any other symptoms in the early stages, so most women do not know that they have an infection.

In women, chlamydia can travel upwards into the Fallopian tubes (the tubes that carry the eggs from the ovaries to the womb), and can eventually affect the tubes, making the woman infertile. For this reason you need treatment, so that you do not pass the infection on to a female partner.

Gonorrhoea is caused by a bacteria called Gonococcus (see page 138). Like NSU, it is caught during sex, and often causes a discharge and pain when you pass urine. The discharge can be any colour – yellow, green, white, cloudy or clear. The symptoms may be so slight that you hardly notice them, or there may be a lot of discharge. Gonorrhoea can spread to the testicles, causing pain, swelling and redness. As with NSU, the woman you caught it from was probably unaware that she was infected; only 10–20% of women with gonorrhoea have a discharge.

Inflammation. Occasionally, the urethra can become inflamed without there being any infection. For example, if you poke anything up the urethra you can damage the lining, which will become inflamed and cause a discharge. Similarly, antiseptics, perfumed bubble baths or strong soaps can inflame the urethra if you are very sensitive to them. And check to make sure the discharge is actually coming from the urethral opening, rather than from a sore area under the foreskin.

What you should do

Any discharge from the penis needs to be checked out by your doctor or, preferably, a doctor at a sexual health clinic. This is because chlamydia and gonorrhoea can be easily treated with the correct antibiotics, but can cause problems to you and your future partners if they are not treated properly. Some types of the bacteria that cause gonorrhoea are resistant to certain antibiotics, but the sexual health clinic will be able to test you to select the correct one.

RED, SORE AND ITCHY

If the head of your penis (glans) is inflamed, you have balanitis. This is a Greek word meaning 'inflammation of the acorn'. Balanitis usually looks more worrying than it is.

- It may simply be a hygiene problem. If you do not wash under the foreskin, a cheesy material, called smegma, accumulates. This can become infected and cause irritation. The solution is to wash carefully with warm water to which you have added enough kitchen salt to make it taste like seawater.
- A milder form of balanitis can appear soon after intercourse, but disappears within about a day. This is probably caused by allergy to thrush in your partner's vagina. If she is treated the problem will usually go.

- Balanitis can sometimes be caused by a skin disease, such as psoriasis. Psoriasis can occur on the penis without you having it anywhere else. On the glans, it looks red and shiny (unlike on other parts of the body where it is silvery and scaly). In this situation antifungal treatment will not have any effect, but your doctor can prescribe a steroid cream.
- Check your soaps and shower gels. Balanitis can sometimes be a sensitivity to perfumes in soaps and detergents. Never put disinfectant in the bath, as this can be very irritating.

What to do about balanitis

- Change to a simple, unperfumed soap. Alternatively, buy 'aqueous cream' from a pharmacy and use it as body-wash cream (i.e. apply a small amount and rinse off).
- Put two handfuls of salt in the bath, but no other additives (no bubble bath, no bath oils, no disinfectants).
- Do not use 'biological' or 'enzyme' powders when washing your underpants.
- Ask your partner to visit her doctor or a sexual health clinic to check for thrush (especially if your balanitis occurs after sex).
- See your doctor – if your balanitis is severe, ask for a diabetes check; if anti-thrush treatment does not work, ask your doctor if it could be psoriasis.

Thrush

If your penis is swollen, intensely itchy and very red, you probably have thrush (also known as Candida, a yeast). Occasionally this can be the first sign of diabetes, so check with your doctor. It is cured with antifungal cream or tablets.

ODD-LOOKING PATCH

It is quite common to notice an area of skin on the penis that looks different from the surrounding skin. It may be red, shiny or scaly, or pale and thin like a scar. If it does not disappear in a week or two, you should have it checked by your family doctor or local sexual health clinic.

- Most skin conditions that can affect other parts of the body, such as psoriasis, can occur on the penis, and sometimes the penis may be the only site.
- If the patch is lumpy, it could be warts (see page 134).
- Very, very rarely, a funny-looking patch is a pre-cancerous condition.
- A pale, thin-looking patch could be a condition called 'balanitis xerotica obliterans', which is usually treated with a steroid cream.

OPENING IN THE WRONG PLACE

Normally, the opening of the urethra (the tube for urine and semen) is at the end of the penis, in the middle of its head (glans). About 1 in every 300 males is born with the opening on the underside, and the middle of the glans just has a blind dimple. This is called hypospadias. It tends to run in families; if one child has hypospadias, his brothers have a 1 in 20 chance of also having it.

In 65% of men with hypospadias, the opening is on the underside of the head of the penis, near where it joins the shaft, but it can be anywhere along the underside of the shaft or even at the root of the penis near the testicles. If the opening is on the shaft, the end of the penis may bend when it is erect; this does not occur if the opening is near the head. The foreskin is often abnormal as well; part of it is missing on the underside of the penis, so it looks like a hood.

Effects of hypospadias

Hypospadias does not make you incontinent because the urine flow is controlled by the neck of the bladder, which is higher up inside the body. However, it can make it difficult to direct the stream of urine accurately, and some men with this condition choose to sit down when they pass urine.

Treatment. Severe hypospadias, where the opening is on the shaft or near the testicles, will have been noticed at birth, and will have been put right by an operation at the age of 12–18 months. Babies with slight hypospadias, where the opening is on the head of the penis, not far from the dimple, do not always have an operation. If you have hypospadias that was not operated on, but which bothers you because of the appearance of the foreskin or because you cannot control the direction of the urine stream, ask your family doctor to refer you to a urological surgeon who will be able to give you more information and discuss the options. Seeing a surgeon does not commit you to having an operation.

CHANGING COLOURS

It is normal for the head of the penis (glans) to change colour. Often it is quite red when aroused, and a more purple colour at other times. This is because the skin of the glans has lots of tiny blood vessels near its surface, so the colour just represents the changes in blood flow. If the skin is sore and itchy as well as red, or looks abnormal in any other way, you might have balanitis (see above), for which you should see your doctor.

SIZE

Most men do not think rationally about penis size.

- Research has shown that men do not have a clear idea of the size of their own penis. Looked at from above, it appears shorter than it really is.
- Men do not have a clear idea of what average is.

What's normal?

According to the Kinsey Institute, many American men mistakenly think the average erect penis is 25 cm (almost 10 inches) long, and worry that they do not measure up. Here are the results of two surveys.

University of California researchers measured the penises of 80 normal men and published their results in the *Journal of Urology* in 1996. They found that:

- without an erection (limp), the average length was 8.8 cm
- the average flaccid penis could be stretched to 12.4 cm
- the average length when erect was 12.9 cm.

Of the men studied, many had penises that were larger or smaller than the average. They also found that the length of the penis when flaccid does not predict the size when erect – smaller penises expand more when erect. So, the researchers found the average erect penis to be about 13 cm long, regardless of whether it is 5 cm or 10 cm long when it is flaccid.

In 2001, the condom manufacturer Durex asked men visiting its website to take part in a penis size survey, and just under 3000 men responded. They measured themselves and reported the results to the website. The average erect length was 16.3 cm, and the average circumference (measured round the penis at its widest point) was 13.3 cm. It is difficult to know how reliable these measurements are – there might have been some wishful thinking involved. The survey also showed that a long penis is not usually thick. Durex says, 'While the "mythical" well-endowed man with a very long and very wide penis does exist, there are not that many of them about.'

Shoe size and penis size

It is a myth that men with large feet have larger penises; researchers have found no correlation (*British Journal of Urology International* 2002;90:586–7).

Lose a paunch

If you are carrying a few excess pounds on your abdomen, the first part (called the root) of your penis will be buried in the fat. This makes it look shorter than it really is. Losing weight will make the penis grow!

Penis enlargement

The shaft of the penis can be made thicker by injecting fat under the skin of the penis. The fat will have been removed by liposuction from another part of the body, usually the thigh or abdomen. The glans (the tip of the penis) stays the same size, and so it may look a bit out of proportion. The fat tends to be absorbed by the body, so the injections have to be repeated two or three times a year. The fat can sometimes form unsightly nodules, and there can be puckering of the skin and scarring.

Another method is dermal grafting. Strips of skin and underlying fat are removed from beneath the buttocks; the upper layer of skin is taken off and the rest of the tissue is implanted along the shaft of the penis under the skin. As a result, there may be some scar tissue along the shaft of the penis.

The penis can be made longer by a surgical operation in which the ligaments that attach the penis to the pubic bone are cut. This makes the penis hang down about 2.5–5 cm further when it is limp, but the size of your erection will not be increased. Also because it no longer has the support of the ligaments, the erect penis will not point as high as before. The operation can be risky, because important nerves that carry sensation can be damaged and infection or bleeding can also occur, and unsightly scarring is common. If you are considering this operation, make sure that you find a reputable surgeon (look at the section on cosmetic surgery on page 339). This may be difficult, because not many surgeons are willing to do this operation, because of the problems associated with it.

A safer approach is to have a 'suprapubic lipectomy' to remove fat from the lower abdomen above the root of the penis. This makes the whole length of the penis more visible.

TIGHT FORESKIN

The foreskin is the hood of skin that covers the head of the penis. If you have been circumcised, you will not have a foreskin.

- In small children the foreskin is tight and stuck to the glans, but normally begins to separate at about the age of 3 or 4. If the hole in the foreskin looks abnormally tiny, ask your doctor to check.
- After the age of 7, it is usually possible to pull the foreskin back over the head (or glans) of the penis, but in some boys this is not possible before the age of 14 or 15. So if you are 13 or 14, do not worry – this is perfectly normal.
- If you are 15 or over and cannot pull your foreskin back, it may be too tight.

A tight foreskin is called phimosis. If you have phimosis, you will not be able to wash under your foreskin properly, so a white, cheesy material called smegma can accumulate. Also, if the condition is severe, it may be painful when the penis is erect.

Some men have phimosis from childhood, but it can also occur late in life, perhaps as a result of several thrush infections affecting the head of the penis. Another common reason is a skin condition called balanitis xerotica obliterans, which makes the foreskin pale and thickened. The cause of this condition is not known; it is not an infection.

Treatment

If it is very tight, there is no point in trying to force the foreskin back: you will only cause painful cracks on the inside of the foreskin, which will scar as they heal and make it worse. NORM-UK suggests that you try gentle stretching, and advises on how to do this (see Useful contacts on page 211). If this does not solve the problem, you probably need an operation.

Circumcision is the most common operation. The surgeon separates the foreskin from the head of the penis (if it is stuck down), cuts the foreskin away and closes the incision with stitches. The glans will seem very sensitive after the operation, because it is not used to being exposed. Most men have erections during their sleep, so for a few weeks after the operation, you may wake in the middle of the night with a sore penis; taking a pain-relieving medication at bedtime will help. Wear loose boxer shorts and use a condom during sex for the first month or two.

If the doctor thinks the cause is balanitis xerotica obliterans, steroid creams will be used first; this often relieves the condition for several years, but eventually circumcision is usually needed.

Preputioplasty is a lesser operation. It involves making a vertical incision in the foreskin and then stitching it crosswise to widen the opening; it usually leaves a very normal appearance.

Useful contacts

Andrology Australia provides access to quality and authenticated information to improve understanding and knowledge of the range, causes and treatment options of male reproductive health disorders. Click onto 'Your health' to access information on Peyronie's disease under 'A–Z topics'.
www.andrologyaustralia.org

The Sexual Dysfunction Association (previously known as the Impotence Association) has a free fact sheet on Peyronie's disease, which is also available on its website.
www.sda.uk.net
www.impotence.org.uk

Peyronies.org is an informative website for men with Peyronie's disease. It explains the disease and gives an overview of treatment, especially surgery.
www.peyronies.org

The Guide to Getting It On by Paul Joannides lives up to its claim to be 'America's coolest and most informative book about sex'. The author says his aim is to help people who would like to be more at ease with themselves and with their partners about sex. It has upbeat information about many penis worries. The website contains some extracts from the book and is not for under-16s.
www.goofyfootpress.com

NORM-UK advises on treatments for phimosis (tight foreskin) that avoid circumcision surgery.
www.norm-uk.co.uk

'Size matters' is a reliable article on penis enlargement written by Dr JC Gingell in the year 2000. It is written for doctors by an expert surgeon. On the website, use the link to the reference section and search for 'size matters'.
www.doctorupdate.net

'Penis Enlargement: fulfillment or fallacy?' is a good article on the US Mayo Clinic website, written in 2003. Use the search facility on the website to find it.
www.mayoclinic.com

Piles

The lining of the anal canal contains three soft, spongy pads of tissue that act as an extra seal to keep the canal closed until you go to the toilet. The lining of the gut is very slimy (so that faeces can pass along easily); the extra seal stops the slime (mucus) from leaking out. The pads contain a network of tiny blood vessels.

What are piles?

People sometimes think that piles (haemorrhoids) are like varicose veins of the legs (i.e. a single vein that has become swollen). This is not the case. A pile is one of the soft pads that has slipped downwards slightly, because the surrounding tissue is not holding it in place properly. When this happens, the small blood vessels within the cushion become engorged with blood, so the cushion swells up. When faeces are passed, the pile may be pushed further down the anal canal to the outside, and this is called a prolapsed pile. Doctors classify piles into three types.

First-degree piles are swollen cushions that always remain within in the anal canal; these are painless.

Second-degree piles are pushed down (prolapsed) when faeces are passed, but return to their starting position afterwards.

Third-degree piles are pushed down (prolapsed) when faeces are passed, or come down at other times. They do not go back by themselves after faeces have been passed.

Who gets piles?

Piles can occur at any age, but are more common in older people. They affect both men and women. In fact, most people suffer from piles at some time, but usually they are nothing more than a temporary problem. Many experts believe that they are caused by continuous high pressure in the veins of the body, which occurs because humans stand upright. They are particularly common in pregnancy because of the additional pressure from the baby, and because of hormonal changes. Sometimes they result from straining hard to pass faeces, which is more likely if you do not eat enough fibre, or lifting heavy weights. They are not caused by sitting on hot radiators or cold, hard surfaces, or by sedentary jobs.

What are the symptoms of piles?

The symptoms of piles can come and go. There are five main symptoms:

- itching and irritation
- aching pain and discomfort
- bleeding
- a lump, which may be tender
- soiling of underwear with slime or faeces ('skid marks').

Itching and irritation probably occur because the lumpy piles stop acting as soft pads to keep the mucus in; instead, a little mucus leaks out and irritates the area around the anus. Pain and discomfort comes from swelling around the pile, and from scratching of the lining of the anal canal by faeces as they pass over the lumpy area. The scratching also causes bleeding, which is a fresh bright red colour and may be seen on faeces or toilet paper or dripping in the pan. A pile that has been pushed down (a second- or third-degree pile) may be felt as a lump at the anus.

How you can help yourself

Most piles get better in a few days without any treatment, but there are several ways of relieving the discomfort.

- Wash the area gently with warm, salty water, to get rid of irritant mucus that has leaked out. Dry carefully with cotton wool and apply petroleum jelly (available from pharmacies) or nappy rash cream to protect your skin if more mucus or moisture leaks out.
- Use soft toilet paper, and dab rather than wipe.
- Wear loose underwear and clothing (i.e. not tight trousers), so that nothing will rub the pile.
- Do not scratch. For more information on dealing with itch, look at the section on anal itching on page 26.
- Avoid constipation by eating lots of fresh fruit and vegetables and bran cereal. Aim for faeces that are soft enough to change their shape as you push them out.
- Drink plenty of fluids.
- After you have passed the faeces, do not strain to finish. People with piles often think there is more to come, but this is a false sensation caused by the swollen spongy pads in the piles themselves. Do not read on the toilet and aim to be out of the toilet within a minute.
- If you can feel a lump, try pushing it gently upwards; try to relax your anus as you do so.
- If you have a lot of discomfort, buy a haemorrhoid cream or gel. A pharmacist will be able to help you choose one that is suitable for you. A haemorrhoid cream or gel does not cure the pile, but will usually relieve the discomfort effectively until the pile goes away of its own accord. Do not use it for longer than a week or two.

To stop piles returning, continue the high-fibre diet to keep your stools soft and do not put off opening your bowels, and avoid straining.

When to see your doctor

See your doctor if the symptoms last longer than a week. You should also see your doctor if you have bleeding, to ensure that there is not some other cause. Your doctor will examine your anus, feel inside the anal canal and may also insert a small metal tube, called a proctoscope, a couple of centimetres or so into the anal canal to give a better view. For more information, look at the section on seeing your doctor about an anal problem on page 338.

What your doctor can do

First- and second-degree piles often go away on their own if constipation is avoided, but your doctor may prescribe a short course of haemorrhoid cream to relieve symptoms. Third-degree piles may also go away on their own, but if they persist, they may need hospital treatment.

Only a few people need an operation; most are treated by banding or phenol injections. There is usually no need for a general anaesthetic or overnight stay in hospital for these procedures. Stretching (anal dilatation) was a popular treatment in the 1970s, but is seldom used now.

Banding involves placing a small rubber band at the base of the pile, so that it pinches the lining of the anal canal. This 'strangles' the pile, so it dies and falls off. It causes some scarring. It is more effective than the other treatments but has some drawbacks, such as severe bleeding in a few cases. Therefore you need to tell the surgeon if you are on blood-thinning medication. Some people feel faint and nauseous just after the bands are put on, and they can be quite painful for the following 48 hours. According to an article in the *British Medical Journal* (2003;327:8847–521), the success rate for banding is:

- 79% of piles are cured
- 18% of piles return so that repeat banding is needed
- for 2% of piles, it does not work at all.

Injection of phenol in almond oil is a method of causing scarring in the area, but produces a permanent cure in only about 25% of cases. It is less commonly used now, because the results are not as good as with banding.

Cryosurgery freezes the pile to destroy it. It is not used much, because it causes a watery discharge afterwards.

Infrared coagulation uses infrared light to destroy the pile. This method is not commonly used, because it is not as effective as other methods.

Surgery. There are several different operations for piles. In the usual operation, the swollen spongy pad that forms the pile is cut away. It is painful for 7–10 days afterwards. A newer operation, called 'stapling', involves cutting away a 2 cm strip of the lining of the rectum and joining the cut edges with a special stapler. People seem to recover quicker from 'stapling' than from the ordinary operation. It is not yet a common operation in the UK, but it is popular in the rest of Europe. Although it is less painful than the ordinary operation, it seems to be less effective in the long term and about 12% of people have a recurrence of the piles within 16 months (*Surgery* 2006;24(4):148–50). However, more research is needed.

Useful contacts

Colorectal Surgical Society of Australasia has some very useful information on haemorrhoids under 'Patient info' on its website. Brochures can also be purchased by completing their online order form.

www.cssa.org.au

American Academy of Family Physicians have two detailed articles on 'Common Anorectal Conditions' on their website. The articles are intended for doctors and explain how doctors

examine the anus. They discuss itching, pain, bleeding, lumps, constipation and incontinence of faeces.
www.aafp.org/afp/20010615/2391.html
www.aafp.org/afp/20010701/77.html

Digestive Disorders Foundation is a UK non-profit organization that provides reliable information about all gut problems. They supply a range of leaflets which are available on the 'Patients info leaflets' section of the website.
www.digestivedisorders.org.uk

National Digestive Diseases Information Clearinghouse is a US government organization. Its website has pages on piles (haemorrhoids/hemorrhoids), constipation and other gut problems.
www.digestive.niddk.nih.gov/ddiseases/a-z.asp

The American Gastroenterological Association is an organization for doctors who specialize in the gut. Look in the 'Patient center' of the website for excellent information about various gut problems including piles and constipation.
www.gastro.org

YourSurgery.com is a US website that gives details of various operations. It has a detailed page about surgery for piles ('hemorrhoidectomy'), but you have to pay to view.
www.yoursurgery.com

Pfizer, the manufacturers of Anusol, have a very pleasant website about piles.
www.pilesadvice.co.uk

Wyeth Pharmaceuticals, the manufacturers of Preparation H for piles, have an informative and entertaining website. Look at the symptoms section, which includes a page on 'Doctor's examination' (rectal examination).
www.preparationh.co.uk

Red face

Some people just naturally have a reddish face. Of course, if you work in the open air, you may acquire a weathered, red, jolly-farmer face, especially if you are naturally fair-skinned. But a red face can mean that you have a skin disorder, and appropriate treatment should solve the problem. And, rarely, it can mean a more serious disorder such as 'systemic lupus erythematosus' that needs to be properly investigated and treated. So do not feel you are wasting your doctor's time by seeking help for a red face.

Questions to ask yourself

Is my face red all the time, or is the problem flushing/blushing? Have a look at the section on blushing and flushing on page 49.

Have I been taking steroids? Steroid tablets can cause a red face in some people. If you think this might be the cause in your case, discuss it with your doctor. Do not simply stop the steroids, because this could make you very ill. Strong steroid creams can also make the face red, and can encourage the formation of thread veins (see page 316) that make the skin look redder.

Am I sensitive to something? Think about whether you have changed your cosmetics or perfume recently, or whether a chemical in your workplace could be responsible. Or have you come into contact with something – some people are very sensitive to certain plants and flowers. Nickel in spectacle frames can cause redness around the eyes and ears.

Is it related to sunlight ('photosensitivity')? This is possible if most of your face is red, but the shaded areas under the nose and chin, and behind the ears are all right, and the redness stops sharply at your collar-line (see below).

Is the redness in a special shape? If the redness is just across your cheeks and nose, in a shape like a butterfly, you need to see your doctor. It could be a disorder called 'systemic lupus erythematosus' (SLE), in which your immune system is not behaving properly.

As well as being red, is my skin scaly, itchy, sore or lumpy? Are there blackheads or pustules? Lots of skin disorders can cause reddening of the skin. You might have ordinary acne (see page 7), rosacea (see below) or dermatitis (eczema).

Photosensitivity

Of course ordinary sunburn will cause a red face, but some people find that exposure to sunlight that is not very bright has a similar effect. Photosensitivity may be the cause if the shaded areas under the nose and chin, under a fringe of hair or behind the ears are unaffected, and the redness stops sharply at the collar-line. This can be a difficult problem for your doctor to sort out, because it is often an interaction between a chemical and sunlight. The chemical might be a drug that you are taking – amiodarone, thiazide diuretics, chlorpromazine, some fluoroquinolone antibiotics and some tetracycline antibiotics occasionally have this effect. Or the chemical could be in a perfume or a sunscreen.

Rosacea

One of the most common causes of a red face is a skin disorder called rosacea (pronounced 'rose-ay sha'). Rosacea affects people of any age, but usually starts in the 30s and 40s. The skin of the nose, cheeks, chin and forehead becomes red. Instead of being smooth, the skin in the red areas may also feel slightly lumpy with acne-like spots. Tiny, spidery thread veins are often visible. There may also be a burning sensation. The eyelids are often inflamed (blepharitis). The eyes may feel dry, gritty and irritable.

Symptoms of rosacea

- Redness of nose, cheeks, chin and forehead
- Small visible thread veins on the face
- Bumps or pimples on the face
- Irritated eyelids and dry, gritty eyes

People with rosacea often say that the problem started with flushing of the face, without sweating. The flushes may be triggered by hot or spicy food, alcohol, coffee, emotional upset, windy weather or exercise. Each flush lasts from a few minutes to an hour, and then goes away. This flushing stage can last for years, but then the face gradually becomes more permanently red, and the flushes lessen. (Of course this does not mean that if you have a tendency to blushing or flushing, you will develop a permanently red face – in most people blushing is not an early stage of rosacea.)

What causes rosacea? It is frustrating that the cause of rosacea has not been discovered. It is certainly not infectious, so you cannot catch it by skin contact with someone who has it. It may be partly genetic, because a rosacea-type red face seems to run in some families, and it is more common in fair-skinned individuals with Irish or Scottish ancestry.

Some researchers think that an allergy to a microscopic mite (Demodex folliculorum) that lives in the hair follicles may be the cause. Other researchers have suggested that a reaction to the bacterium Helicobacter pylori, which many people carry in their stomach, is involved. Stress may be a factor, but no one really knows. In the past, 'lifestyle' factors, such as too much alcohol, were blamed, but there is no evidence for this at all.

Is it really rosacea? Your doctor is the best person to decide whether you really have rosacea. There is no laboratory test for it. Acne (see page 7) can sometimes look similar, but blackheads and big lumpy cysts do not occur in rosacea. Some types of dermatitis can also look similar, but the skin has tiny scales that are not seen in rosacea.

Does rosacea go away? Rosacea is a problem that you are likely to have for a long time, and it is unlikely to go away completely. Like other skin problems, there will be periods when it improves and is less troublesome. Fortunately, there are some effective treatments. After a few years, some people with rosacea develop thickening of the skin, especially on the nose, but this can now be dealt with by laser treatment.

What you can do

- It is common sense to avoid hot drinks, spicy foods or alcohol if they make the flushing worse. The National Rosacea Society website (see Useful contacts below) has a 'diary checklist' to help you identify situations or substances that may worsen your rosacea.
- Some people find rosacea flares up in the summer in response to ultraviolet light; if so, use a sunscreen (at least 15) and keep out of the sun.
- Avoid strong winds and sudden temperature changes.
- Chlorinated water (e.g. in swimming pools) can make rosacea worse.
- Treat your skin kindly. Avoid perfumed soaps, alcohol-containing preparations (such as aftershave lotions) and exfoliating skin cleansers.
- Do not put strong steroid creams on your face, because these usually worsen rosacea.
- Special make-up to disguise the thread veins and redness is available – cosmetic camouflage. In the UK, some hospital dermatology departments provide advice about cosmetic camouflage from volunteers trained by the Red Cross, using products available on prescription. You will need a referral letter from your family doctor (see Useful contacts below).
- See your doctor immediately if you experience severe eye pain or blurring of vision. This could mean that the cornea at the front of the eye is inflamed.
- It is worth remembering that your skin is sure to look much worse to you than to anyone else. Specialists on rosacea always say that the distress it causes is out of proportion to the actual appearance. This is because we are the worst critics of our own faces.

What your doctor can do

- For many years antibiotics (usually metronidazole or tetracycline and sometimes doxycycline), taken as tablets, have been the standard treatment for rosacea. No one knows why antibiotics work, because rosacea does not seem to be an infection. They are particularly helpful for the lumpiness of the skin. It may be more than 3 weeks before you notice any improvement, so be patient. If you are pregnant or breastfeeding, you should not take tetracycline or doxycycline; your doctor may prescribe erythromycin instead.
- A gel or cream containing an antibiotic (usually metronidazole, sometimes erythromycin) is an alternative treatment, but takes even longer to work (often about 8 weeks). The gel needs to be applied twice a day, is difficult to cover with make-up and seems to leave a sticky film on the face, whereas the cream is used only once a day.
- Azelaic acid gel is another effective treatment. It is applied twice daily. It may sting when you first start to use it (*New England Journal of Medicine* 2005;352:793–803).

When the treatment has had an effect, it is usually continued for another month or two and then stopped. It is possible that the rosacea will come back again, in which case you can have another course of treatment.

If your rosacea is severe, and these treatments are ineffective, your doctor can refer you to a skin specialist (dermatologist) for other treatments such as isotretinoin. The specialist can also organize laser treatment if skin thickening or thread veins are very noticeable.

Private clinics. Some private clinics advertise costly treatments for rosacea, such as 'intense pulsed light'. This uses light to destroy the tiny blood vessels in the skin that cause the redness. Several treatments may be needed. Some small studies suggest that this treatment reduces redness and flushing, and improves skin texture (*Journal of Drugs and Dermatology* 2003; 2:254–9, *Dermatological Surgery* 2003; 29: 600–4), but it has not yet been tested in large trials. Therefore we do not really know how effective it really is. Before going to any private clinic, think carefully, be cautious and discuss it with your doctor, and look at the section on cosmetic surgery (see page 339).

Useful contacts

The Australasian College of Dermatologists website contains basic information about various skin diseases and problems. It has a helpful section on rosacea under 'A–Z of skin'.
www.dermcoll.asn.au

National Rosacea Society is a US organization. Their excellent website has lots of information, including a section on coping with rosacea, a comprehensive FAQ section, a patient diary checklist, a list of common triggers and links to other sites.
www.rosacea.org

American Academy of Dermatology has information about rosacea in the Public Resource Center A–Z on its website.
www.aad.org/public

Acne Support Group offers support and information for people with rosacea, even though rosacea is different to acne.
www.m2w3.com/acne/what_is.html

American Family Physician has a detailed article on rosacea on its website, written for doctors, dated 2002. Some of the illustrations show a severe form (rhinophyma) which may worry you, but this is unlikely to occur. There is a link to an information sheet for the general public.
www.aafp.org/afp/20020801/435.html

Changing Faces is a non-profit organization giving help and support to people with any type of unusual facial appearance, and provides excellent information about cover-up make-up.
www.changingfaces.org.uk/

British Red Cross Skin Camouflage Services are provided free (but a donation is welcome) at a number of hospitals. They use volunteers trained by the Red Cross. You will need a referral letter from your family doctor.
www.timewarp.demon.co.uk/redcross.htm
www.redcross.org.uk

Restless legs

Restless legs is a very unpleasant feeling in the legs that is difficult to describe. You feel you must move them to get rid of the sensation. It is not pins-and-needles, but is more like a crawling, prickling and tingling irritation just under the skin (*Sleep Medicine* 2004;4:101–9).

Restless legs usually comes on when you have been sitting or lying still for a while, especially in bed just as you are getting off to sleep or when you wake in the night. It may also come on when you have to sit in a confined space, such as a cinema or plane.

It is very unusual to have it in one leg – usually both legs are affected, mainly the calves, but sometimes the thighs or feet. Some people also have it in their arms.

The only way to get rid of the feeling is to move your legs or get up and walk, which can be awkward if you are sitting at a public function, and annoying for your partner when you are in bed. If you try to keep still, the feeling becomes stronger and stronger, and more like a painful ache until you simply have to move.

Causes of restless legs

No one knows what causes restless legs, but researchers think it is probably due to a lack of availability of dopamine (a chemical transmitter) in a small area of the brain or spinal cord, rather than a problem in the legs themselves.

- In three-quarters of sufferers, the tendency to restless legs is inherited.
- In a few people (usually elderly), it is due to a shortage of iron.
- Some people have restless legs only when they are pregnant or find that pregnancy worsens it.
- Sometimes a similar feeling occurs in people who have illnesses that affect small nerves in the skin (such as diabetes or rheumatoid arthritis).
- Stress, fatigue, smoking, caffeine and alcohol can all make it worse.
- Some medications (e.g. antidepressants and calcium channel blocker drugs for blood pressure) can cause or worsen restless legs.

What you can do

Stop smoking. Restless legs is another good reason for stopping smoking.

Consider reducing coffee, tea, alcohol. You may have to do some detective work to decide if these causes apply in your case. The caffeine in coffee and strong tea makes restless legs more likely, as well as interfering with sleep. Try cutting them out and see if the problem improves. Likewise, try to work out if alcohol might be a factor in your case.

Deal with stress. This is easier said than done but, if you have noticed that the problem is worse when you are tense, consult your public library for books or tapes on relaxation.

Do not nap during the day. This can make it more difficult to sleep at night.

Cool your legs. Some people find that cooling the legs helps to prevent attacks, or relieves the sensation. Make sure your bedroom is cool and airy. Try putting your feet in cold water for 5 minutes before going to bed, and avoid using a hot water bottle or electric blanket in the winter. During an attack, remove the bedclothes from your feet and legs to allow them to cool down.

Massaging the legs with a mint or herbal leg cream or gel gives some relief.

Try a painkiller. Some people find that a painkiller such as paracetamol (acetaminophen) or ibuprofen gets rid of the unpleasant feeling.

The symptoms of restless legs had been noted by Dr Thomas Willis as far back as 1685

What your doctor can do

Check your iron levels. Your doctor can do a blood test to check your iron stores. If these are low, an iron supplement might help.

Check the medication you are taking. Your doctor can review any medication that you are taking, as some medications can worsen or cause restless legs.

Look for other causes. Your doctor can also decide whether you have ordinary restless legs, or whether it is due to some condition such as rheumatoid arthritis.

Discuss treatment. Some prescription drugs can help restless legs, but they all have some side effects. You will need to decide whether the discomfort in your legs and disturbance of your sleep is bad enough to warrant them.

If you are pregnant, or trying to become pregnant, you will just have to put up with the problem until after the pregnancy – you should not take any of the drugs used to treat restless legs. The problem will probably disappear within a few weeks after the birth of your baby.

Dopamine drugs are becoming very important treatments for restless legs. They compensate for the lack of availability of dopamine in specific areas of the brain.

- Ropinirole (Ardartrel) is a dopamine drug that seems to be very effective for restless legs with minimal side effects, though headache, nausea and dizziness occasionally occur. It is taken as a single dose in the evening..
- Pramipexole (Mirapexin) is another dopamine drug that is effective for restless legs. Like pergolide, it has been tested on only a small number of people, but seems to be an even more effective drug. It can cause drowsiness in the day and also nausea and insomnia.
- Pergolide is another dopamine drug. Researchers in America tested it in patients with restless legs and found that it was effective in relieving the problem. At present pergolide has been tried in only a small number of people with restless legs. Side effects include nausea, constipation and low blood pressure, so it is started at a low dose. There have been worries that, in rare cases, it could damage the valves of the heart.

- Levodopa with carbidopa (the drugs are combined in one tablet) is a dopamine drug for Parkinson's disease that has been used for severe cases of restless legs. The major drawback is that the symptoms initially improve, but tend to come back after a few months and are even worse than before. This occurs in about 80% of people. For this reason it is not used much.

Tranquillizers. Clonazepam is a tranquillizer that has been used for many years for restless legs. It can help if the problem is not too severe, but you may find you are drowsy in the day. If you are elderly, it is not a good choice, because you might become confused or have a fall.

Anti-epilepsy drugs, such as carbamazepine or gabapentin, are sometimes used to treat restless legs.

Restless legs is also known as Ekbom's syndrome, because Dr Ekbom, a Swedish neurologist, wrote about it in the 1940s

Useful contacts

RLS Australia is a sub-group of Sleep Disorders Australia. It is relatively new, operated by a small group of volunteers. The website is regularly updated with the most current information on research and treatments. The organization is currently developing a database of patient-recommended doctors.
www.rls.org.au

Restless Legs Syndrome Foundation is a US organization that provides information and support to sufferers. Its informative website tells you everything you could ever want to know about restless legs. Remember that some of the drugs mentioned might not be available in the UK, or might not be appropriate in your case.
www.rls.org

Ekbom Support Group is a UK non-profit organization to help people with restless legs. The newsletter section has tips for members.
www.ekbom.org.uk

RLS:UK is a group of doctors and other specialists who are interested in RLS. Its website is clear and simple, and contains reliable information. Some of its funding comes from the pharmaceutical company GlaxoSmithKline.
www.restlesslegs.org.uk/

Southern California RLS Support Group has an interesting 'Patient letters' section on its website, in which people explain how they cope with restless legs.
www.rlshelp.org

Bandolier RLS is an organisation related to Oxford University, UK. It looks at the best scientific evidence for health care. It now has a special website on restless legs, sponsored by the pharmaceutical company GlaxoSmithKline. The information on the site is independent, and it is brilliant for anyone who wants detailed scientific information about treatment options.
www.jr2.ox.ac.uk/bandolier/booth/booths/RLS.html

Scars

Most injuries to the skin result in scars – tattoos are one of the few exceptions. We all have some scars and, of course, anyone who has been damaged in an accident or had a surgical operation will be left with a scar.

We tend to scar worst on the shoulder and chest

Why scars occur

After injury to the skin, our body's priority is to make a rapid and strong repair. This would have been particularly important for primitive man, living in dirty and dangerous conditions. Although scars may look unattractive, they are an efficient way of healing. To regenerate tissue that was the same as before would take longer, with the wound remaining vulnerable during the process.

Surgeons are very keen to minimize scarring after their operations, because they know that scars can be distressing. Whenever possible, they make their incisions along lines in the skin that will heal best. They also take great care with 'sewing up' the skin. But sometimes a nasty scar cannot be avoided.

In northern countries, there are 80 million surgical operations a year, and almost all will result in some scarring. In addition, there are about 4 million burn scars a year

Questions to ask yourself if you are bothered by a scar

How recent is the scar? A recent scar will probably become less noticeable in time. Most scars take 2–3 years to become pale. If you see a doctor for advice about a scar that is less than a year old, you will probably be advised just to wait and see.

What is really bothering me? Is the appearance of the scar the main problem? Or does the scar interfere with movements (which may happen with a large scar over a joint, especially a burn scar)? Is the scar causing any other problems such as itching or discomfort?

How much trouble and expense am I prepared to go to? There are lots of treatments for scars. The simplest are creams and oils, or 'scar plasters' (special adhesive strips). You can buy these treatments from pharmacies, but you have to use them for some time, and it is uncertain whether there will be any result. So you could spend a lot of money for nothing. At the other end of the spectrum, doctors might advise cutting the scar out, which is a surgical operation.

What type of scar do I have? Not all scars are the same! Different types of scar need different types of treatment, so try to work out what type you have.

- Stretch marks are common after pregnancy (see page 253).

- Stretched scars can also occur after surgery. The original scar is satisfactory, but over a few weeks it gradually widens to become a pale, soft scar. These scars are not usually uncomfortable, but the appearance may bother you.
- Keloids are large, bulky, raised scars. They can be very unsightly. Unlike other scars, they gradually grow bigger. They are most common in black skin.
- Other raised scars (not all raised scars are keloids) can occur after burns or surgery but, unlike keloids, they do not keep growing. They are often red and itchy.
- Chickenpox and acne (see page 7) scars are flat, small and slightly sunken.
- Shrunken scars are common after burns and can cause problems if they lie across joints. The medical term for these scars is 'contractures'.

What can I expect from treatment? Whatever treatment you go for, it is best not to have too high expectations. Do not expect that any treatment will get rid of the scar completely, and then you will not be disappointed.

Adolescents and young adults tend to scar worse than the elderly

Treatments for scars

Creams and massage may help. Any sort of moisturizing cream will do; 'cocoa butter' cream is a popular choice. Apply the cream and then gently massage it into the scarred area with a circular movement. Do this for about 5 minutes twice a day. Do not use steroid cream; it will not help (*British Medical Journal* 2004;328:1329–30).

Sunblock is important if the scar is on exposed skin. Scars do not contain the normal pigments that protect skin, so burn easily.

Silicone gel can be bought from pharmacies. Silicone gel sheeting is used in hospitals to soften and flatten scars, but it is questionable whether the gel has an equivalent effect (*British Medical Journal* 2004;328:1329–30). It is also very expensive.

'Scar plasters' are sticking plasters that claim to reduce or soften the scar, but scientific evidence for their effect is scanty.

Consider camouflage with special make-up (see Useful contacts below).

We scar least inside the mouth

Specialist treatments. If simple treatments do not help, discuss the matter with your doctor. Explain clearly to your doctor what the problem is – whether it is the appearance of the scar, or discomfort, or perhaps interference with movement of a joint if it is near the scar. Your doctor can then refer you to an appropriate specialist. For example, acne scars might be best dealt with by a dermatologist, while a plastic surgeon would be the best person to deal with keloid scars.

Different scars need different treatments. The specialist might recommend compression therapy, laser therapy, steroid injections, or application of a special silicone sheet. A wide, stretched scar could be cut out by a surgeon to leave a thin, neat line. Keloid scars are particularly difficult to treat, because if they are cut away another keloid often forms in the new scar.

Do not be surprised if the specialist advises leaving the scar alone, and just waiting for it to become less noticeable; this might be the right thing to do.

Private treatment. If you decide to see a cosmetic surgeon privately, be very careful. Ask your family doctor for advice, and look at the section on choosing a cosmetic surgeon on page 339.

Acknowledgement

Special thanks to Dr A Bayat and Professors D A McGrouther and M J W Ferguson for their excellent article from which I obtained many of my facts on this topic (Bayat A, McGrouther DA, Ferguson MJW. Clinical review: skin scarring. *British Medical Journal* 2003;326:88–92).

If they are injured, lower vertebrates (such as salamanders) and invertebrates can grow new skin tissue without any scarring. Mammals cannot do this

Useful contacts

The Australasian College of Dermatologists website contains basic information about various skin diseases and problems. It has a helpful section on cosmetic dermatology under 'A–Z of skin'.
www.dermcoll.asn.au
www.dermcoll.asn.au/public/a-z_of_skin.asp#Cosmetic_Dermatology

Health*Insite* is an Australian government initiative aimed to improve the health of Australians by providing easy access to quality information about human health. The following link provides information about body image and how it affects your health and lifestyle.
www.healthinsite.gov.au/topics/Body_Image

Changing Faces is a non-profit organization giving help and support to people with any type of unusual facial appearance, and provides excellent information about cover-up make-up.
www.changingfaces.org.uk

British Red Cross Skin Camouflage Services are provided free (but a donation is welcome) at a number of hospitals. They use volunteers trained by the Red Cross. You will need a referral letter from your family doctor.
www.redcross.org.uk

Sexual worries

SEX – NO INTEREST

Sexual appetite (libido) tends to wax and wane – there are periods in our lives when we have little desire for sex, and other periods when sex assumes an overriding importance. Most of the time we are somewhere in between. So losing interest in sex is probably a temporary phase, and not a disaster. In fact it is only a problem if it means there is an imbalance between our desires and those of our partner, if it makes our partner feel unloved and frustrated, or if we ourselves feel unhappy because of it. It is also important to remember that most people are having much less sex than everyone else thinks, as has been shown by many surveys. All the same, there may be a reason for lack of sexual desire that can be remedied.

'All this fuss about sleeping together. For physical pleasure I'd sooner go to the dentist any day.' (Evelyn Waugh, British writer)

Reasons in both men and women

Depression is one of the most common reasons. Surveys show that about 2 out of 3 people with depression lose interest in sex, as a result of imbalances in brain biochemistry. So it is not something that you should blame yourself for.

Medications, such as antidepressants, tranquillizers and beta-blockers, can damp down sex drive.

Sexual side effects of various antidepressant drugs

Women

- Loss of desire
- Vaginal dryness (so intercourse is uncomfortable)
- Difficulty having an orgasm

Men

- Loss of desire
- Erection problems (see page 111)
- Delayed ejaculation (see page 107)

Stress and physical illnesses take their toll on every aspect of life, including sexuality. It is difficult to be enthusiastic about sex if you are worried, tired, in pain or generally under par.

Relationship problems of any kind can depress libido (although some couples find their sex life improves when other aspects of their relationship are rocky).

Something in the past can affect the present, such as memories of sexual abuse, or a demoralizing sexual relationship.

'I know it does make people happy, but to me it's just like having a cup of tea.'
(Cynthia Payne, after her acquittal on a charge of controlling prostitutes in a famous case in 1987)

Reasons in women

Infection and contraception. Worries about infection or a contraceptive method you are not comfortable with can trigger a loss of interest in sex. For example, you may have noticed some vaginal discharge or something about your partner's genitals, and are worrying that you or your partner could have a sexually transmitted disease. Some contraceptive pills, particularly those with a high progesterone content, can reduce sexual desire.

A new baby is very demanding of time and energy, hormone balances are changing and there may be soreness from stitches. So it is not surprising that 50% of women do not have much interest in sex for many months after childbirth (although 1 in 5 women feels more sexual than before). The American sexologists Masters and Johnson found that 47% of women had little desire for sex for at least 3 months after having a baby. Another survey asked women about their sex life 30 weeks after having a baby: only 25% were as sexually active as before; most said their sexual desire was much reduced; and 22% had almost stopped having any sex at all.

Breastfeeding causes temporary vaginal dryness and discomfort (because of the high levels of the breastfeeding hormone, prolactin), making sex seem even less attractive.

Painful intercourse is obviously a turn-off (see page 228). This can happen because the vagina is dry (see page 232) or for various other reasons. In some women, the pelvic and nearby muscles clamp up so strongly when intercourse is attempted that it is uncomfortable, painful or even downright impossible; this is called vaginismus.

Reasons in men

Pressure to perform well in bed seems to be increasing – fuelled by media images of the ever-potent, ever-ready male. A man is expected always to be able to perform sexually. At the same time, modern society expects him to deal with increasing stresses in the workplace, to do his share of household tasks, to be an intellectual companion and emotional support to his partner, and to be a perfect father. It is no wonder that he finds he cannot perform sexually. Over the past decade, the number of couples coming to Relate (a relationship counselling organization in the UK) with difficulties blamed on lack of sexual desire in the male partner has doubled.

Heavy drinking is a common cause of loss of interest in sex (and problems with erections). This is because alcohol eventually reduces the production of testosterone by the testes, interferes with processing of testosterone (male hormone) by the cells of the body, and affects the parts of the brain that control hormone balance.

A low testosterone level is seldom the reason for a loss of sex drive, but your doctor can check this quite easily.

Questions to ask yourself

Is this really a problem, are my expectations unrealistic, what do I really want, is it affecting my relationship? You and your partner may feel the situation is quite acceptable. On the other hand, it may be affecting your self-esteem and your relationship.

Am I depressed? Feelings of sadness, hopelessness and helplessness, with lack of energy and disturbed sleep, and an inability to find anything enjoyable are symptoms of depression. Modern antidepressants are very effective at treating depression, and are not addictive. As your depression gradually lifts, your sex life will improve. If this does not happen, it may be that the tablets are curing the depression, but their side effect is making the sex problem worse. Do not stop taking the medication; mention the problem to your doctor, who will be able to change the dose or use a different antidepressant.

Am I drinking too much? If so, try to cut down.

Have I started taking any new medications? A drug is unlikely to be the cause if you had already gone off sex before starting it, but otherwise it is worth checking with your doctor to see if any medication could be responsible.

Is there any other physical reason? If you are tired or physically unwell, it is quite reasonable to wish to put your sex life on hold for a while.

Is there any specific aspect of our sex life that is putting me off? A relatively simple problem, such as the type of contraception or pain during sex (see below), can be dealt with by a visit to your doctor or family planning clinic. However, there may be a problem that is easy to identify, but less easy to deal with. This could be anything – your partner's standards of cleanliness, the type of sexual activities your partner wants, lack of privacy, a suspicion that your partner has a sexually transmitted disease, or a triggering of unpleasant memories of sexual abuse. Unfortunately, this type of problem does not usually go away on its own, but a counsellor (see Useful contacts on page 235) will be able to help you find the best way of dealing with it.

Is my loss of interest in sex really because I am unhappy about other aspects of the relationship? If so, tackle these issues, perhaps with the help of a counsellor.

37% of men have sex less than once a fortnight
(MORI/Esquire poll of 800 men aged 18–45, 1992)

PAINFUL SEX

There are lots of reasons why sex may become painful, and even when the problem has been sorted out, it can take a long time before sex becomes enjoyable again. You definitely need help from your doctor for this symptom – it is not something you can sort out on your own.

Before you see your doctor, try to be clear in your mind whether the pain occurs:

- when your partner attempts to put his penis into your vagina (superficial pain)
- when the erect penis is fully inserted and during thrusting (deep pain)
- in the hours after sex
- in another part of the body, such as the hip joints.

Causes of pain at the entrance of the vagina during sex

Lack of arousal and a dry vagina is one of the most common reasons (see page 232).

After childbirth, some women experience pain when they start having sex again. It is more likely after the first baby. Sometimes it is due to an episiotomy (that is, the cut made during the delivery) that has not healed properly. The pain almost always goes away after about 3 months.

Infections, such as thrush or herpes, cause soreness of the vulva (the lips round the opening of the vagina). Vaginal discharge causes chafing of the skin, which makes the problem worse.

Blocked Bartholin's glands. Bartholin's glands are just inside the opening of the vagina, one on each side. They help produce lubrication for sex. If the opening of a Bartholin's gland becomes blocked, it swells up into a cyst. Bacteria may enter the cyst, turning it into a painful abscess.

Skin irritants such as perfumed soaps, bubble baths, biological (which means that they contain enzymes) washing powders, 'intimate' deodorants and spermicides can all make the vulva sore.

When sex causes pain deep inside

Pelvic inflammatory disease is an infection of the Fallopian tubes (the tubes, one on each side, that carry the egg from the ovaries to the uterus). These tubes lie close to the top of the vagina, so sex causes a deep pain.

Endometriosis is a peculiar condition, in which some of the tissue that normally lines the uterus (the womb) lies outside the uterus, in the pelvic cavity. No one knows why it occurs, though it seems to be quite common. Many women have no symptoms from it, but if the tissue is lying behind the uterus it can cause painful sex, especially on deep thrusting. A sign of endometriosis is bad period pains – especially if they last throughout the period.

Pelvic pain syndrome. For 2 out of every 3 women with deep pain during sex, no cause can be found; you may have to accept that you have pelvic pain syndrome. This syndrome is not fully understood, but it is related to stress. One possible, but not proven, explanation is that, in some women, chronic stress alters the flow of blood in the veins of the pelvis, so that the pelvis becomes congested. If you are easily aroused during sex, but have difficulty reaching orgasm, the problem becomes worse because the pelvic congestion is not relieved. You may then experience a pain that persists after sex for some hours.

Lack of arousal. Intercourse will be uncomfortable if penetration occurs before you are aroused. This is partly because of lack of lubrication, but also because with sexual arousal the upper part of the vagina balloons open. This helps to lift the womb up and away from the thrusts of the penis. If penetration occurs too early, there may be a pain or discomfort felt deep in the middle of the pelvis with each thrust.

Other causes include irritable bowel syndrome (IBS) and cystitis – both the bladder and bowel lie close to the vagina.

VAGINA TOO TIGHT

The vagina itself is never too small to accommodate a penis – remember that its walls are stretchy enough to allow a full-sized baby to pass along it. But it can seem too small for sex if the muscles at its entrance go into a spasm when your partner tries to insert his penis. This is a fairly rare condition called vaginismus.

Some women with vaginismus can insert a tampon without any problem, but others find that trying to insert anything – a tampon, a finger or a penis – makes the muscles contract. Women with vaginismus often avoid having cervical smears, because they think it will be painful or impossible.

Very occasionally, the penis cannot be inserted because the hymen (which is the membrane at the entrance to the vagina) is unusually tough, but this is very rare indeed.

How the woman feels. Vaginismus is a very distressing condition. It is very painful if your partner attempts to push his way in, and you may feel wary that he may do this. You may also have feelings of anger, guilt and inadequacy, and fear that your partner may leave you. Some women withdraw from all physical contact – even holding hands – in case it leads to sex.

How the partner feels. Partners are usually confused and worried. Your partner will hate the idea of causing you any pain. He may think that his sexual technique is at fault.

What causes vaginismus?

It is really a deep-rooted phobia of penetration, and perhaps of pregnancy or childbirth. The reason is different for each woman: it can result from some unresolved sexual conflict, from sexual abuse or from a belief that sexual activity is undesirable. You may have had a painful vaginal condition that has left you with a conditioned fear of sex.

Vaginismus should not be confused with frigidity; women with vaginismus are often sexually responsive, but can not tolerate penetration.

Treatment

Vaginismus can be helped. Relate, a counselling organization in the UK, reports that of 3693 women seen over a 2-year period, 80% improved with therapy.

Psychosexual counselling. The therapy is not at all frightening. You will be taught how to relax your vaginal muscles and eventually to insert a small tampon. In due course you will learn to insert larger tampons. If you have a partner, the therapist will start by telling you not to attempt sex. Instead, you will be encouraged to resume non-genital physical contact in very small steps, such as holding hands, sitting close together or putting an arm round each other. Quite late in the programme, you and your partner will be shown how you can insert his penis yourself, as if it were a tampon; he lies on his back and is not allowed to move at this stage. Only at the very end of the therapy programme will you be encouraged to have actual sex.

What your doctor can do. To get this psychosexual therapy, it is best to talk to your doctor. Explain that you have a problem with sex, and that this problem means that you have not been able to have sex at all. Your doctor will be able to check that there is no physical problem (such as a tough hymen) and will then arrange for psychosexual counselling as outlined above. A few doctors are specially trained in this area and will do the therapy themselves.

In the UK, if you do not want your doctor to be involved you can contact Relate (see Useful contacts on page 235 or look in your phone book for your local branch). Relate provides very good psychosexual counselling, but there may be a waiting list.

SEX AND AGEING

No one is too old for an enjoyable sex life, and many surveys have confirmed that older people continue to enjoy sexual activity into their 80s and 90s. According to a report in the *Independent* newspaper (19 May 2000), a survey has shown that over-65s in the UK spend more time making love than younger people. Some 44% of the over-65s said that they spent more than 2 hours a week making love, compared with 15% of those aged 16–25 years and fewer than 26% of those aged 25–64 years.

On the other hand, for many older people, sex assumes less importance than it did during their younger years.

How ageing can affect sex

Good points

- Reduced frequency of sexual desire
- Likely to have more leisurely lifestyle, with more time for sex
- Likely to know each other very well, so greater understanding of each other's sexuality
- Although less frequent, sex may be more enjoyable

Bad points

- Reduced frequency of sexual desire
- Arousal takes longer, and needs more genital stimulation
- Reduced lubrication (women)
- Poor body image (a feeling of being unattractive and undesirable)
- Erections less hard and ejaculations less powerful (men)
- More likely to be taking medication for other medical conditions (e.g. blood pressure) which may affect erections (men)
- More likely to have conditions that can affect sexual activity or cause anxiety about having sex
- Emotional 'baggage'
- Lack of privacy if not living in own home
- More difficult to find a new relationship

Common problems as you get older

Problems for women

Vaginal dryness and soreness is the most common physical problem for women and makes intercourse uncomfortable (see page 228 and 311). Sexual stimulation no longer causes a sudden increase in lubricating secretions. And because more and more older men are now using effective medications for impotence, many older women are having sex again after a break of several years. This can be problematic, as the vagina can feel uncomfortable and sore. Thrush (see page 139) is another possible reason for vaginal soreness.

Tenderness of the clitoris, so that friction easily makes it sore, is another common problem.

Symptoms of cystitis. Bruising of the urethra (the opening through which urination occurs) during sex is more likely in older women because their skin tissue is thinner. This can lead to a burning sensation when urine is passed after sex, and the woman may also feel she needs to pass small amounts of urine frequently. This is known as 'urethral syndrome'. Although it feels like cystitis, it is not caused by an infection.

Less desire for sex occurs in some women after the menopause. In all premenopausal women, the ovary secretes 'female' hormone (oestrogen), and also a small amount of 'male' hormone (androgen). The androgen is important for sexual desire (libido). After the menopause, the levels of both types of hormone fall. The fall in androgen level may be one reason why some women feel less desire for sex in later life.

Loss of self-esteem may also lead to less desire for sex. If you feel despair over lost youth and slimness, and believe that some of your sexual attractiveness has gone, it may be hard to respond to a partner.

Worries about your partner. You may also worry that your partner is not really up to it, particularly if he has angina or has had a heart attack – some women are terrified that their partner will die during sex and this, unsurprisingly, puts them off.

Problems for men. Men have different problems to contend with as they get older. Some sexual slowing down is natural.

- For older men to become aroused, the penis needs to be fondled – sexy thoughts are not enough.
- Waking with an erection becomes less common.
- Erections may take longer to develop and be less hard.
- If the erection is lost before ejaculation, it is less easy to regain.
- Ejaculation becomes less powerful, with a smaller volume of semen produced, and more difficult to control.
- It usually takes longer to become aroused again after orgasm.

This slowing down is a long way from impotence, but it can cause panic. You may fear that you are going into a speedy sexual decline and will soon be unable to perform at all. Some men take any slight reduction in their body's response – however marginal, and whatever its cause – as the first sign of the onset of impotence. In fact, almost any illness will interfere with sexuality for a while, but the danger is that this 'performance anxiety' will take over, so the fear becomes a self-fulfilling prophecy.

With increasing age, men are more likely to be taking drugs for high blood pressure (hypertension); many of these can cause problems with erections. You are also more likely to have a condition, such as diabetes, which can affect erection and ejaculation.

Some men also have a fixed idea that sex means vigorous, thrusting intercourse with the man on top (the 'missionary position'). But as a man gets older, he may find this more and more difficult, or a heart condition may make him frightened to try. So he may start to regard himself as a sexual failure and give up, instead of experimenting with new positions and new ways of gaining satisfaction.

Problems for both men and women

Other illnesses. For both men and women, other illnesses can interfere with sexual enjoyment. For example, breathlessness from a chronic chest problem, lack of mobility from arthritis or from a stroke, or simply obesity can make sex difficult.

Emotional 'baggage'. A relationship that has been poor for years may become worse as the older couple find themselves spending more time together.

Finding a partner. Older people are often on their own, and finding a partner may be difficult.

How you can help yourself

Remember that a sex life is not compulsory. The point of your sex life is to bring greater happiness to you and your partner. If you both feel happy and relieved not to continue with your sex life, that is fine. But equally, if you both wish to have an enjoyable sex life there is no reason why you should not. Sex is not just for the young and beautiful!

Share your expectations. If one partner has needs or expectations that are not being met by the other, sort the problem out rather than let resentment, anger or guilt take over. Counselling (see Useful contacts on page 235) can be very helpful in this situation.

Try to avoid becoming 'performance conscious'. Do not interpret natural sexual 'slowing down' as being near to impotence. In fact, the natural slowing down of your sexual responses may make you more in tune with your partner's needs, because it may mean that stroking and cuddling become more important.

Sort out relationship problems. You may feel that your relationship with your partner has been unsatisfactory for so many years that it is pointless to try to do anything about it. In fact, it is never too late to try to improve things, particularly as you and your partner may have many years ahead in which you will be increasingly in each other's company.

Ignore setbacks. If you have a sexual setback, do not assume it is the 'beginning of the end' of your sex life. It is natural for an illness, or a period of depression, to make you lose the desire for sex, the ability to perform sexually or the ability to respond to your partner. When you or your partner feel better, your sex life will improve again. If it does not, talk to your doctor as there may be a simple explanation (for example, you may have been put on some medication that is affecting your sexuality).

If you are worried that sex could damage your heart, or that you or your partner might have a heart attack during sex, talk to your doctor. If you have had a heart attack or heart surgery the hospital should have given you advice about when to resume your sex life.

If impotence is the problem, see your doctor. Do not accept impotence as being just a normal part of growing old. If you can not get an erection that is sufficient for intercourse, discuss it with your doctor, no matter how old you are. There may be a reason that can be put right and there are various methods of improving erections (see the section on impotence on page 111). Viagra is as safe in elderly men as it is in younger men. A study of Viagra in the over-65s reported a 69% improvement (*Journal of Gerontology* 2001;56:M113–M119).

Use lubricants. Whatever a woman's age, sex should not be painful. If it is, it is important to find out why. If a dry vagina is making sex uncomfortable, special lubricants or hormone treatment will help (even if it is many years since the menopause). Apply the lubricant generously over and around the clitoris and urethra, as well as the vagina, to relieve clitoral soreness and prevent urethral syndrome.

Similarly, if you are using a hormone cream, apply a small amount to the clitoris and around the urethra. For further information, look at the section on vaginal dryness on pages 232 and 311.

Try more foreplay. Remember that older women need more foreplay to become aroused. Inserting the penis before the woman is fully lubricated (perhaps because the man secretly worries that he will lose his erection) will cause discomfort or even pain.

New partners. If you have a new partner, be aware that you need to practise safe sex to avoid the risk of sexually transmitted infection, whatever your age. In the past 5 years in the UK, the numbers of people with chlamydia, gonorrhoea and syphilis have increased three-fold in the over-65s.

SEX DURING PERIODS

- Sex during a period is really a matter of culture (in some cultures menstruation is considered 'unclean') and personal preference.
- Menstrual fluid consists of blood and tissue from the lining of the uterus (womb), with some of the normal 'friendly' bacteria from the vagina. It contains nothing dirty or harmful, so contact with menstrual fluid will not cause irritation of the penis or any other problems.
- Sex at this time will not harm the woman. The menstrual fluid seeps out of the normal small opening in the cervix (see page 189). This hole does not become any larger during a period, so there is no need to worry that the penis might poke up into the uterus.

The period is the least fertile time of the woman's cycle, so it is one of the safest times for avoiding pregnancy. However, it is possible to conceive at this time – sperm can live for several days, and ovulation could occur earlier than usual, so it might be possible for the sperm to meet up with an egg. To be safe, use contraception.

Remember to remove a tampon beforehand, otherwise it might become pushed up into a corner of the vagina during sex, and then forgotten.

Useful contacts

Andrology Australia provides access to quality and authenticated information to improve understanding and knowledge of the range, causes and treatment options of male reproductive health disorders. Click onto 'Your health' to access a range of information on sexual disorders.
www.andrologyaustralia.org

Health*Insite* is an Australian government initiative aimed to improve the health of Australians by providing easy access to quality information about human health. By following the links below, you will find information on issues about sex and growing older, as well as individual link to sexual health for men and women.
www.healthinsite.gov.au/topics/Sexual_Health_for_Men
www.healthinsite.gov.au/topics/Sexual_Health_for_Women
www.healthinsite.gov.au/topics/Sex_in_Later_Years

Impotence Australia is a non-profit organization that was set up to decrease the suffering of men with impotence and their partners by providing quality telephone counselling and information fact sheets on many sexual issues. On the 'Get the facts' section of the website there is a number of topics on impotence-related treatments.
www.impotenceaustralia.com.au

Relate counsels couples of all ages and in all types of relationship (you do not have to be married). To find out about counselling or sex therapy in your area, contact your local branch of Relate in your telephone directory, or look at the 'Want advice' section on their website or contact the national office.
www.relate.org.uk

The British Heart Foundation has information about sexual activity and heart disease in the 'Any questions' section of their website. The foundation also supplies a video called 'Sex and heart disease: a guide for patients and their partners', which has advice and information from heart specialists and couples who have been in a similar situation.
www.bhf.org.uk

Arthritis Care provides practical information for people with arthritis, including publications, support networks and discussion forums.
www.arthritiscare.org.uk

The British Association for Sexual and Relationship Therapy has a list of psychosexual clinics and qualified sex therapists throughout the UK. These therapists work privately, so they will charge.
www.basrt.org.uk

The Sexual Dysfunction Association provides information for men suffering from impotence, and women experiencing problems with arousal and/or reaching orgasm.
www.sda.uk.net

Diabetes UK (formerly the British Diabetic Association) has information on all aspects of diabetes, including sexual problems.
www.diabetes.org.uk

Cruse Bereavement Care provides counselling for anyone who has been bereaved, practical advice and social contacts.
www.crusebereavementcare.org.uk

CRY-SIS offers support to parents of babies who cry excessively or will not sleep. The website list some useful publications, as well as a contact for helpline support.
www.crys-sis.org.uk

Depression Alliance is a self-help group for people suffering from depression. They have a wide range of publications covering various aspects of depression, which can downloaded free from the website.
www.depressionalliance.org

Parentline is a confidential service offering help and support to anyone in a parenting role. The website has a FAQ section and you can email them for further help. A variety of their free publications can also be downloaded from their website.
www.parentlineplus.org.uk

National Endometriosis Society gives information about pelvic pain, and provides support to women with endometriosis.
www.endo.org.uk

Institute of Psychosexual Medicine is a training organization for doctors, but it does have some information for patients on its website. www.ipm.org.uk

Shaky hands

Normally, our hands shake very, very slightly all the time we are awake. This is because the tiny muscle fibres in our hands and arms constantly contract and relax at random. It is only when shakiness of our hands begins to interfere with writing, holding a cup of coffee or using a knife and fork that it becomes a problem. When people notice their hands are shaky, they often start to worry that they have Parkinson's disease, but this is usually not the case.

If you are worried about shakiness, consult your doctor rather than try to work out the cause yourself. There are many varieties of shakiness that are difficult to describe, but doctors can recognize the common types easily from experience. Also, some simple tests, such as a blood test for thyroid overactivity, might be appropriate. Your doctor may use the word 'tremor' to describe shakiness that consists of small movements.

Common causes

Anxiety. We all become trembly if we are angry, stressed, anxious ('shaking with nerves') or very tired.

Low blood sugar causes shakiness because the nerves and muscles are deprived of fuel. The adrenaline system responds by kicking in, and this can make the shakiness worse for a while. The circumstances will make it obvious if this is what is happening in your case. A low blood sugar is most likely to occur if you eat a lot of sugary snack foods; these raise the blood sugar sharply, but then it plummets down again. The answer is to eat more slowly digested carbohydrates, such as porridge for breakfast instead of a sweet cereal and fruit instead of sweet puddings. Low blood sugar can also occur after excessive exercise.

Too much coffee and tea can make you a bit shaky, particularly in combination with a low blood sugar. So cut down your intake of coffee or strong tea, and avoid snack 'meals' that are mainly sweet foods.

'Essential tremor' is one of the most common types of shakiness. Instead of contracting at random, the tiny muscle fibres contract and relax together ('synchronization'), resulting in more noticeable movements. (In medicine, the word 'essential' has a special meaning – it is used to describe a condition that is not caused by any other medical condition or disease, but simply exists on its own.)

- Essential tremor is unusual in young people, but affects 1 in 20 of the population over the age of 40.
- It tends to run in families, so some of your close relatives may also have it.
- It usually affects the hands, often the head, and sometimes the voice and other parts of the body as well.
- It becomes worse when you use your hands to do something, such as picking up a small object, or if you try to maintain a position, such as holding a cup steady. If you rest your hands quietly on your lap, the shaking usually stops.

- It is uncontrollable and does not mean you are 'nervy' or 'neurotic' (although, frustratingly, it becomes worse when you are anxious).
- An alcoholic drink often improves it, but obviously you should not overdo this remedy.
- If the shaking is really troublesome, your doctor can prescribe a drug such as a beta-blocker or primidone. Avoid too much coffee and strong tea.

Less common causes

Medications can sometimes be responsible, in particular some asthma medications, some antidepressants and lithium. A few medications, such as some tranquillizers, can cause shakiness if you stop taking them suddenly. Similarly, a heavy drinker may get 'the shakes' the morning after a binge.

Parkinson's disease is much less common than essential tremor. It does cause shaking of the hands but, unlike essential tremor, the shaking is worse when you are resting and not using the hand. The shaking in Parkinson's disease is called 'pill rolling' because it is like rolling a small pill between your thumb and the side of your index finger.

Overactive thyroid is more common in women than in men, and occurs most commonly in people in their 20s and 30s. If your thyroid is overactive, shakiness will not be the only symptom; for example, you usually lose weight even though you are eating well. Your doctor can do a blood test to check your thyroid hormone levels.

Useful contacts

Health*Insite* is an Australian government initiative aimed to improve the health of Australians by providing easy access to quality information about human health. Follow the link to find information on Parkinson's disease.
www.healthinsite.gov.au/topics/Parkinson_s_Disease

Parkinson's Australia (PA) is the country's peak body representing all of the state organizations, which offer support to people with Parkinson's disease and their carers. The website has some good general information about the disease as well as link to other national and international-related websites on Parkinson's disease.
www.parkinsons.org.au

Parkinson's Disease Society is a UK non-profit organization. The website has an A–Z of information about Parkinson's disease.
www.parkinsons.org.uk

National Parkinson Foundation is a US non-profit organization with a very informative website about Parkinson's disease. The website has a 'Tremor' questionnaire to help you decide what sort of shakiness you have.
www.parkinson.org

The American Academy of Family Physicians has a fact sheet about 'essential tremor' on its website. There is also a link to a detailed article for doctors written in 2003.
www.aafp.org/20031015/1553ph.html

Shaving rash

Shaving rash is a common problem for men with curly hair, or for women who shave their bikini-line pubic hair. (Pubic hair is naturally more curly than head hair.) The medical term is 'pseudofolliculitis barbae' or 'sycosis barbae'; it is a syndrome also called 'barber's itch' or 'razor lumps'.

Normally, the weight of each individual hair straightens it slightly. When you shave, a remnant of hair is left in the hair follicle. As this starts to grow out of the follicle, it may immediately curve round into the surrounding skin, because there is nothing to keep it straight. The ingrowing hair irritates the skin and can cause a lumpy reaction, especially in black skin (*Journal of the American Academy of Dermatology* 2002;46(2 Suppl):5113–9). The next time you shave, you will nick the tops of the lumps, worsening the inflammation and perhaps allowing an infection to occur.

Since 1957, all Disney workers had to be clean shaven (although Walt Disney himself had a moustache). This ban was lifted in 2000, allowing workers to grow moustaches, but not beards

How to prevent shaving rash

Do not pull on the skin. Hairs are most likely to ingrow if you pull the skin while you are shaving, to get a close shave. This makes the hairs pop out of the follicle. Afterwards, the cut tip retracts into the follicle and then turns into the wall of the follicle.

Shave in the direction of the growth of the hairs. If the hairs naturally grow downwards, pull the razor downwards.

Avoid a close shave. The aim is to shave the hairs just above the skin, when they have already emerged from the hair follicle. Use an electric razor or an ordinary single-blade razor. Double-blade or triple-blade razors give too close a shave.

Prepare your skin before shaving, by using a good shaving gel, oil or foam, and thoroughly wet it into the hairs.

Police authorities in Assam, India have paid a monthly bonus to an officer who grows a moustache. One officer said 'Having a big moustache is a symbol of masculinity and that helps you to excel in your professional duties as people are afraid to challenge you' (UK Daily Telegraph*)*

How to deal with shaving rash. Curing shaving rash is tedious and will leave you with stubble for a few weeks.

Analyse the problem. Inspect the area with the help of a magnifying mirror. You may be able to see the hairs curling inwards. Have a good look for tiny yellow pustules, and redness and inflammation around the hair follicles or the tips of the ingrowing hairs – this could mean infection with staphylococci bacteria.

Beards grow faster in spring, possibly indicating a seasonal variation in androgen (male hormone) production

If you can see them, try to get the tips of the ingrowing hairs out of the skin. Soak a towel in hot water and put it on the skin for a few minutes to soften the hairs. Then very carefully, using clean tweezers, pull the end of the hair out of the bump. Do not pull the whole hair out of the skin – just the loose end. Then with small scissors cut off the end of the hair that is curling back, quite close to the skin.

Stop shaving. Grow a beard and cut off the hair close to the skin with nail scissors (designer stubble look). As the hair grows, it should grow slightly straighter, and not grow back into the skin. If the problem is in the pubic area, stop shaving and remove the hair after a few weeks with a depilatory cream if you wish.

Sharing electric razors has been blamed for spreading diseases such as viral hepatitis

If you think the rash is infected, dab on a mild antiseptic such as tea-tree oil. The infection may clear up on its own if you stop shaving. If it does not improve after a few days, see your doctor again; you might have a fungal infection.

Exfoliants remove the dead cells from the surface of the skin. They will not prevent the hairs turning in, but they may help to flatten the bumps. So if the bumps are slow to settle, exfoliants might be worth trying. Do not use them if your skin is inflamed or infected. There are various types of exfoliants. Facial scrubs usually contain tiny particles of pumice. Alpha hydroxy acids (fruit acids), in creams and face washes, have an exfoliant action. Alpha hydroxy acid creams are often labelled as 'anti-ageing'; check the ingredients label.

There have been cases of men who fail to grow a beard on one side of the face, but this is very rare

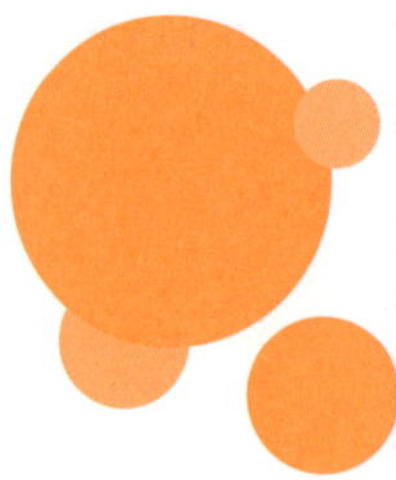

Shyness – excessive

Many people think they are shyer than they actually are. According to psychologists at Stanford University in California, 30–40% of people say they are shy, but when their behaviour is observed only 15–20% behave in a shy manner (but of course they may still be feeling shy inside).

An extreme form of shyness, known as 'social anxiety disorder' or 'social phobia', affects 1–2% of men and 2–3% of women.

What social anxiety disorder feels like

- You are terrified of being the centre of attention. You worry that everyone is looking at you and judging you, and that you will make a fool of yourself.
- In a social situation, you may experience blushing, sweating, trembling or palpitations.
- You fear being introduced to other people. At a party, you hover round the edge of the room or stay in the kitchen, avoiding being involved.
- Even the thought of socializing may bring on your anxiety.
- Afterwards, the unpleasant feelings may remain as you worry about what other people thought of you.
- It is not that you prefer to be alone – in fact, you want to connect with others, but intense self-consciousness makes this impossible for you.
- Eating and drinking in public may be very stressful.
- You may be able to interact with new people on a one-to-one basis, but go into a total panic if you have to speak or perform in front of a number of people.
- You may drink too much, in an attempt to give yourself extra confidence.

What causes social anxiety?

About 70% of people with social anxiety disorder are female. It usually starts at about 11–15 years of age, and onset after 25 years of age is rare. It seems to run in families, but the cause is not really understood. Recent research has suggested that you are more likely to have social phobia if your parents were overprotective or rejecting.

How to help yourself

Opting out of social situations is not the answer. You have to face your fears. A helpful strategy is to join a club that focuses on a specific hobby that interests you; take a friend with you to the first meeting.

If you are troubled by blushing or sweating, look at the sections on blushing and flushing (see page 49) and sweating (see page 255).

Do not drink too much alcohol trying to make yourself relax. People with social anxiety can develop serious alcohol problems. Instead, seek help from your doctor.

Treatments for shyness

Treatments for shyness are increasingly available, especially for social anxiety disorder. The first step is to recognize that your excessive shyness is a real disability that needs help. You then need to explain to your doctor that it is affecting your life, and that you think it is beyond ordinary shyness. The very fact that you have social anxiety will make it difficult for you to ask for help. One way round this difficulty is to take some information about social anxiety disorder with you (see Useful contacts on page 243) and say to your doctor, 'I've been reading this, and I think I have this problem.' Alternatively, you could write a letter to your doctor beforehand to prepare the ground.

Social skills training is one possibility. This will teach you simple social skills, such as how to start a conversation.

Cognitive therapy teaches you to think of the social situation in a new way, instead of focusing on your own inadequacies. It is helpful to more than 50% of sufferers (*Archives of General Psychiatry* 2004;61:1005–13). In some parts of the UK, it is available under the NHS.

Cognitive therapy for social anxiety disorder (social phobia)

A person with social anxiety has very negative thoughts, such as:

- 'If the conversation stops, it will be my fault'
- 'I won't be able to think of anything to say'
- 'I'm boring'
- 'I'm a social failure'

Cognitive therapy teaches the person to test out and then to correct these thoughts, for example by:

- deliberately pausing during a conversation and seeing what happens
- looking for real signs (rather than imaginary ones) of whether the other person actually is bored
- recognizing that a conversation may dry up because the other person has nothing to say – in general, concentrate on past successes rather than failures.

Medication can helpful

- 'Selective serotonin-reuptake inhibitors', or SSRIs for short, help to ease the anxiety symptoms and panic feelings that go with social anxiety.
- In the past, tranquillizing drugs, such as diazepam, were given to people who were over-anxious in social situations. They are now used mainly for people who do not benefit from SSRIs. They can become addictive.
- 'Inhibitors of monoamine oxidase' can make you feel more able to participate socially.
- Beta-blockers control the physical signs of anxiety, such as shakiness, so they can make you calmer for a specific event, such as public speaking.
- Gabapentin is a medication used for epilepsy, but it can help people with social anxiety.

Useful contacts

Social Anxiety Australia is an Australia-wide service empowering people in Australia who live with social anxiety disorder by providing information and education, common Q&As, treatments and therapies available to overcome this disorder.
www.socialanxiety.com.au

beyondblue is a national, independent, non-profit organization working to address issues associated with depression, anxiety and related substance-misuse disorders in Australia. The website provides a national list of medical practitioners and clinical psychologists with expertise in the recognition and treatment of depression, anxiety and related substance-misuse disorders.
www.beyondblue.org.au

National Phobics Society provides help with anxiety and panic attacks, and its website has a good section on social anxiety disorder (social phobia).
www.phobics-society.org.uk

Social Anxiety UK is an organization that aims to raise awareness of social anxiety and give help and information to sufferers.
www.social-anxiety.org.uk

Royal College of Psychiatrists has a free leaflet on social phobia on its website.
www.rcpsych.ac.uk/info/help/socphob/index.htm

Triumph Over Phobia runs a national network of self-help groups, and its website gives help and advice about phobias. .
www.triumphoverphobia.com

At ease is an excellent website for stressed teenagers and young adults.
www.rethink.org/at-ease/

BBC Health has a mental health website with information about many mental health problems and their treatments.
www.bbc.co.uk/health/conditions/mental_health/index.shtml

Snoring

Snoring is very common and is more likely the older you are.

- Among 30–35 year-olds, about 20% of men and 5% of women snore regularly.
- By the age of 60 years, about 60% of men and 40% of women snore regularly.

Snoring may be a sign of disturbed sleep, meaning you are less alert during the day. Lots of couples row about snoring, and often sleep in separate rooms because of it. Sharing a bed with a snorer can seriously affect the partner's sleep; this was proved by a study in the US (reported in the *Mayo Clinic Proceedings* 1999;74:939–66), which showed that when snoring was eliminated, the bed partners got an extra hour of sleep each night.

41.5% of the UK population snore (British Snoring and Sleep Apnoea Association)

What causes snoring?

When we are awake, the muscles of the throat hold the throat open, so that air passes in smoothly as we breathe. During sleep, these muscles relax and the throat sags inwards, causing air turbulence, particularly as we breathe in. Snoring occurs when the roof of the mouth (soft palate and uvula – the uvula is the piece of tissue that dangles at the back of the throat), and sometimes the base of the tongue as well, starts to vibrate intermittently as a result of excessive turbulence. (Interestingly, astronauts hardly ever snore in space, because without the pull of gravity, the throat and tongue will not sag in.)

Snoring is particularly likely to happen if you:

- have a small jaw and narrow throat and/or a large uvula and base of tongue
- drink alcohol or take sleeping pills, because both of these make the throat muscles very relaxed, and so worsen turbulence in the throat
- are overweight, particularly if you have a fat neck (collar size over 43 cm or 17 inches) (This is because more muscle power is needed to hold the throat open if the neck is fat, and so the throat will become more narrow as the muscles relax during sleep.)

Snoring is said to have been useful to primitive man, frightening away predators at night

- breathe through your mouth rather than your nose (When you breathe through your mouth the air hits the back of the throat head-on, increasing turbulence, whereas in nose breathing, it enters the throat in parallel with it. This is why any blockage of the nose will cause snoring; we all snore when we have a cold. Some people have a permanent blockage from polyps in the nose or because the wall between the two sides of the nose – nasal septum – is shifted to one side.)

A study at the University of Erlangen, Germany, found that many young people snore; 61% of medical students (both male and female) have been told so by their partners

- smoke, because smoking may cause swelling and inflammation of the lining of the throat
- sleep on your back, because when the muscles are relaxed, the throat is particularly narrow in this position
- eat a large meal before bed, because a full stomach presses upwards on the diaphragm and can lead to laboured breathing
- have relatives who snore as snoring tends to run in families.
- have a round-shaped head rather than a long, thin head (In round-headed people, the tissue has to fall back a shorter distance to narrow the throat.) (*Sleep and Breathing* 2001;5:79-91).

Is snoring dangerous?

Snoring is not a disease. In fact, it is so common that one could argue that it is almost normal.

Sleep apnoea. Loud snoring, however, may be a sign that the relaxed throat muscles are allowing the throat to become excessively narrow during sleep, and not enough air is getting through with each breath (*Chest* 2003;124:2309–23). Sometimes breathing stops altogether for 10 seconds or more, until the body's arousal system makes it start again – this is called sleep apnoea syndrome. It is nine times more common in men than in women, particularly those who are overweight, and most sufferers are loud snorers. Men with a collar size of 43 cm (17 inches) have a 30% chance of suffering from sleep apnoea syndrome.

In sleep apnoea, you may wake up quickly with a feeling of choking or shortness of breath, or you may hardly wake at all, but just enough for the throat muscles to tone up and pull the throat open again. This can happen hundreds of times a night without you being aware of it. Not surprisingly, you will feel tired during the day because of the disturbed sleep and may be aware that sleep is not a refreshing experience. Your bed partner may notice that you are very restless during your sleep or that you seem to stop breathing for a few moments, with resumption of breathing signalled by sudden loud snoring.

To see if you are excessively sleepy in the day, check your score on the Epworth Sleepiness Scale (see below). A total score between 0 and 8 is normal.

A doctor at the University of Minnesota, US, found that the snores of 12% of people referred to his clinic exceeded 55 decibels – the maximum legal outdoor night-time noise in Minnesota. 'They could get arrested for disturbing the peace – that's how loud the noise is,' he said

Epworth Sleepiness Scale

For each situation

- Score 0 if you would never doze off
- Score 1 for a slight chance of dozing
- Score 2 for a moderate chance of dozing
- Score 3 for a high chance of dozing

Situation	Chance of dozing score
Sitting reading	________
Watching TV	________
Sitting (inactive) in a public place (e.g. at the theatre, at a meeting)	________
As a passenger in a car for an hour	________
Lying down to rest in the afternoon if circumstances would permit	________
Sitting talking to someone	________
Sitting quietly after lunch (no alcohol)	________
In a car, while stopped for a few minutes in traffic	________

If you think sleep apnoea syndrome is a possibility, consult your doctor, who may refer you to a laboratory that has equipment for assessing disordered breathing during sleep.

High blood pressure (hypertension) and heart disease are more likely in people who snore – both men and women (*Journal of American College of Cardiology* 2000;35:308–13). This may partly be because many snorers are overweight. Another reason may be that with even moderate snoring your breathing is obstructed and you are not getting quite enough oxygen during sleep, and this has a knock-on effect on your cardiovascular system. Whatever the reason, if you are a snorer ask your doctor to check your blood pressure.

Daytime functioning. If you snore, you may be disturbing your own sleep (as well as the sleep of others). This can affect how well you function in the day. For example, students who snore tend to do badly in exams (*Student British Medical Journal* 1998;6:182).

Headache. People who have daily headaches are more likely to be snorers (*Neurology* 2003;60:1366-8). The reason for this is not clear.

What you can do

There is no shortage of 'cures', for snoring (over 300 anti-snoring devices have been registered at the US patent office alone), but in many cases self-help is effective.

- Lose weight if you are overweight.
- Avoid alcohol, tranquillizers and sleeping pills within 4 hours of bedtime.
- You could try a herbal remedy from a health shop or pharmacy but, according to *Health Which?* (December 2001), there is little evidence that they are effective despite the claims on the packaging. There are gargles or throat sprays that you use at bedtime,

which contain peppermint, thyme, pine and eucalyptus oils. They may help by leaving a thin friction-reducing layer on the palate and uvula. They are also the most pleasant of the anti-snoring remedies for your sleeping partner.

- Put a walnut, cork or even a tennis ball into a sock and pin it to the back of your pyjamas (use a safety pin). This will encourage you to sleep sideways rather than on your back.
- Tilt the head of your bed up 10 cm (4 inches) by putting bricks under the legs to lessen the effect of gravity on the throat muscles. Do not use a thick, hard pillow; this will kink your neck and make the problem worse.
- Try sleeping in a whiplash foam collar, to stop the neck kinking.
- Have a coffee or cola drink at night, so that your partner gets to sleep first.
- Nostril dilators encourage nasal breathing and help to prevent mouth breathing. To decide if nasal dilators might help, stand in front of a mirror and close one nostril with your hand. Breathe in through the other and see if the nostril tends to get sucked in. If it does, support it with the clean end of a match and see if breathing is easier. Check the other nostril in the same way. If this does improve your breathing, then nasal dilators might be helpful (only 10% of snorers are in this category). There are various types of nasal dilator (see Useful contacts on page 249). Some are inserted into the nostrils and some are self-adhesive strips that you apply to the outside of the nose to widen the nostrils. You can buy them from pharmacies.
- You may be snoring mainly because you sleep with your mouth open. To test this, open your mouth and make a snoring noise. Now try again with your mouth closed. If you snore only with your mouth open, a device to keep your mouth closed may help (see Useful contacts on page 249). A reader of Dr Le Fanu's *Daily Telegraph* column suggests a do-it-yourself version – take a lady's stocking and bind it tightly under the jaw and over the head with a reef knot.
- Plastic mouth devices (technically called mandibular advancement splints, because the mandible is the bone of the lower jaw) are available to hold the jaw slightly forward while you sleep; when the jaw is in this forward position the airway opens wider. There are various different types (see Useful contacts on page 249), and some can be moulded to fit by placing them in hot water. These devices may be difficult to get used to, but are said to help 70% of snorers. They are, however, inferior to the type properly fitted by dentists.

In the UK, there are about 15 million snorers – 10.4 million males and 4.5 million females (British Snoring and Sleep Apnoea Association)

What your doctor and dentist can do

- Consult your doctor and dentist if you have tried the self-help approaches without success.
- You should also see your doctor if nostril dilators have relieved the problem, because it could mean that you have nasal obstruction that could be dealt with by surgery.
- You should also see your doctor if you have any of the symptoms of sleep apnoea.

Your dentist can advise you about 'mandibular advancement splints' that you place in your mouth for sleeping. Made-to-measure splints are better than the types you buy over the counter. They consist of splints that fit closely over the upper and lower teeth, and are linked by a tension band to pull the lower jaw forward. But they are expensive, costing several hundred pounds in the UK, and will probably have to be replaced after 18 months. Also, they do not always work (they reduce snoring in about 75% of people), and they may make your jaw ache and cause dry mouth or excessive saliva production. A few dentists have been trained to fit them. If your dentist has not had this training, he or she can refer you to a specialist orthodontist.

Churchill and Mussolini were both famous snorers

Your doctor can advise you about other treatments.

Uvulopalato-pharyngo-plasty. In the 1980s, an uvulopalato-pharyngo-plasty operation was a common treatment for people who could not lead normal lives because of their snoring. In this procedure, a 1-cm strip is removed from along the entire free edge of the soft palate, including the uvula. As it heals, it scars, and this stiffens the palate so that it cannot vibrate. The disadvantages are that it is very painful, recovery takes several weeks, it will not cure the problem if the base of the tongue vibrates as well as the palate, the voice may change (which is especially noticeable in singers) and cure may not be permanent. After the operation, 5–10% of people find that fluid goes up into the nose when they drink.

Laser surgery. In the 1990s, laser treatment became popular. This burns away part of the uvula and soft palate to produce the desired scarring. It takes about 15–20 minutes and can usually be done under a local anaesthetic. This technique (laser palatoplasty) has fewer side effects; there will be pain and discomfort in the throat for about 2 weeks afterwards, and some people have a slight feeling of dryness in the throat for several months. These operations improve snoring in about 85% of cases, but the cure is not always permanent, so the long-term success rate is about 66%. A similar technique uses a fine, heated needle (diathermy palatoplasty).

Radiofrequency ablation (somnoplasty) is another method of stiffening the fleshy soft palate. It uses radio waves to heat, stiffen and shrink the tissue. Each treatment takes about 20 minutes and about 10 treatments are needed. It is done under a local anaesthetic. It may not be very effective in the long term; 18 months after the treatment, 78% of patients said that they were still snoring heavily (*Journal of Laryngology and Otology* 2002;116:116–8).

Other methods of stiffening the soft palate have been tried. 'Chemical snoreplasty' involves injecting a chemical called tetradecyl sulphate into the soft palate to cause scarring and stiffening; after about a year, the scar may soften, so another injection may be needed. Implants of Dacron threads are a more recent idea. These methods are not generally available.

Mask and air pressure treatment. The other approach is nasal CPAP, which stands for 'continuous positive airways pressure'. This involves wearing a mask at night, which is attached to a machine that delivers air under pressure to keep the throat open. Some people cannot get used to the noise of the machine, or the claustrophobic feeling of wearing a mask. In the UK, each machine costs the NHS about £600, with a further £200 each year for filters and masks, so the treatment is available only for people whose snoring is part of the sleep apnoea syndrome.

Useful contacts

www.snoring.com.au is a free online resource for medical practitioners, patients and snoring sufferers dealing with snoring, snoring-related illness such as apnea (apnoea) and treatments for snoring.
www.snoring.com.au

Health*Insite* is an Australian government initiative aimed to improve the health of Australians by providing easy access to quality information about human health. Follow the link below to find information on sleep apnoea.
www.healthinsite.gov.au/topics/Sleep_Apnoea

British Snoring and Sleep Apnoea Association is a mine of information. It publishes leaflets on all aspects of snoring and sleep apnoea on its website. The website also gives details about anti-snoring products and services, and the Association sells many by mail order.
www.britishsnoring.com

American Sleep Apnea Association is a non-profit organization. It is mainly about sleep apnoea, but also provides information about snoring on its website.
Email: asaa@sleepapnea.org.
www.sleepapnea.org/snoring.html

Health Which? is no longer published, but back issues should be available in local libraries in the UK. The December 2001 issue contained an excellent report on so-called snoring cures.

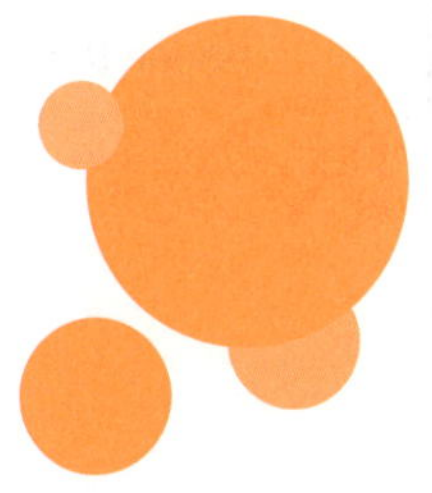

Stammering

About 9% (almost 1 in 10) of the UK population stammers. It is about 3 times more common in males than females. It usually starts in childhood – between the ages of 2 and 5 – but most children grow out of it without any specific therapy.

Why stammering occurs

Putting thoughts into words and then organizing speech so that the words flow well is a very complex task for the human brain. It is amazing that we do not all stammer. No one understands why stammering occurs, but a lot of research is being done to find out.

Stammering seldom occurs when a single word is being spoken or read, but it usually occurs at the beginning of a sentence or idea. Different parts of the brain deal with language processing and the formation of speech, and scientists are looking at the coordination between these processes. One study suggests that, in stammerers, speech formation jumps the gun before the language processing has been completed. Other researchers are looking at the roles of chemicals in the brain that transmit messages between brain cells.

More men than women stammer

How to help yourself

There are various ways in which you can help yourself. The British Stammering Association suggests the following approach.

Define the problem. What do you actually do when you stammer?

- Do you repeat sounds (s...s...s...supper) or syllables (su...su...su...supper)?
- Do you prolong sounds (sssssssupper)?
- Do you get blocked in speech so that you are unable to make any sound (s...upper)?
- Do you close your eyes or rush through speech?
- Do you try to avoid the word by changing it for another that is easier to say?
- Do you give up speaking altogether?

You also need to consider what you feel about your stammer.

- Do you think it is severe or quite mild?
- Do you think it is holding you back in your social life or at work?
- Is it better in some situations and with some people?
- How do you feel when you stammer: embarrassed? annoyed? frustrated?
- Do you get angry with other people, with yourself, or both?

Tackle the problem piece by piece. Having analysed your stammer, tackle it one element at a time, starting with something you feel you might be able to change. For example, you might take one sentence of your speech two or three times a day and make a special effort to say that sentence slowly and calmly. Do not allow yourself to rush or panic; when speaking more slowly, most people stammer less. Or perhaps you might try to concentrate on not looking away from people, or not closing your eyes when you stammer.

There is a 20% greater chance of you stammering if a close relative has a stammer

Do not try to hide your stammer. You have probably adopted some 'avoidance behaviours' to hide or avoid your stammer. The problem is that the more you avoid, the more you need to go on avoiding. If you are avoiding very successfully, you may be thought to be fluent by workmates, partner and friends, but you have to be constantly vigilant to maintain this fluency. Your stammer does not improve or go away because you hide it.

Try to reduce the number of times that you avoid saying a particular word or talking to a particular person or speaking in a particular situation. As well as experimenting with stammering more openly, you may find it useful to try to talk about your stammer to one or two people who are close to you. You will start to learn that people are not as critical as you thought.

Be aware of degrees of fluency. You may think there are only two possibilities – either you stammer or you are fluent. Watch and listen carefully when people are speaking on buses, on radio phone-ins, at home and in shops. Is everyone as fluent, concise and articulate as you imagined? You may discover that many apparently fluent speakers are, in fact, quite hesitant when speaking, and that there is not such a clear division between speaking fluently and stammering. You may then begin to accept that you do not have to be fluent all the time.

Famous stammerers include Moses, Aristotle, Aesop, Virgil, King Charles I, Charles Darwin, Marilyn Monroe and Napoleon

Speech therapy

You should get the help of a speech and language therapist, preferably one who specializes in the treatment of stammering. Your doctor can refer you, or you can get in touch with a therapist yourself. The therapy may be on an individual basis, or may be in a group. If you have already had speech therapy and feel that you were not helped, try again because therapy may have changed and you may have changed.

Helping a stammerer

- Do not give unhelpful advice, such as 'slow down' or 'take a deep breath'. Just accept that the person stammers.
- Do be patient and maintain eye contact with the stammerer when he or she speaks.
- Do not interrupt or finish words or sentences for the stammerer. This is frustrating for the stammerer and you may guess wrongly.
- Concentrate on what is being said, rather than how it is being said.

There is no difference between stammering and stuttering; they are two words with the same meaning

Acknowledgement

The information in this section is taken from a leaflet called *The Adult Who Stammers* published by the British Stammering Association.

People who stammer can usually whisper and sing without stammering, like Pop Idol Gareth Gates

Useful contacts

Australian Stuttering Research Centre (ASRC) was established to disseminate knowledge about stuttering and its treatment. A list of the ASRC publications can be found at the Publications link on its website.
www3.fhs.usyd.edu.au/asrcwww/

British Stammering Association provides advice and information about all aspects of stammering.
www.stammering.org

Michael Palin Centre for Stammering Children is a joint initiative between the non-profit Association for Research into Stammering and the UK NHS. It is named for the actor Michael Palin who played a stammerer in the film *A Fish Called Wanda*. The website has plenty of useful information on stammering, including a 'Top tips' section for stammerers, their friends, families and teachers.
www.stammeringcentre.org

Stammering. A Practical Guide for Teachers and Other Professionals is a book written by Rustin, Cook, Botherill, Hughes and Kelman (ISBN 1-853467-14-6) mainly for teachers, but parents of children who stammer will find it informative. Hughes is the Schools Liaison Officer for the British Stammering Association, and the other authors are speech and language therapists for the Michael Palin Centre for Stammering Children.

Stretch marks

What are they?

Stretch marks look like thin, stretched tissue, and that is more or less what they are. They appear in people who put on or lose weight rapidly. The upper layer of the skin is normal, but in the lower layer the collagen and elastin, which give the skin its strength and elasticity, have become thinner and broken. At first, the marks look reddish-purple. This is because the stretched skin is more transparent and the small blood vessels that lie deep in the skin show through. Later, the blood vessels contract. The purplish colour then fades to white, which is simply fat under the skin showing through.

Who gets them?

- Stretch marks often appear on the breast and abdomen during pregnancy. The reason is partly hormonal. During pregnancy, hormones have the job of softening the collagen ligaments of the pelvis, so that the tissues can stretch easily during childbirth. Unfortunately, the skin collagen softens as well, allowing stretch marks to form easily.
- Some women have weaker collagen than others, so are more likely to get stretch marks. Recent research suggests that if you have stretch marks, your pelvic floor ligaments may be slightly weak, so it is very important to do pelvic floor exercises (see page 288) after childbirth to prevent incontinence of urine.
- 'Yo-yo dieters' and bodybuilders can get stretch marks on the upper arms, chest and thighs.
- Growing adolescents can get them on their backs, where they look like a series of horizontal lines.

Preventing stretch marks

Try to avoid 'yo-yo dieting'. If you are overweight, aim to lose weight slowly (do not aim to lose more than 0.5 kg or 1 lb a week.

If you are pregnant, there is not much you can do except keep your fingers crossed and think, 'This is a small price to pay for a beautiful baby!' Rubbing baby oil into the abdomen each night might help. Various special creams and oils are promoted for preventing stretch marks, but there is no proof that they are effective.

Curing stretch marks

Stretch marks are permanent in the sense that the skin in these areas will never be completely normal. However, after a time they contract down into much less obvious, thin, whitish scars.

Collagen creams claim that they will improve stretch marks. There is no evidence that they do so. In fact, collagen and elastin put onto the surface of the skin can not penetrate into the deeper layers.

Cocoa butter cream, which is available from pharmacies, is often recommended to soften scars, so might be worth a try.

Lasers can be used to treat stretch marks at an early stage, when they are still red. The red blood cells in the small blood vessels absorb the energy from the laser beam and convert it into heat, which then seals the blood vessels. This gets rid of the red colour and might speed up the contracting process, but is uncertain whether it will make any difference in the long run.

It is quite costly, and can not be done under the NHS in the UK. As with any cosmetic treatment, check that the clinic is reputable; your doctor can probably advise you, and look at the section on cosmetic surgery on page 339.

Tretinoin is another approach to the treatment of early stretch marks. There have been claims that this produces improvement, but other researchers have not found any effect (*Cutis* 1994;54:121–4).

Surgery is a possibility for tummy stretch marks if you also have a lot of loose skin on the tummy. The operation is a 'tummy tuck' (removal of the skin and the fatty tissue beneath). You will be left with scars around the belly button and across the lower stomach. This is not a minor operation and, like all operations, it carries risks. Recovery takes several weeks. Look at the section on cosmetic surgery on page 339.

Sweating

Men are sweatier than women, even when you take body size into account. Scientists tested volunteers in a laboratory mock-up of a sweltering car. Men lost 250 g of sweat per hour, which was 70 g more than the women (*New Scientist* 1 June 2002)

About 3% of people say that they sweat excessively. Of course, we all sweat more when we are hot or anxious (see page 49), but excessive sweating may be partly caused by genes – 1 in 3 sufferers says that others in their family have the same problem. Sweating, accompanying hot flushes (see page 50), is common in women at the menopause. Occasionally, excessive sweating can signify a medical problem (such as an overactive thyroid gland). Antidepressant drugs can also cause sweating especially of the head and neck (*Dermatology in Practice* 2005;13(1):24–6).

Each person has 3–4 million sweat glands

The uses of sweating

- Sweating is one of the ways we regulate our body temperature – humans rely on the evaporation of sweat to protect the body against a hot environment (most other animals rely on insulation or panting).
- Sweat helps to keep our skin moist.
- Sweating of the body and hands when we are anxious may occur for a reason – to help us escape from enemies if they try to grab us.
- Sweat from some areas of the body contains scents ('pheromones') that send secret signals to other people.
- According to *New Scientist* magazine (10 November 2001), sweat contains a natural antibiotic, dermicidin, that helps to destroy bacteria on the skin.

There are two sorts of sweat glands.

- Apocrine glands are found mainly in the armpits and near the anus. We each have about 1 million of these glands. They are really scent glands. The sweat that comes from them has a particular smell in each person, and probably includes 'pheromone' scents that send messages to other people.
- Eccrine glands are responsible for sweating when we are hot. We each have about 3 million of these glands. Every 1 cm^2 of the back has about 60 sweat glands. On the palms and soles, there are about 600 glands per cm^2.

The sweat glands are capable of producing 12 litres of sweat in 24 hours

If you sweat excessively, it is not because you have too many sweat glands or that they are abnormally large. It is probably because there is a lot of activity in the tiny nerves that control them.

At rest in a cool environment, a normal person loses about half a litre of sweat in a day

Worries about sweating

Excessive sweating can be annoying in two ways.

- The sweat may show on your clothes (for example at the armpits) or give you embarrassingly sweaty palms.
- You may be worried about the smell of the sweat. Sweat is not smelly itself (except the pheromones, which are so subtle that we are not consciously aware of smelling them), but it quickly becomes a breeding ground for bacteria. These bacteria break down sweat to produce fatty acids. It is these fatty acids that have the acrid, penetrating, pungent, 'stale sweat' smell. Arm and groin sweat is particularly rich in protein – a favourite of bacteria. Sweat from other parts of the body is saltier and less hospitable to bacteria. This problem can be approached in two ways: sweating itself can be prevented; or the bacteria that cause the smell can be attacked.

Doctors are now becoming more sympathetic to people troubled by excessive sweating. They are realizing that excessive sweating can affect your work and social life (*British Journal of Dermatology* 2002;147:1218–26).

*We can smell the sweat of a giraffe from a quarter of a mile away. The smell repels ticks (*New Scientist *1 February 2003)*

SWEATY ARMPITS

What you can do for sweaty armpits

Avoid pungent foods such as onions, fish, garlic and spicy meals. These foods can be smelt in sweat and make it more noticeable.

Malt vinegar is an old-fashioned remedy that might be worth a try. Apply some to your armpits at night. Wash it off in the morning and then use your normal deodorant or antiperspirant.

Victorians sponged their armpits with sulphuric acid, a potentially dangerous treatment

Commercial antiperspirants. You have probably tried most commercial deodorants and antiperspirants, but check the labels and look for one with a different active ingredient. If you have heard a rumour about antiperspirants or deodorants and breast cancer, take a look at the section on antiperspirants and breast cancer on page 264.

Shave your armpits. Hair holds sweat and gives the bacteria more to work on.

20% aluminium chloride is the next thing to try if ordinary antiperspirants have not done the trick, but it can damage clothing. It can be bought from the pharmacist (ask for Drichlor, Anhydrol Forte, Odaban or Perspirex) and should be used as follows.

- Before going to bed, wash and dry your armpits thoroughly. If you apply the solution to wet skin, a chemical reaction produces hydrochloric acid, which can irritate skin and tarnish jewellery. If necessary, use a hair dyer to ensure your skin is absolutely dry.
- Apply the solution when you are lying down in bed. This sounds odd, but armpit sweating switches off when you lie flat, and the solution will be more effective if applied then. The solution works by passing into the openings of the sweat glands, causing them to swell up and block, but if sweat is pouring out of the glands when you apply the solution, it will not be able to get in.
- It works best if the area is covered with plastic cling-film (food wrap). Unfortunately, the armpit is an awkward shape. Use tape (such as Micropore, which you can buy from a pharmacy) to hold the plastic wrap in place, then put on a tight-fitting T-shirt to help keep it in position.
- Do not apply the solution directly after shaving, or the skin may become sore.
- Wash off the solution in the morning, and do not reapply until bedtime.
- If it proves effective reduce the application to every other night, and then to once or twice a week. Do not use it every day, because it can irritate the skin.
- If it causes irritation, applying 1% hydrocortisone cream twice a day for not more than 2 weeks can help.

In the 1950s, you might have been sedated with barbiturates or given a course of X-ray treatment for this embarrassing problem

What doctors can do for sweaty armpits

Botulinum toxin (Botox, Dysport) is a powerful poison, but injections of very tiny doses into the skin stop excessive sweating.

- The injections are painful, but the pain is tolerable. Treatment takes about 30–45 minutes.
- Botulinum toxin works by inactivating the nerves that trigger sweat-gland activity.
- One treatment of about 12 tiny injections stops or substantially reduces armpit sweating for 2–8 months. After that, a repeat session will be needed.
- This is a fairly new treatment, and is not available in all hospitals, but your doctor will be able to find out the location of the nearest specialist treatment centre.
- It does not work for everyone, but about 9 out of 10 people respond (*Drug and Therapeutics Bulletin* 2005;43:77–80).
- People who have had this treatment say that it greatly improves their quality of life (*British Journal of Dermatology* 2004;151:1115–22).
- As you would expect, this treatment also reduces the smelliness of the armpits (*Archives of Dermatology* 2003;139:57–9).

According to the French newspaper Le Figaro, *only 47% of French people shower or bathe every day compared with 70% of Britons and 80% of Dutch, Germans and Scandinavians. But the French are Europe's biggest consumers of perfume and deodorants*

A sympathectomy operation to destroy the sympathetic nerves that control sweating, often by keyhole surgery, is almost the last resort.

- A general anaesthetic is required.
- The sympathetic nerves lie in the chest just under the second, third and fourth ribs on each side. The surgeon operates through an incision in the chest wall and cuts the nerves or destroys them using an electrical current.
- After the operation, you can return to a sedentary job after 1–2 weeks, and to a manual job after 2–3 weeks.
- The immediate success rate is almost 80%, but after a few years only one-third of people who have had the operation are satisfied (*Drug and Therapeutics Bulletin* 2005;43:77–80).
- The main drawback is that the body may compensate by increasing sweating elsewhere – usually the trunk, but sometimes the feet – so you may end up swapping sweaty armpits for a sweaty abdomen. This happens in between one-third and three-quarters of people who have had the operation. In 1 in 100, this 'compensatory' sweating is very severe, and they regret they had the operation. Unfortunately, the operation cannot be reversed.

Liposuction and subcutaneous curettage are methods of removing sweat glands from the deep layer of skin. They do not always work, and there may be bruising or scarring.

Surgical removal of some skin from the armpit is the final option. It can be dramatically effective, but can cause scarring so is rarely performed nowadays. Under a local anaesthetic, the surgeon removes a section of skin about 4 x 1.5 cm in size, taking away the most troublesome sweat glands.

SWEATY FEET

Because we normally wear shoes, the sweat from the foot cannot evaporate normally. This sweat rapidly becomes smelly, because bacteria work on it to produce smelly fatty acids. Warm moisture also encourages the growth of the fungi that cause 'athlete's foot', and this can add to the cheesy smell, as well as being unpleasant in itself.

One of the main causes of sweaty, smelly feet is wearing the wrong socks or footwear. Shoes with plastic or other synthetic fabric linings don't allow any sweat to evaporate and don't absorb it either, so the foot stays wet. Synthetic socks have the same effect, particularly if they're tight.

Every square cetimetre of the sole of the foot (and the palm of the hand) has about 600 sweat glands – more than other part of the body

What you can do for sweaty feet

Deal with your socks

- Throw out all your nylon socks. Replace them with socks that are 60–70% wool combined with 40–30% man-made fibre. Socks that are all cotton are not as good because they do not hold as much moisture without becoming sodden, and all-wool socks become clammy. Make sure your socks are not too tight. Some sports socks have ventilation panels and are designed to transport moisture away from the foot. If necessary, wear a second pair of the correct socks over the first pair to increase absorbency.
- Wear clean socks every day. Wash socks on the hottest cycle. After washing, rinse your socks in antiseptic, diluted 20 times, and let them dry naturally.

Deal with your shoes

- Check the linings of your shoes. Leather shoes often have a plastic lining, so be sure to choose all-leather shoes without a lining or ones that are lined with leather.
- Buy some washable insoles for your shoes, and wash them every day.
- Every couple of weeks, use the nozzle of a vacuum cleaner to clean the inside of your shoes. This will help to remove dried old sweat. You can also wipe the inside of your shoes with surgical spirit, which you can buy from a pharmacy.
- Avoid wearing trainers for long periods. Most trainers are insulating and synthetic – ideal conditions for cheesy feet.

An average male foot exudes a quarter of a litre of sweat a day

Deal with your feet

- Check the soles of your feet for hard skin. Hard skin is dead skin, and it becomes soggy when damp, providing an ideal environment for bacteria. Remove it with a pumice stone.
- Bathe your feet in warm water with a few drops of tea-tree oil added. Tea-tree oil has antibacterial properties. Dry your feet thoroughly.
- Alternatively, soak your feet daily in black tea, which contains tannic acid. Boil 2 tea bags in half a litre of water for 15 minutes. Add this to 2 litres of cool water and soak your feet for 20–30 minutes. Dry thoroughly.
- Try wiping your feet with surgical spirit (available from a pharmacy) each day. Stop if it irritates your skin.
- Check between your toes for fungal infections such as athlete's foot. Fungi thrive when the feet are warm and moist. The skin between the toes will look red and soggy. Buy an antifungal foot spray, which is more effective than antifungal foot powders. Keep using the spray for 10 days after the symptoms have gone. If the problem persists, see your doctor.
- If you notice lots of small pits in the skin of your soles – almost a honeycomb appearance – and a very pungent smell, you may have an infection called 'pitted keratolysis'. This is caused by a bacterium and is common in soldiers who wear boots in humid conditions (called 'Mekong foot' by US troops in Vietnam). It needs to be treated with antibiotics, so see your doctor.

Other measures. You could also try using a special foot antiperspirant or deodorant or a 20% aluminium chloride solution (see Useful contacts on page 265). It is important to use the aluminium chloride solution correctly. Use it at night. Wash and dry your feet first and then apply the solution when you are lying in bed. Do not miss between your toes. Allow it to dry naturally and wash it off in the morning. Apply it every night until the problem is under control – usually 3 or 4 days – and then twice a week. Do not use it if you think you might have an infection, such as athlete's foot, or if you have any sores on your feet.

If you are really bothered by sweatiness of your feet, and the measures described above have not dealt with the problem, it would be worth talking to your doctor. If you feel too shy to talk to your doctor, see a chiropodist (see Useful contacts on page 265). Chiropodists are experts on all foot problems, including sweatiness, and give very useful advice.

*A man with sweaty feet who removed his shoes in a university library was fined 250 euros by magistrates in The Netherlands. The court ruled that his feet smelled so badly that he constituted a public nuisance (*Guardian *6 July 2002)*

What doctors can do for sweaty feet

Iontophoresis is a treatment available through some hospital physiotherapy departments. It used to be difficult to obtain this treatment, but more hospitals now have the equipment – your doctor can find out if it is available locally.

- It involves placing your feet in a bath of tap water, through which a very small electrical current is passed for about 30–40 minutes.
- You may find it a slightly uncomfortable, tingling or burning sensation, and skin irritation can occur.
- It is not suitable if you could be pregnant or have a heart pacemaker.
- At first, treatment is every few days, so it is time consuming, but it is gradually decreased to once every 3 or 4 weeks.
- If you find it works well, you might consider buying the equipment to use at home – ask the physiotherapist's advice. (Obviously, you should not try to make homemade equipment, because you could electrocute yourself.)

Botulinum toxin injections (Botox; see page 257) are probably the best treatment for seriously sweaty feet. It is tedious and uncomfortable because you may need about 36 tiny injections into the soles of the feet and the skin of the feet is very sensitive. This is a new treatment so it may not be available in your local hospital, but your doctor can find out the location of the nearest specialist treatment centre.

Anticholinergic drugs block the action of the nerves responsible for sweating, and are fairly effective. However, their side effects – drying of the mouth, blurring of vision, constipation, sedation – are probably worse than the sweating! Propantheline bromide can be prescribed by your doctor. In the UK, glycopyrronium bromide is available only through a specialist dermatologist (because it has to be imported from the US); this drug has lesser side effects than propantheline bromide.

A sympathectomy operation to destroy the nerves that control sweating of the feet is possible, but is not to be recommended because it causes impotence in men and probably also interferes with sexual function in women.

SWEATY HANDS

Sweaty hands are annoying and embarrassing, particularly if you use a computer keyboard or your sweat smudges ink and wets paper. You can disguise sweaty hands to some extent by smoothing back your hair – so that you wipe your hands on your hair – before you shake hands with anyone. But it can be embarrassing if you leave sweaty handprints on anything you touch.

The palms of the hands have about 600 sweat glands per square centimetre

What you can do for sweaty hands

First ask yourself whether your sweaty hands mean that you are excessively anxious in certain situations. If this is the case, dealing with the anxiety will lessen the problem (see below and the section on shyness on page 241).

You may not be excessively anxious – it may simply be that even slight, normal anxiety triggers your hands to produce too much sweat. If this is the case, you can try rubbing your palms with astringent oils, such as cypress or geranium (from health stores). You can also buy a special powder to keep your hands dry, designed for use in sports to keep a grip on the ball or racquet (available from sports shops). You apply it as a liquid, which changes into a fine dry powder.

Alternatively, try 20% aluminium chloride, painting it onto your hands as described for armpits (see page 257). You can buy aluminium chloride from chemists without a prescription (ask for Drichlor, Anhydrol Forte or Perspirex Hand and Foot Lotion). Unfortunately, it is not as effective for hands as for armpits. If this does not work, you need to see your doctor.

What doctors can do for sweaty hands

Help for anxiety is the obvious solution if the sweating is caused by anxiety and stress. Your doctor can discuss your anxieties, suggest ways to deal with them and might suggest beta-blocker tablets to take a couple of hours before an anxiety-provoking situation.

Iontophoresis is a treatment available through some hospital physiotherapy departments. It used to be difficult to obtain this treatment, but more hospitals now have the equipment (your doctor can find out if it is available locally).

- It involves placing your hands in a bath of tap water, through which a very small electrical current is passed for about 15 minutes.
- You may find it a slightly uncomfortable, tingling or burning sensation, and skin irritation can occur.
- It is not suitable if you could be pregnant or have a heart pacemaker.

- At first, treatment is every few days, so it is time consuming, but it is gradually decreased to once every 3 or 4 weeks.
- If you find it works well, you might consider buying the equipment to use at home (see Useful contacts page 265). It is expensive, so you should ask the physiotherapist's advice. (Obviously, you should not try to make homemade equipment, because you could electrocute yourself.)

*UK government scientists are working on technology to identify each person's sweat odour profile, to use as a possible form of identification (ID). You would hold your palm against a sensor, and the details would be stored on your ID Smart Card (*Observer *29 December 2003)*

Botulinum toxin injections (Botox; see page 257) will stop or substantially reduce sweating of the palms for about 6 months. After that, repeat injections are needed. However, there is a major problem with this treatment when used for hand sweating – some people notice weakness of their hand muscles for some weeks afterwards. For this reason specialists are reluctant to use this treatment on hands.

A sympathectomy operation is probably the most effective treatment for seriously sweaty hands. This is often done to control excessive sweating under the arms, but it is 95% successful for sweating of the hands. The result is immediate; you wake from the anaesthetic with dry, warm hands. The long-term results seem good; after about 14 years about 73% of people are still satisfied with the result (*Drug and Therapeutics Bulletin* 2005;43:77–80). For more information, see the section on sweaty armpits on page 256.

NIGHT SWEATS

Nights sweats are a surprisingly common problem, especially in middle-aged people. (*Journal of Family Practice* 2002;51:452–6).

The most common reason is the menopause in women (see page 50 on flushing). Alcohol seems to be a common cause, so it might be worth seeing whether stopping alcohol altogether would solve the problem. If you are overweight and a snorer, you may have 'sleep apnoea', which causes restless sleep and, in some cases, night sweats (see page 244 on snoring). Some people with restless legs syndrome (see page 220) wake with sweating as well as with the discomfort or jerking of the legs (*Annals of Family Medicine* 2006;4:423–6). If the sweats are a new problem that has followed a sore throat, you might have glandular fever (infectious mononucleosis), which is a common viral infection that usually clears up in 1–2 weeks.

You should discuss this problem with your doctor, who will wish to rule out an overactive thyroid, so will ask you about nervousness, palpitations and weight loss. It is also worth checking whether medication might be the cause. Aspirin or acetaminophen (paracetamol) are the most common culprits; propranolol, pilocarpine and some antidepressants (tricyclics, vanlafaxine, fluoxetine) can also encourage sweating. People taking treatment for diabetes can have night sweats if their blood sugar falls too low in the night, so if you are diabetic you should certainly report the sweats to your diabetes doctor.

All doctors were taught in medical school that night sweats can be a symptom of tuberculosis. Therefore, when a patient says they have night sweats, doctors always consider tuberculosis, but this is actually a very unusual cause. Other serious causes include HIV infection and lymphoma.

PHEROMONES

Pheromones are body scents that we cannot smell. Everyone has over 3 million sweat glands on their skin that are able to put out pheromones. Although we are not consciously aware of them, there is evidence that pheromones from other people affect our behaviour, our feelings about the other person and even the physiology of our bodies. For example, pheromones would explain why women who live together are likely to menstruate at the same time.

Many scientists believe that some pheromones convey a sexual message to other people – such as 'I am available' or 'I am attracted to you' – or help women to spot a man whose immune system would be the best match for her own if she became pregnant by him.

- Researchers asked women to rate some photos of men for attractiveness. When secretly exposed to men's sweat chemicals, the women rated the men as more attractive – especially the ugly men. Unknowingly, the women may have been responding to pheromone chemicals in the sweat.
- In a different experiment, researchers asked men to smell T-shirts worn by young women, and to rate them for attractiveness of the smell. A T-shirt worn by a woman during her fertile phase of the menstrual cycle was rated as more pleasant and sexy than a T-shirt worn by the same woman during her non-fertile phase. So maybe women have a pheromone that reveals when they are fertile (*Proceedings of the Royal Society*, May 2001).

What are the chemicals in pheromones?

Researchers have not yet managed to identify the actual chemicals that would produce instant sex appeal although, in the US, products claiming to contain copies of human male and female pheromones are marketed as sexual attractants.

How do we smell pheromones?

A few scientists think we smell pheromones with two tiny pits in the nose known as 'vomeronasal organs' (VNOs). (Sometimes they are called 'Jacobson's organ', because a Danish doctor called Jacobson first noticed them in the early 1800s.) They suggest that the VNOs have a direct connection to an older, more primal, part of the brain than the area that processes normal smells.

Most scientists argue that the pits in the nose have no function at all in humans, and are just leftovers from the dinosaur age. They say that we detect pheromones in the same way that we smell ordinary smells.

ANTIPERSPIRANTS AND BREAST CANCER

Rumours have been spread on the internet that using antiperspirants in the armpit might cause breast cancer and that shaving under the arm opens up pathways for harmful chemicals. Aluminium or paraben chemicals, used as preservatives, are blamed. On the label, parabens may be listed as methyl paraben, ethyl paraben, propyl paraben, butyl paraben, isobutyl paraben or E216.

Why do some people think that antiperspirants might cause breast cancer? Most cancers occur in the area of the breast closest to the armpit. Also, breast cancer is slightly more common in the left breast, which could be because right-handed people tend to be more heavy-handed with deodorant when using that hand. Breast cancer is more common in countries where a lot of antiperspirant is used. One study found paraben chemicals within breast tumours (*Journal of Applied Toxicology* 2004;24:5–13), and other research suggest aluminium may affect breast cells (*Journal of Inorganic Biochemistry* 2005;99:1912–9).

What do cancer experts think? Cancer experts are not convinced by these arguments. They point out that the reason most cancers occur towards the armpit is because there is more actual breast tissue in that area. Breast cancer is more common in richer countries, but this could be due to diet rather than use of deodorants. If there is an effect from parabens or aluminium, it must be very small.

Has any research been done?

Researchers in Seattle, US, asked 813 women with breast cancer about their use of antiperspirants and deodorants, and whether they applied them within an hour of underarm shaving. They also asked the same questions of 793 women who did not have breast cancer. They found that women who used antiperspirants or deodorants and women who shaved their underarms did not have a greater risk of breast cancer (*Journal of the National Cancer Institute* 2002;94:1578–80). So the research shows that antiperspirants or deodorants are safe.

Another study of breast cancer patients found that those who shaved their armpits most often and applied deodorant tended to have developed their cancer at a younger age. But this does not prove anything, because there was no 'control group' of women without cancer. The reason for the result could simply be that younger women shave and use deodorants more often than older women (*European Journal of Cancer Prevention* 2003;12:479–85).

No research has proved a link between antiperspirants or deodorants and breast cancer.

Do all antiperspirants or deodorants contain parabens or aluminium? Most antiperspirants and deodorants are now paraben free and aluminium-free deodorants are also available. To be sure, check the list of ingredients on the label. Alternatively, use vinegar or bicarbonate of soda. Just put some in your hand and rub it on. These preparations do not stop sweating, but they inhibit the bacteria that cause the smell.

Useful contacts

myDr is an Australian healthcare website compiled by a team of experienced Australian healthcare writers, with contributions from practising Australian healthcare practitioners and recognized Australian health organizations. The website has an interesting article on the treatment of sweating. Type in 'excessive sweating' in the Quick search form fill for a list of related articles.
www.mydr.com.au

Health*Insite* is an Australian government initiative aimed to improve the health of Australians by providing easy access to quality information about human health. Follow the link to find information on skin diseases and sweating.
www.healthinsite.gov.au/topics/Skin_Diseases

Cosmetic Medical Centre is a fully accredited and licensed day surgery centre in Sydney, NSW. The website contains interesting information on the treatment of excessive sweating.
www.cosmeticmedical.com.au/proc/sweat.html

International Hyperhidrosis Society is a US organization with an excellent and informative website. (Hyperhidrosis is the medical term for excessive sweating.) The website has practical suggestions for dealing with excessive sweating, and a special section for teenagers. There is also a facility to view the website in four other languages.
Email: info@SweatHelp.org
www.sweathelp.org

Hyperhidrosis Patient Support Group is a UK organization that offers support to people suffering from excessive sweating (hyperhidrosis).
www.hyperhidrosisuk.org

www.sweatfree.org.uk is a website run by two UK surgeons. It has information about various types of excessive sweating.
www.sweatfree.org.uk

The Society of Chiropodists and Podiatrists has a website with lots of useful advice about caring for feet.
www.feetforlife.org

The American Cancer Society website has a section (updated in 2006) explaining that there is no reason to believe that deodorants can cause breast cancer.
www.cancer.org/docroot/MED/content/MED_6_1x_Antiperspirants.asp?sitearea=MED

www.snopes.com is a hoax-busting website that has a section on underarm deodorants and breast cancer.
www.snopes.com/medical/toxins/antiperspirant.asp

Cancer Research UK has an excellent section (updated in 2006) on 'Does antiperspirant cause breast cancer?'
www.cancerhelp.org.uk/help/default.asp?page=3943

Antiperspirantsinfo is a website that aims to give accurate information about antiperspirants and health. Note that it is funded by Unilever, who manufacture antiperspirants. There are

sections on myths and facts, as well as a FAQ section.
www.antiperspirantsinfo.com/english/index.php

The Seeing, Hearing and Smelling website from the Howard Hughes Medical Institute gives more information about pheromones.
www.hhmi.org/senses/d210.html

Perspirex Hand & Foot Antiperspirant Lotion. The manufacturer's website has information about stockists and how to use the product.
www.perspirex.co.uk

Iontophoresis machines for home use can be bought in the UK from STD Pharmaceuticals.
Email: enquiries@stdpharm.co.uk
www.stdpharm.co.uk/iontophoresis/index.html

The American Academy of Family Physicians has an interesting article, 'Diagnosing night sweats' on its website. The article was written in 2003 and is intended for doctors.
www.aafp.org/afp/20030301/1019.html

US National Cancer Institute has a fact sheet on antiperspirants or deodorants and breast cancer.
www.cancer.gov/cancertopics/factsheet/Risk/AP-Deo

Tattoos

Having a tattoo you hate used to be a real problem. Until lasers became widely accessible, it was very difficult to remove them.

How tattoos are done

To understand tattoos, you have to know about the structure of your skin. It has two layers.

The outer layer is the epidermis. This is the layer that is constantly being shed and renewing itself. The new cells are formed deep in this layer. They then take about 14 days to move gradually to the surface, pushed upwards by even newer cells forming beneath them. They remain for about another 14 days at the surface before being shed. So it takes roughly a month for the epidermis to renew itself completely.

The under layer is the dermis. This contains elastic tissue, blood vessels, sweat glands, nerve fibres and hair follicles. The dermis is relatively static, and does not renew itself like the epidermis.

Tattooists use a machine with one or more needles connected to tubes containing dye. As the tattooist guides the machine over the skin, the needles move up and down, penetrating the skin a couple of millimetres and depositing particles of dye in the under layer of the skin (dermis). Over time, the body seals the dye particles with a protective wall of collagen protein. Because the dermis does not renew itself, the dye will remain there forever.

'Five-year tattoos' are offered by some hairdressing salons and market stalls. (Professional tattoo studios will not have anything to do with them.) They claim that they place the ink only in the epidermis, and that they will be shed in 3–5 years.

It is unlikely that they will disappear in 5 years. If the ink really was only in the epidermis, it would be shed in a few weeks and the tattoo would be gone. In fact, some of the ink will be placed in the more static tissue of the dermis like any other tattoo, and is likely to be permanent.

Problems with tattoos

Allergy. Very occasionally, an individual is allergic to one of the pigments used. There will be swelling and itching, often in the red part of the tattoo. Allergy may not occur immediately and may develop months or even years after the tattoo was done.

The dyes used in tattooing are industrial pigments that were originally produced for other purposes, such as car paints and writing inks. Their safety in skin has never been properly investigated.

Infection. Cases of hepatitis B infection as a result of tattooing have been reported. Theoretically, HIV and hepatitis C could be caught if contaminated needles were used. This is why, in the UK, you cannot donate blood for a year after having a tattoo.

Wishing you had not had it done. There is now a greater appreciation of the real distress that an inappropriate tattoo can cause – having an obvious tattoo can be a real disadvantage in the job market. When doctors in Wales questioned patients who wanted tattoos removed, they found that a quarter had regretted their tattoo within a month of having it. Over 70% had been below the legal age of 18 when it was done and, on average, they had endured 14 years of embarrassment before deciding to get it removed.

Ways of removing tattoos

In some areas of the UK, you cannot have your tattoos removed under the NHS. In a few parts of the UK, the NHS will remove tattoos if they are on exposed skin (such as the hands and face), and are interfering with your chance of getting a job. Private treatment is most likely and, as with all cosmetic procedures, take care when you choose a private clinic (see page 339).

Laser removal of tattoos breaks the ink down into tiny particles that scavenger cells in the skin can digest. A special type of laser that emits light energy in very brief pulses, each lasting only nanoseconds, is used. This keeps heating of the surrounding skin to a minimum, making scarring less likely. Each session will take 15–45 minutes, depending on the size of the tattoo. Afterwards, the area may ooze some blood for several hours and need to be covered with a dressing. Treatments are usually given every 6–8 weeks, and more than 20 treatments will usually be needed if the tattoo was done professionally. (Amateur tattoos can often be removed with only one or two treatments.) The cost is likely to be quite expensive.

It is quite rare for the tattoo to be completely removed by laser treatment and traces of it will probably remain. Successful removal depends partly on the colour of the tattoo – complicated multicoloured tattoos are more difficult to deal with.

- The 'ruby laser' works best against blue-black and green tattoos, but is not much help against red, yellow and orange.
- The 'Nd-YAG' laser is used against blue-black and red tattoos, but green and light blue colours do not respond well.
- The alexandrite laser is used for blue-black and green tattoos.

Excision involves cutting out the area of skin that bears the tattoo, and is a good way to deal with a small tattoo. It may be the only way of removing a deep, clumsy tattoo not done by a professional tattooist. Surgery for large tattoos is likely to cause scarring and may need skin grafts.

In some cases, the surgeon may use a technique called 'tissue expansion'. Inflatable balloons are placed under the skin to stretch it before removing the tattoo. This procedure can take several months (*Pulse* 2004;63(5):48–9).

Salabrasion. A salt solution can be rubbed into the tattoo to damage the skin, until the pigment is extruded. This technique is seldom used nowadays. It sounds homely, but do not try it yourself – it must be done by someone experienced in the technique.

Useful contacts

The Australasian College of Dermatologists website contains basic information about various skin diseases and problems. It has a small section on tattoos and pigment laser therapy under 'A–Z of skin'.
www.dermcoll.asn.au
www.dermcoll.asn.au/public/a-z_of_skin-chemical_peels_etc.asp#11

Lasercare are a chain of clinics providing laser treatments in the UK. They are private, but some are based in NHS hospitals. Their website has information about tattoo removal.
www.lasercare-clinics.co.uk

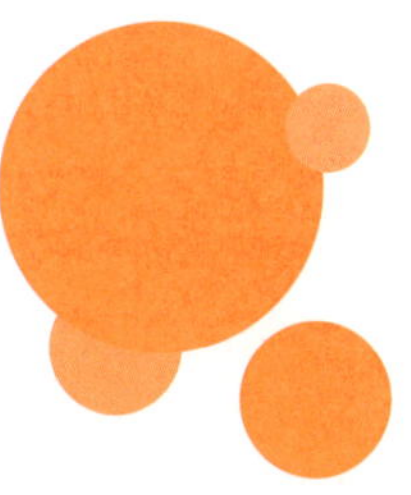

Teeth grinding

Grinding your teeth together when you are asleep is surprisingly common. Most teeth-grinders are unaware that they do it, and find out only because their partner complains. When they wake up, they may feel discomfort or pain in the jaw, shoulders or neck, or have a headache, but they will not know the cause.

Causes of teeth grinding

Teeth grinding is sometimes caused by the upper and lower teeth not fitting together properly – dentists call this 'malocclusion'. The grinding may be a subconscious attempt to grind the teeth down until they fit. Some people who grind their teeth have a problem with the joint of their jaw (where the jaw hinges onto the skull). Clicking or grating of the joint, or occasional locking of the jaw, suggests a joint problem.

Another possibility is stress. Dentists say that teeth grinding is becoming increasingly common, which may be a sign that we live in a stressful society. Apparently teeth grinding usually occurs during the dreaming phases of sleep.

What you can do

Your dentist should be your first port of call. The dentist will tell you if there is abnormal wear and tear of your teeth, and whether the grinding has damaged the enamel. Serious damage to the enamel is fairly unlikely. Unfortunately, enamel does not repair itself (a design fault of the human body), so teeth might need to be crowned if the enamel has been damaged.

To help you break the grinding habit, your dentist may make a night-guard for you to wear. This is a plastic appliance that keeps the teeth apart and allows your muscles to relax into a normal position. Sometimes a dentist can relieve the problem by slightly grinding down some of your teeth, so they meet correctly – doing the job you were trying to do in your sleep.

If you think stress is a factor, work out ways of reducing it or coping. Look in your local library for self-help books on stress. Anything that helps to relax you, such as massage, yoga or exercise, would be worth trying.

Useful contact

Teeth-grinding resource. If you want to know more, there is a nice little website about teeth grinding
www.teethgrinding.org/html/understanding_bruxism.html

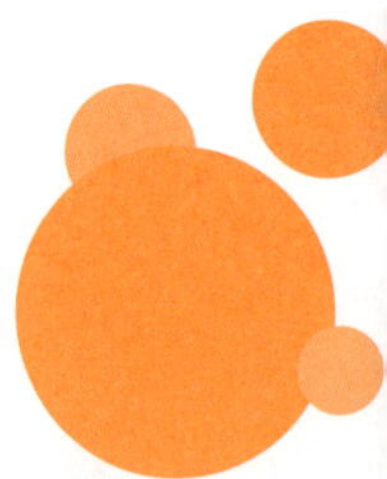

Testicle problems

It is a good idea to examine your testicles regularly, so that you become familiar with your own anatomy. Then you will be able to tell if anything unusual develops.

- The testicles make sperm. They are oval in shape, and are usually about 4–5 cm long, 3 cm wide and 2 cm thick. One is often slightly larger than the other.
- The epididymis is a sausage-shaped lump stuck onto the back and top of each testicle. It is actually a coil of tiny tubes, which carry and store the sperm. If uncoiled, they would be about 6 metres long.
- The spermatic cords lead upwards from behind the epididymis. They carry the sperm towards the penis, and also contain blood vessels.
- The scrotum is the skin sac that contains the testicles and the epididymis.

How to examine your testicles

- The best time is after a warm bath or shower, when the skin of the scrotum is relaxed.
- Support the scrotum and testicles in the palm of your hand, to feel their weight. One testicle may be slightly larger than the other, but they should be about the same weight.
- Hold a testicle between the thumb and fingers, with your thumb on top and first and second fingers underneath. Roll the testicle gently, feeling for any hard lumps. A normal testicle is oval in shape; it feels firm but not hard and is smooth with no lumps.
- Feel the epididymis, a sausage-shaped lump at the top and back of each testicle. It will feel soft and perhaps slightly tender.
- Feel the spermatic cords which lead upwards from the epididymis and behind the testicles. They are firm, smooth tubes.
- Do the same with the other testicle.

If you are worried about lumpiness of the skin of the scrotum, look at the section on lumps on the scrotum on page 188. If you feel a lump within the scrotum, on or alongside your testicle, you must see your doctor straightaway. Also see your doctor if one testicle feels enlarged and heavy, or if when you squeeze it gently it feels much firmer than the other side. In all these cases, it could be a cancer of the testicle. This is the most common type of cancer to affect young men in their 20s and 30s (but it can occur at any age). The good news is that cancer of the testicle can be completely cured in 96% of cases. The earlier it is picked up, the better.

In fact, most swellings in the scrotum turn out to be non-cancerous. For example, it is common to have small lumps and cysts in the epididymis and in the spermatic cord. Surgeons do not usually remove these non-cancerous cysts unless they are large and troublesome. It is important that all lumps in the scrotum are examined by a doctor, so even if you think the swelling is non-cancerous have it checked anyway. If your doctor is not sure, he or she will arrange for you to have an ultrasound scan (which is painless).

'Bag of worms' or varicocele

If you feel something in your scrotum like a bag of worms (most obvious when you are standing), you probably have a varicocele.

What a varicocele is. The 'spermatic cord' that leads upwards from the scrotum carries a tube for sperms to reach the penis, and also veins and arteries. The veins of the spermatic cord can become swollen, elongated and looped, similar to varicose veins in the leg – this is a varicocele. If the veins are only slightly swollen they will be unnoticeable, but moderately swollen veins can often be felt. A varicocele does not usually cause any symptoms, although some men report discomfort or may feel embarrassed if the swollen veins are visible under the skin. About 15% of normal healthy young men have a varicocele, usually on the left side.

Varicocele and fertility. Doctors have been arguing for years about whether a varicocele affects fertility, by damaging the development of sperm in the testicle (*British Medical Journal* 2004;328:967–8). For example, the blood in the swollen veins could act like a hot water bottle, keeping the testicle too warm. Developing sperm like to be cool, which is why the scrotum hangs outside the body. In fact, varicocele is only slightly more common in men with sperm problems and, if it does affect fertility, it is only a small effect.

Treating a varicocele will probably not improve fertility. In 2001, the Cochrane Collaboration, an international network of experts who look at every scrap of scientific evidence about medical problems, investigated varicocele treatment for fertility. They concluded that routinely treating varicoceles in men who are having fertility problems is 'ill-advised', because there is not enough evidence that it does any good. A more recent survey came to the same conclusion (*The Lancet* 2003;361:1849–52).

Missing testicle

Some people have a testicle on only one side. On the other side, the testicle is completely missing or it may be felt as a lump in the groin. In either case, it is called 'undescended testicle'.

How undescended testicle occurs. Your testicles started to develop when you were a tiny fetus (a few weeks after you were conceived). They began high inside your abdomen, near the kidneys at the back. About 6 months before you were born, they started to journey forwards and downwards towards the groin. Meanwhile, your scrotum was developing ready to receive them. About a month or two before birth, the testicles normally complete the journey by descending into the scrotum.

In about 5% of boys, one testicle doesn't make the journey from the back of the abdomen to the scrotum before birth. Instead, it becomes stuck inside the abdomen or at the groin. This why it is called an 'undescended testicle'. No one knows why it happens. For unknown reasons, it is most common in babies born in March or April. It is also common in premature babies (*Surgery* 2004;22:252–5).

Most babies with an undescended testicle do not need any treatment – in 2 out of 3 cases the testicle will come down naturally before the baby is 3 months old. If not, the baby will usually need an operation to bring the testicle down.

What to do if you have only one testicle. If you are a teenager or an adult with an undescended testicle you should definitely see your doctor. Your doctor should refer you to a hospital specialist (urologist). There is no need to feel at all embarrassed, because all doctors know this is a problem that needs attention. There are at least three issues that you will need to discuss with the urologist.

- Firstly, an undescended testicle is slightly more likely to develop cancer than a normal testicle. The risk is roughly 1 in 2000. (The risk of testicular cancer in all men is about 1 in 100,000.) In fact, cancer of the testicle is almost always curable, partly because men easily notice a lump on their testicle and therefore it is caught at an early stage. But if the cancer develops in a testicle that is hidden up in the abdomen, it will be difficult to detect. A testicle that has become stuck in the abdomen is unlikely to be producing sperm, so the urologist may suggest that you have an operation to remove it, to prevent it becoming cancerous in the future. This is a complicated decision, which you will have to discuss in detail with the urologist. It may depend partly on your age; cancer of the testicle is most common in young men, so after the age of about 32 years the risk of the operation may outweigh the likelihood of getting cancer and it might be better to do nothing, but your urologist will advise you.
- Secondly, if you have only one testicle you may be worrying about fertility. Although the undescended testicle probably isn't doing much, you need not be too worried because your other normal testicle is likely to be producing many millions of sperms.
- Thirdly, an undescended testicle is not firmly anchored, and can become twisted on the tissues that surround it. This is called 'torsion'. Episodes of torsion are very painful. So if you have abdominal pain as well as an undescended testicle stuck in the abdomen, your doctor will need to consider the possibility of torsion.
- Fourthly, if having an empty scrotum on one side bothers you, you can ask the urologist about having an artificial implant to give the appearance and feel of a normal testicle. These are either silicone, or a silicone bag filled with saline (similar to a breast implant).

Useful contacts

Andrology Australia provides access to quality and authenticated information to improve understanding and knowledge of the range, causes and treatment options of male reproductive health disorders. The website contains a wide range of information on testicular cancer.
www.andrologyaustralia.org

Institute of Cancer Research is the research arm of the Royal Marsden Hospital, London, UK. Its website has a page on testicular cancer, which has photographs showing how to examine your testicles.
www.icr.ac.uk/everyman/about/testicular.html

Orchid Cancer Appeal has information and diagrams explaining testicular cancer on its website.
www.orchid-cancer.org.uk

Undescended testicle. If you want to know more, look at an excellent article by top expert Professor Steven Docimo, Director of Pediatric Urology at the Children's Hospital of Pittsburgh, US.
www.chp.edu/clinical/03_urosurg_undescend.php

The American Academy of Family Physicians has a fact sheet on undescended testicle.
www.aafp.org/afp/20001101/2047ph.html

Toenail infection

- Nails are made of keratin, the same protein as horses' hooves.
- It takes 12–18 months for a toenail to grow from root to tip.
- If you are right-handed, the nails on your right hand grow faster than on your left, but toenails grow at the same rate on each foot.
- Nails grow faster in summer than winter.
- Toenail problems have strange medical words. Onychogryphosis (*on-ee-co-gry-foe-sis*) is the thickened, hard toenails that old people often have: onychomycosis (*on-ee-co-my-co-sis*) means fungal nail infection.
- In the UK, the NHS spends more than £15 million a year on treatments for fungal nail infection.

Thickened, ugly nails are common – up to 10% of the population have infected toenails – but can be very upsetting. A doctor at Massachusetts General Hospital, US, questioned over 500 people with the condition, and discovered that it led to embarrassment, loss of confidence and self-esteem, and even depression and social isolation (*Journal of the American Academy of Dermatology* 1999;41:189–96). Fortunately, there are now some fairly effective treatments available from your doctor that can help even if you have had the problem for years.

Causes of thickened toenails

Physical damage to your toenail may cause it to be thick until the damaged area grows out. This is why thickening of the big toenails is common in young men, particularly football players. Old people also often have thickened, hard toenails, probably because of the damage they have sustained over the years, and because their nails grow more slowly, it takes longer to repair the damage.

Fungal infection can make your nails thick. The commonest infection is with *Trichophyton rubrum*, the same fungus that causes athlete's foot. Occasionally, other types of fungus, such as yeasts, are responsible, and people who have been abroad may have some quite exotic fungi.

Psoriasis, a skin condition, can make nails thick, with tiny pits on their surface.

How a fungal infection occurs

It is easy to pick up fungi – they are particularly common on the floors of communal showers and changing rooms – and many of us probably already have fungi on our skin. They cause problems only when conditions are ripe for them to thrive, which means warmth and moisture. When human beings started wearing enclosed shoes, which trap sweat and heat, we created ideal conditions for fungi. This is why only 1% of people in Zaire, Africa, have fungal toenails compared with 10% of people in the UK. It is not surprising that fungal toenail infections (and also athlete's foot) are five times as common in people who have to wear work boots for long periods in wet conditions.

The fungi shelter under the tip of the nail and start to get a hold. This is particularly likely to happen if:

- the end of the nail has been damaged (e.g. by ill-fitting shoes) and is already slightly separated from its toe
- you have a condition such as diabetes or an immune deficiency
- you are elderly
- the fungus is already multiplying between the toes (athlete's foot).

The fungus very gradually spreads towards the base of the nail and down the sides, loosening the nail from the underlying toe and filling the separated area with crumbly, yellowish-white gunk. The nail itself becomes thicker and yellowish brown in colour. This can take months or years.

Sometimes the infection starts at the base of the nail, giving a whitish area near the half moon, or it may just affect the surface of the middle of the nail, where it will appear as a white patch.

What you can do

Be patient. For any treatment to be successful, one of the most important elements is patience. You will have to use the treatment for at least 3 months, and some treatments take even longer to work. Nails grow from the base to the tip, as anyone who has used nail varnish knows. Because it can take 18 months for a nail to be replaced completely by a new one, it may be a long time before you see a result.

Try tea-tree oil. The antifungal treatments that you can buy from the chemist, designed for thrush or for athlete's foot, do not penetrate nails and are not worth trying. However, if you really do not want to go to your doctor, you could try tea-tree oil, which is available from health shops and chemists. It has some natural antifungal properties and one study found that it improved or cured 60% of cases of toenail infection. Apply it generously twice a day with a cotton-wool bud, wiping it under the tip of the nail and on the surrounding skin. Because it is an oil, it may discolour leather shoes. At night, soak a small piece of cotton wool with the oil, and tape it to the end of your toe.

Care for your feet sensibly by following these rules.

- Give your feet plenty of air, because warmth and sweat encourage the fungi; so follow the advice given for sweaty feet on page 258. When you are at home, go barefoot whenever possible, and if you don't want to expose your toenails, search for some strappy sandals that cover the toes.
- Choose shoes that give your toes plenty of room.
- Dry your feet very thoroughly after washing, using a tissue to dab underneath the end of the nail to make it as dry as possible.

- It is tempting to use nail varnish to disguise the nail, but nails need to breathe so use it for short periods only, removing it as soon as possible.

Treat athlete's foot promptly. If you ever develop athlete's foot in the future, treat it so it does not spread to the nails.

How a chiropodist can help

For any problem with your feet, particularly the toenails, it is well worth seeing a registered chiropodist – in the UK, they will have the letters SRCh after their name (see Useful contacts on page 298). The chiropodist will be able to advise you on foot care, and will be able to tell you if your thickened toenail is likely to be a fungal infection or due to some other cause. The chiropodist can also thin down the thickened nail so that other treatments such as paints or tablets will be more effective. Chiropodists cannot prescribe antifungal tablets or the most effective antifungal paints – you will have to see your family doctor for these.

How your doctor can help

There are now some quite effective treatments for fungal nail infections – on the downside, they have to be taken for a long time, can have side effects and do not work for all types of fungi. So before starting treatment, your doctor will usually take a sample by scraping under the nail (this may be slightly uncomfortable but not painful) and sending it to the laboratory to identify your particular fungus. It can take over 3 weeks for the laboratory to grow and identify the fungus.

Antifungal nail paints. If only the end of the nail is affected, and the nail is not too thick, and the cause is a *Trichophyton* fungus, your doctor may prescribe a nail paint. There are various types of nail paint.

- 28% tioconazole is applied twice a day for 6 months.
- Amorolfine is applied once a week for 9–12 months.
- Ciclopirox is used in the US, but is not available in the UK.

You need a doctor's prescription for these nail paints – you cannot buy them over the counter. They are inconvenient and it is important to use them continually because if you stop, even for a short period, the new nail that has grown will become infected by the fungus, and you are back to square one. These antifungal paints are not suitable if you are pregnant. Success rates are not very high – about 22% for tioconazole, possibly 40% for amorolfine and about 12% for ciclopirox. However, they do have an important plus point; you apply the drug only to the part of the body where it is needed, rather than taking a tablet that could have side effects.

Medications that you swallow. Your doctor may prescribe terbinafine, fluconazole or itraconazole for certain types of suitable fungus shown on the laboratory test.

- Terbinafine is taken every day for about 3 months.
- Itraconazole is taken twice daily for a week, followed by a 3-week medication-free period. The treatment saturates the nail, and continues to work during the medication-free period. Repeat the treatment cycle two more times.

The treatment does not have an immediate effect. The drug stays in the nail and continues to act for long afterwards, and the result shows when the new, healthy nail grows.

Experts are arguing about how effective these drugs are. Some claim that they have an 80–95% likelihood of cure, but the true figure may be lower – probably about 25–40% for itraconazole and 35–50% for terbinafine (*Archives of Dermatology* 1998;134:1551–4).

Like any drug, these medications can have unwanted side effects. There have been rare cases of severe reactions, and each of these drugs can affect the liver. You should not take itraconazole if you are taking erythromycin (an antibiotic), or if you are taking calcium-channel blocking drugs (for angina or blood pressure). Also, itraconazole may weaken the force of the heart's contractions, so you should not take it if you have a heart problem (see Useful contacts below).

Useful contacts

The Australasian Podiatry Council is the national professional body with which State Associations and Podiatry New Zealand are affiliated. Follow the link to publications and brochures which discuss specific areas of foot care, podiatry and how your podiatrist can contribute to maintaining your foot health.
www.feet.org.au/publications.htm

Health*Insite* is an Australian government initiative aimed to improve the health of Australians by providing easy access to quality information about human health. Follow the link to find information on foot care and foot conditions and diseases.
www.healthinsite.gov.au/topics/Foot_Care

The Society of Chiropodists and Podiatrists is the main society of state-registered chiropodists in the UK. (Some chiropodists use the title 'podiatrist', which is the international name for a chiropodist.) They can help you to find a chiropodist near you. Their website also contains useful information about caring for your feet, and about foot problems including fungal infections.
www.feetforlife.org

The American Podiatric Medical Association has a website page that gives sensible general information about fungal nails, but does not discuss drug treatments in detail.
www.apma.org

Mayo Clinic is a US organization with several pages about fungal infections on their website.
www.mayoclinic.com/invoke.cfm?id=DS00084

US Food and Drug Administration. Safety warnings about drugs for fungal nail infections can be found on the administration's website.
www.fda.gov/cder/drug/advisory/sporanox-lamisil

Tongue problems

In the olden days doctors were very keen on asking patients to put out their tongue, and made all sorts of diagnoses from its appearance. It is true that some conditions can alter the appearance of the tongue (for example, a smooth, red, sore tongue may be a sign of anaemia), but the appearance of the tongue normally varies a lot between individuals.

We each probably have about 10 000 tastebuds on our tongues

'Bald' tongue

The tiny projections that cover the surface of the tongue are called 'papillae'. If you could examine them under a microscope you would see that the papillae are tiny folds of the surface of the tongue. Each is surrounded by a trench, rather like a castle surrounded by a moat. In each trench, there are several clusters of cells sensitive to various tastes; these are the actual taste buds. If we did not have any papillae, the tongue would be very smooth and slippery, and not very efficient at moving food round the mouth. Some animals (such as cats) have very prominent papillae, which is why their tongues feel so rasping.

There are two different sorts of papillae on the tongue – flat ones and slender ones. The slender type are paler in colour. The flat type are bright red in colour and slightly shiny.

Bald sides of the tongue. It is normal for the sides of the tongue to look balder than the middle. The main surface of the tongue is covered by the pale, slender papillae. The flat, shiny papillae cover the sides and tip of the tongue (with a few scattered on the main surface of the tongue, looking like small red spots). Therefore it is normal for the edges of the tongue to look flatter and more shiny.

Patchy tongue

About 2% of people have a patchy appearance of the tongue, called 'geographic tongue'. This sometimes runs in families. The patches are red areas with a distinct margin, and in these areas the slender papillae are reduced. It looks a bit like a map, which is how it got the name 'geographic'. In some people, the papillae are lost only from the sides of the tongue, or the sides and tip. The papillae usually grow again but this can take a long time and, meanwhile, a new patch may be occurring on another part of the tongue. Geographic tongue is not a sign of disease – it is normal and nothing to worry about.

Furred tongue

Instead of looking pink, your tongue may seem to have a greyish-white coating. This is not a sign of disease. It is more common in heavy smokers, people who breathe through their mouth rather than their nose (look at the section on snoring on page 244) and people who eat mainly soft foods (perhaps because they do not want to wear their false teeth). Debris, bacteria and dead cells collect between the papillae and build up into a coating. Eating more high-fibre foods such as vegetables can help or you can discuss it with your dentist, who may suggest that you obtain a tongue scraper (see bad breath on page 33).

Very occasionally, the tongue appears to be black and hairy. This is caused by the papillae of the tongue growing longer than usual and becoming brown in colour. No one knows exactly why this occurs, but it may be made worse by taking antibiotics, using antiseptic mouthwashes, smoking and poor oral hygiene. Try using a tongue scraper and, if it persists, ask your dentist for advice.

White patches

There are two main causes of white patches.

- White patches on the tongue and inside of the cheeks may be caused by thrush, a fungal infection that is common in babies and also in adults who have been taking antibiotics or have been unwell. These patches can be scraped off to leave red, sore areas underneath, and can be improved by special lozenges from your doctor.
- White patches that are not sore, cannot be scraped away and do not go away on their own (leukoplakia) are sometimes an early warning sign that the area could become cancerous in the future. These patches should be checked by your doctor so they can be dealt with before they develop further.

Ulcers and lumps on the tongue

Most people have ulcers on their tongue from time to time. Usually they are very sore, but so small that they are difficult to see. They are harmless, and clear up in a day or two without any treatment. However, you must not ignore a lump on the tongue or an ulcer that doesn't heal, even if it is painless, because it could be a cancer. Get it checked by your doctor if it is still there after 2 weeks. Cancer of the tongue is unlikely under the age of 50.

Tastebuds on the tongue can detect only four tastes – sweetness and saltiness at its tip and centre, acidity at the sides and bitterness at the back. Sense of smell helps to increase our range of tastes, which is why we lose our sense of taste when we have a cold

Tongue piercing

Tongue piercing is normally safe, but it is theoretically possible that it could lead to infection with hepatitis B, hepatitis C or HIV, and it can cause other health problems. So think very carefully about the risks before having it done.

Obviously you must make sure that the person doing the piercing is experienced and that the piercing parlour is hygienic. This may be difficult, because there are no official qualifications or training standards for body piercers in the UK. Check the piercer uses clean needles for each person, disposable gloves and antiseptics, and has a 'sharps' box (as in a doctor's surgery) for disposing of each used needle. The jewellery is not sterile, so ideally the piercer should sterilize it in an 'autoclave' (as in a doctor's surgery). Usually, however, the jewellery is wiped with antiseptic or boiled before insertion; this lessens the risk of infection but not as absolutely as autoclaving. Ask about all of this before you decide to have it done.

The tongue is one of the most touch-sensitive organs in the body; for example, it can detect tiny hairs that our fingers are unable to feel

Bleeding. There is a very slight risk of serious bleeding when you have the piercing done. This is because the tongue contains lots of blood vessels. Because you naturally swallow the blood, you may not realize how much you are bleeding. Doctors at the London Hospital, UK, have given the following advice to anyone having a tongue piercing (*British Dental Journal* 2000;188:657–8).

- Reduce the risk of swelling by sucking ice cubes hourly for the rest of the day.
- If your tongue swells, making it difficult to swallow or breathe, go to the nearest Accident and Emergency Department straight away.
- Every 4 hours, and after eating, give yourself a salt-water mouth bath to help prevent infection. This means dissolving 1 teaspoonful of salt in a glass of hot water, and immersing the site of the piercing for at least 2 minutes. This is awkward but possible – you have to fill the glass fairly full.
- If the area round the jewellery becomes red and tender, you may have an infection. Go to your doctor or an Accident and Emergency Department.
- If part of the jewellery becomes dislodged and you may have swallowed or inhaled it, go to your nearest Accident and Emergency Department.
- If the piercing bleeds, press it firmly with a clean cloth (e.g. a clean handkerchief) for half an hour. If it continues to bleed, go immediately to the Accident and Emergency Department.

Without our tongues, we would not be able to chew, swallow, taste or talk

Other problems. Bleeding is the most serious, but tongue piercing can cause other problems.

- The jewellery may damage your teeth and gums. A study from Ohio State University found that almost half the people wearing a tongue stud for more than 4 years had chipped teeth, and 35% had receding gums because of the stud banging against the gum (*Journal of Periodontology* 2002;73:289–97). The longer the stud had been present, the worse the damage.
- The pierced site could become infected, but this seems to be fairly unusual in the tongue compared with other parts of the body (maybe because of its good blood supply). Resist the temptation to fiddle with the newly inserted stud.
- Because different parts of the tongue are sensitive to different tastes, some people find that a piercing affects their sense of taste. It can also cause slight difficulty in speaking

clearly. If you need an operation, you will be asked to remove the tongue jewellery, because it can cause difficulties with the anaesthetic.

The tongue doubles in length, width and thickness between birth and adolescence

- Allergy is another problem, because the metal may not be pure. You may think that you have pure gold or steel jewellery, but it may contain substantial amounts of nickel, which can cause a sensitivity. When scientists in Finland tested body jewellery, they found that 11 of the 12 items they tested exceeded the EU safety limits for nickel. Surgical stainless steel with the mark 316L is of good quality and is unlikely to cause sensitivities. Niobium is an expensive metal, but is least likely to cause sensitivities.
- The piercing can allow bacteria to enter the bloodstream. In a recent case in the US, the bacteria from a tongue piercing damaged the valves of the heart.

Urinary incontinence

- Of every 10 women, 4 have suffered from incontinence at some time in their adult life.
- Incontinence costs the UK National Health Service about £242 million a year.
- In the US, 20 million people have incontinence of urine. The annual cost is about $12.4 billion for women and $3.8 billion for men.
- In the US, at least $4.5 billion is spent on incontinence pads alone.

Incontinence is leakage of urine from the bladder. It may be just a few drops or a dribble, or may be a stream.

How common is urinary incontinence?

People often keep the problem to themselves, so incontinence is much more common than most people realize. A few years ago the broadcaster Claire Rayner spoke on TV about incontinence; afterwards, the programme received more than 12,000 letters asking for more information. In fact, there are probably about 3 million people in the UK with this problem. In 1995, the Royal College of Physicians estimated that the following numbers of women were affected:

- 5–7% of women aged 15–44 years
- 8–15% of women aged 45–64 years
- about 15% of women aged 65 years or over.

The true numbers are probably much higher. For example, in 1999, a survey in Sweden found that 1 in 8 women under the age of 30 has urinary incontinence. And when a family doctor in the UK sent a questionnaire to 1000 women in his practice aged 44–65 years, he found that 22% had moderate urinary incontinence and 9% had a severe problem. A huge study in the US (the Nurses' Health study) found that 34% of women aged 50–70 years leaked urine at least once a month (*American Journal of Obstetrics and Gynecology* 2002;100:719–23).

Sadly, most women simply put up with it and do not get the help they need. One survey showed that over 1.1 million women are using sanitary towels or panty liners just to cope with leakage of urine. A quarter of women with incontinence wait at least 5 years before going to their doctor.

Incontinence is not a personal failure, nor is it something that 'women should expect'; it can often be cured. A survey in the US found that 6 out of 10 women with urinary incontinence had never talked to their doctor about it (*Journal of Women's Health* 2003;12:687–98).

How the bladder works

- On average, about 1–2 litres (2–3.5 pints) of urine are produced by the kidneys a day.
- Most people do not feel an urge to pass urine until there is about 150–200 mL (about a quarter of a pint) in the bladder.
- The normal adult bladder can hold about 500 mL (1 pint) of urine.

The two kidneys (one on each side) make urine from fluids and dissolved waste matter in the blood. Each day, the kidneys empty about 1.5 litres (3 pints) of urine into the bladder. The wall of the bladder is made of stretchy muscle, so that the bladder stretches like a balloon as it fills with urine.

A ring of muscle at the 'neck' of the bladder acts like a tap, keeping the urine in. This muscle is strengthened greatly by the muscles and ligaments of the pelvic floor that stretch backwards from the pubic bone to the backbone. Imagine a springy trampoline with tubes passing through it – three tubes in women, but only two in men.

- The pelvic floor muscle is like the trampoline.
- In women, the three tubes passing through the pelvic floor muscle are the bowel, the vagina and the bladder neck.
- In men, the two tubes passing through the pelvic floor muscle are the bowel and the bladder neck.

In women, the bladder and womb lie on top of the pelvic floor. The pelvic floor is stronger in men because they do not have a vagina passing through it.

It is unsurprising that incontinence (leakage of urine) is common. As humans, we walk upright and our bladder system is not really suited for it – it is like holding halfe a litre of urine in a floppy bag that is open at the bottom. If we walked on all fours, this would not be a problem. In fact, without the help of the pelvic floor muscles, the bladder neck would not be able to keep the bladder closed.

When the bladder contains about 500 mL (1 pint) of urine, it sends signals to the brain that you need to urinate. When it is convenient to do so, the bladder muscle stops stretching and begins to contract, squeezing the urine out. At the same time, the bladder and pelvic floor muscles relax, allowing the urine to come out. The urine then passes down a tube, called the urethra, to the outside. In women, the urethra is short. In men, the urethra is long; it passes through the prostate gland, and then along the penis to the hole at the end.

Types of incontinence and why it happens

Incontinence is leakage of urine from the bladder. It can happen to anyone at any age, but is more common in women. The idea that it affects only the elderly is completely out of date – the popularity of active sports, such as jogging, has caused more younger women to notice the problem.

What type of incontinence do you have?

There are two main types of incontinence – 'stress incontinence' and 'overactive bladder' (urge incontinence). Many women have both types together and this is called 'mixed incontinence'. Look at the box below to see what type you have. About 1 in 4 women with incontinence of urine also have faecal incontinence (see page 123; *Obstetrics and Gynaecology* 2002;100:17–23).

Questions to ask yourself	***Stress incontinence***	***Overactive bladder***	***Mixed incontinence***
Do you go to the toilet to pass urine more than 7 times a day?	No	Yes	Sometimes
Do you go to the toilet to pass urine more than once during the night?	Not usually	Most nights	Most nights
Do you ever have to hurry to reach the toilet in time (for urine)?	No	Yes	Yes
Do you ever not reach the toilet in time (for urine)?	No	Often	Often
Do you ever leak urine when you laugh, sneeze, cough, run or jump?	Always	No	Always
If you leak urine, is it just a drop or is it sometimes quite a bit more?	Small	Large (usually)	Large
Are you able to hold your urine all right, but you need to pass it more than 7 times a day, in small or large amounts each time?	See your doctor, because you might have a urine infection (small amounts) or diabetes (large amounts and you are thirsty).		

Reasons for stress incontinence

Leakage of urine when you cough, laugh or bend over, or with exercise such as jumping or jogging, is called stress incontinence. It is most common in young women (25–49 years of age). It occurs if the muscles at the neck of the bladder are not strong enough to hold the urine in when the pressure in the abdomen is increased (as happens when you laugh or cough). No one knows exactly why these muscles may become weak; some women notice the problem after childbirth or the menopause. Women with stress incontinence often have leakage of urine during sex (see page 299), usually at penetration (when the penis enters).

Genes are now thought to be a very important cause of stress incontinence, which explains why this type of incontinence tends to run in families (*Obstetrics and Gynecology* 2005;106: 1253–8). Because of their genes, some women are born with a weak pelvic floor. It is probably a weakness of collagen, the tiny strengthening fibres of muscles.

Childbirth is probably an important cause of stress incontinence. The actual birth is mostly responsible, not just the pregnancy – women who have had Caesarean sections do not usually develop incontinence later. It seems that the nerves can be stretched and bruised during the delivery, and they are unable to make the pelvic floor work after the birth. As a result, the muscles become lazy and weak. However, some research suggests that women who have had children are not more likely to have incontinence (*Obstetrics and Gynecology* 2005; 106: 1253–8), so it seems that more research is necessary.

Hysterectomy. A woman who has had a hysterectomy is more likely to develop incontinence in middle age than a woman who has not had the operation.

Menopause may be another reason, perhaps because the lowering levels of oestrogen make the pelvic floor muscles less efficient. However, recent research shows that although the likelihood of incontinence increases in middle-age, the hormone changes of the menopause may not be the cause. The reason may be that middle-aged women are more likely to be overweight and to have had a gynaecological operation, such as a hysterectomy.

High impact sports, such as jogging on hard pavements, are probably not good for the pelvic floor. Sports such as swimming and cycling are fine. Interestingly, women parachutists in the US Air Force have developed incontinence because the impact of landing has damaged their pelvic floor.

Lifting heavy objects strains the pelvic floor. If you have to lift anything heavy (such as a baby or small child!), get into the habit of doing it in the right way. Place your feet firmly apart in the standing position, and bend at the knees and hip but keep your back straight. Tighten your pelvic floor muscles, hold the heavy object close to you and then lift by straightening your legs.

Obesity. Being overweight is a major cause of incontinence. It puts stress on the pelvic floor muscles.

Smoking 20 cigarettes a day (now or in the past) doubles your likelihood of urinary incontinence – another reason for never smoking.

Drugs can relax the pelvic floor around the ring of muscles at the neck of the bladder, making leakage more likely. The most common culprits are some blood pressure medications (particularly alpha-blockers such as prazosin and doxazosin). If your incontinence problem seems to be related to starting treatment for blood pressure, ask your doctor if you are taking an alpha-blocker. Medications for other conditions, such as fluoxetine (Prozac) and muscle-relaxant drugs, can also promote urine leakage.

Reasons for overactive bladder

The sudden need to pass urine desperately, and maybe not being able to reach the toilet in time, is a slightly different sort of incontinence called overactive bladder. The cause is misbehaviour of the bladder muscle; it starts to contract when it should be stretching to hold more urine. This is called an overactive or irritable bladder (the medical term is detrusor instability, because the bladder muscle is called the detrusor muscle). It means that people with urge incontinence have to pass urine often (probably more than 8 times a day and also during the night), but may not pass much each time. Women with urge incontinence often have leakage of urine during sex (see page 299), usually at orgasm.

Reasons for mixed incontinence

Some people with incontinence have both stress incontinence and an overactive bladder. The 'stress' symptoms may be more prominent than the 'urge' symptoms, or vice versa.

IN WOMEN

You may think that if you have leakage of urine then you just have to put up with the problem, and maybe spend a fortune on pads. This is not generally true.

Decide what type of incontinence you have

It is helpful to work out whether you have stress incontinence or overactive bladder, or both, because they have different treatments. There are some simple questions (see page 285) to ask yourself to find out.

What you can do for stress incontinence

There are no effective medications for stress incontinence, but there is a lot you can do to help yourself.

Check whether you are taking an alpha-blocker for raised blood pressure (hypertension). Alpha-blockers can cause stress incontinence, and your doctor could probably prescribe a different type of blood pressure medication instead.

Lose weight. Being overweight puts stress on your pelvic floor muscles and losing weight can reduce leakage by 60% (*Journal of Urology* 2005;174:190–5).

Cross your legs when you feel a cough or sneeze coming on. This sounds ridiculously simple, but a scientific study found that it helped prevent leakage in 73% of women.

Squeeze before you sneeze. Just before you cough or sneeze, tighten your pelvic floor muscles and hold them tight to prevent leakage.

Strengthen your pelvic floor muscles with pelvic floor exercises or vaginal cones.

Pelvic floor exercises are especially useful for stress incontinence and reduce episodes of leakage by 50%. You may have to do them for a few months before you notice any improvement, so patience is essential. Ideally, these should be taught by a continence adviser as it is easy to do them incorrectly. One advantage is that they are invisible, so you can do them at anytime – at bus stops, in the supermarket queue or while talking on the phone! Once you have learnt to tighten your pelvic floor muscles, you can squeeze them and hold when you sneeze, lift or jump. This will protect them from more damage.

Learning pelvic floor exercises

- Stand, sit or lie with your knees slightly apart (sitting is easiest). Now imagine that you are trying to stop yourself passing wind from the back passage; to do this, you must tighten the muscles round the back passage. Squeeze and lift those muscles as if you really do have wind: you should be able to feel the muscles move and the skin round the back passage tightening. Your legs and buttocks should not move at all.
- Next, imagine that you are sitting on the toilet passing urine. Imagine yourself trying to stop the stream of urine (the stop test) – really try hard. You will be using the same group of muscles as in the first exercise, but you will find it more difficult.
- Next time you go to the toilet to pass urine, try the stop test about half way through emptying your bladder. (If the flow of urine speeds up, you are using the wrong muscles.) Once you have stopped the flow of urine, relax and allow the bladder to empty completely. Do not worry if you find you can only slow the stream, and cannot stop it completely.
- If you are unsure you are exercising the right muscles, put one or two fingers in the vagina and try the exercise to check. You should feel a gentle squeeze if you are exercising the pelvic floor. A common mistake is to just clench your buttocks and hold your breath; if you can not hold a conversation at the same time, you are doing the exercises wrongly. Counting aloud while you do the exercises will stop you holding your breath. Do not tighten the tummy, thigh or buttock muscles or cross your legs. Only use your pelvic floor muscles.

Using pelvic floor exercises

- Stand, sit or lie with your knees slightly apart. Slowly tighten and pull up the pelvic floor muscles as hard as possible. Hold tightened for at least 5 seconds if you can, then relax (slow pull-up). Repeat at least 5 times. Now pull the muscles up quickly and tightly, then relax immediately (fast pull-up). Repeat at least 5 times. Do these exercises – 5 slow and 5 fast – at least 10 times every day.
- Suck your thumb at the same time – you will find it helps to lift the pelvic floor.

Vaginal cones are an easier way of toning up the pelvic floor, though they are not as effective as the exercises. The cones can be bought as a set (Aquaflex) consisting of several different weights with directions for using them (see Useful contacts on page 297). You insert a cone into your vagina and hold it there by contracting the pelvic muscles. The cones have a rounded shape and are comfortable to use. The only problem is that it can be difficult to hold the cone in – a continence adviser can show you how to contract the correct muscles, which is similar to doing the pelvic floor exercises. You should start with the cone that you can hold for 1 minute. By using it twice a day, you will find that you can gradually hold it in for longer and longer. When you can hold it for 15 minutes, progress to the next weight of cone. The aim is to use the heaviest cone in the set for 15 minutes twice a day.

Which is better – pelvic floor exercises or vaginal cones?

A study in Norway (*British Medical Journal* 1999;318:487–93) gave the following results.

	Some improvement	*Almost cured*	*Completely cured*	*No effect*
Pelvic floor exercises for 6 months	8%	44%	40%	8%
Vaginal cones for 20 minutes/day for 6 months	0%	37%	44%	19%

Support your bladder neck to keep the bladder closed. You may find that simply inserting a large-size ('super') tampon before sport of vigorous activity is all you need. (Remember to remove it afterwards.) There are some specially designed vaginal devices that do a similar job, such as Contiguard, Contrelle, Contiform and Introl. Some women find them uncomfortable and they are not effective for everyone. Before buying one, get advice from a continence advisor.

What you can do for an overactive bladder

- Does it sting when you pass urine? If so, you probably have cystitis. See your doctor – the urge incontinence will disappear or improve when the infection is treated.
- Use mental tricks to take your mind off the urge. For example, concentrate on the mental image of a tight knot in a balloon. Or distract yourself by thinking of as many words as you can beginning with the letter A, and then work your way through the alphabet.
- Empty your bladder properly each time you pass urine. Do not 'hover' over the toilet seat. Sit down and bend forward at the waist, and take your time.
- The bladder can be 'retrained' to hold larger amounts of urine, so that the muscle does not start to contract until you are ready. This 'bladder retraining drill' (see page 290) is tedious but does work, particularly for urge incontinence.
- Do pelvic floor exercises. They will not cure the bladder contractions that cause the urge, but stronger pelvic floor muscles will minimize any leakages.

- It is natural to think that by cutting the amount you drink, you will have more control and research backs up this idea (*Journal of Urology* 2005;174:187–9). However, it could make the problem worse by increasing your susceptibility to irritating bladder infections (cystitis) and encouraging the bladder to empty when it does not contain much urine.
- Cut out coffee and strong tea – caffeine encourages overactivity of the bladder muscle.
- Stop smoking – nicotine irritates the bladder.
- Eat plenty of fresh fruit, vegetables and fibre to avoid constipation, which can press on the bladder and the urethra.

Bladder retraining drill

Bladder retraining is based on passing urine by the clock at regular intervals. If holding on is difficult, distract yourself by watching TV or making a phone call

Days 1 and 2

Start by choosing an interval you feel fairly confident you can achieve, such as 1–2 hours. Continue this for 2 days.

Days 3 and 4

Increase the interval between emptying by 15 minutes. Continue with this interval for 2 days.

Day 5 onwards

When you are comfortable with the extra 15 minutes, increase it again. As each interval becomes manageable, increase it again.

Seeing your doctor or continence advisor

You can ask your doctor for advice or, in the UK, you can get help from a continence adviser. Continence advisers are specially trained nurses or physiotherapists. They are expert at working out what type of incontinence (see page 285) you have and the best way to deal with it. They can teach you how to do pelvic floor exercises properly, and tell you whether it is worth buying aids and devices such as vaginal cones.

Your doctor or continence advisor will also be able to check that you do not have a urinary infection or an unusual type of incontinence. For example, you might have a prolapsed womb (see page 190) that is pressing on the bladder. The doctor may wish to do a vaginal examination, inserting a speculum (like when you have a smear) to check for prolapse of the womb.

If you discuss your problem with your doctor, it is quite likely that your doctor will put you in touch with a continence adviser. But you do not have to go through your doctor – you can arrange to see a continence adviser yourself. In the UK, your local Citizens' Advice Bureau should be able to give you details, or you can find out more from The Continence Foundation or Incontact (see Useful contacts on page 297).

Things you can do before visiting your doctor or continence adviser. Make a urine chart for a few days before your appointment to record how your bladder is actually behaving.

Get a jug (marked in millilitres or fluid ounces) – one that you can easily pass urine into – and use it to measure how much urine you pass on each occasion. Note down the time and the volume on a chart. Also make a record of the occasions when leakage occurs. You can print off a chart from the National Kidney and Urologic Diseases Information Clearinghouse website (see Useful contacts on page 297).

Be prepared for questions: your doctor or continence adviser may ask you some of the following, so you might want to think about the answers in advance.

- What medicines are you taking? Take a list with you, and include medicines you buy 'over the counter', as well as prescription medicines.
- When did you start having bladder trouble?
- If you have had the menopause, when did your periods stop?
- Have you had any operations?
- Do you have any pain or burning feeling when you pass urine?
- Do you often have a really strong urge to pass urine immediately?
- Do you leak when you cough or sneeze?
- How do you cope? Do you sometimes wear a sanitary pad because you are worried about leakage?
- How is the problem affecting your life? Do you avoid going out or doing certain activities because of bladder control problems? Are you always on the lookout for the nearest toilet?

What your doctor can do

Your doctor or continence advisor may suggest any of the following options.

Medication for stress incontinence. If your main problem is stress incontinence, there is now a specialist medication, Duloxetine, which is taken twice daily. Duloxetine halves the number of leakage episodes, and 1 in 10 women taking it becomes completely dry. Nausea is the most common side effect (*British Journal of Obstetrics and Gynaecology* 2004;111: 249–57). Other side effects include dry mouth, fatigue and constipation. There have been concerns (but no proof) that it could lead to suicidal thoughts either during treatment or if it is suddenly stopped (*Current Problems in Pharmacovigilance* 2006; 31:2).

Another new medication, solifenacin (see page 292), may also help stress incontinence, though its main use is for overactive bladder.

Medicines for overactive bladder. If you have an overactive bladder, there are some drugs your doctor can prescribe that may help. However, all these drugs have side effects – some make you less alert, so you have to be careful about driving or operating dangerous machinery while taking them. The medication may take some time to work, so persist with it.

- The most common medications for overactive bladder are oxybutynin and tolterodine. These drugs are very similar and work in the same way, by calming the bladder muscle. Their side effects are dry mouth, constipation and blurring of vision. Doctors now usually prescribe 'extended-release' types of these drugs, which you need to take only once a day and which are less likely to have side effects. Extended-release tolterodine seems to have slightly fewer side effects than extended-release oxybutynin (*Mayo Clinic* Proceedings 2003;78:687–95). Oxybutynin is also available as a skin patch; this has fewer side effects than the tablet form, but some people are allergic to the active patch.

- Solifenacin and darifenacin are newer medications which are taken daily to calm bladder muscle. Their main side effects are dry mouth and constipation. It is not yet clear whether they are better than the older medications (though a study has shown solifenacin to be more effective than tolterodine). One benefit of darifenacin is that it does not cause confusion in elderly people, which can occur with some bladder-calming drugs.
- Propiverine and trospium chloride also work in a similar way to oxybutynin, but have to be taken several times a day. Flavoxate has less severe side effects than oxybutynin, but is less effective.
- In the past, propantheline was often used, but this has more side effects than other drugs.
- Imipramine and amitriptyline help urge incontinence by a different action from their antidepressant effect, and are particularly useful for women whose main problem is incontinence during orgasm (see urinating during sex on page 299) or having to pass urine at night.
- Desmopressin is sometimes used for people whose main problem is constantly having to get up and pass urine at night.

Special devices. A number of special devices to help keep the urethra (pee hole) closed are available.

- Devices such as Miniguard, FemAssist and Capsure are tiny caps that are placed over the urethra. They stay in place by suction or the use of an adhesive. They can irritate, but can be helpful for some women with mild incontinence.
- Appliances such as the Urethral Plug, Reliance Insert and Femsoft are inserted into the urethra to plug it. They are tricky to use, and you have to be shown how by a continence adviser or doctor. They are suitable only for short periods, such as during exercise. The main problems are discomfort and infection, or the device may move up inside and be impossible to remove without specialist medical help.

Hormone replacement therapy (HRT). In the past, doctors thought that HRT might help stress incontinence and overactive bladder. This has now been disproved by a study in the US of more than 25 000 women. In fact, women taking HRT were more likely to develop stress incontinence or overactive bladder. If they already had a leakage problem, HRT made it worse (*Journal of the American Medical Association* 2004;172:1919–24).

Botulinum toxin (Botox). Tiny injections of botox into the wall of the bladder are being investigated as another method of calming the bladder muscle in urge incontinence. The effects last for about 8 months and then the procedure has to be repeated.

Special hospital tests. If the cause of your incontinence is not obvious to your doctor, you may be referred to a hospital for urodynamic tests to obtain an accurate diagnosis. These may cause some discomfort – a small tube (1 mm in diameter) is inserted into the bladder to measure pressures, and sometimes a small tube is also inserted into the back passage.

Referral for a surgical operation is a last resort, and you would need to have urodynamic tests first, to be absolutely sure what type of incontinence you have. This is because surgery is usually only for stress incontinence – it cannot really help overactive bladder.

There are many different operations for stress incontinence (more than 200 at the last count). If the pelvic floor muscles have become weak (see page 285–6), the bladder neck and top of the urethra (see page 284) will not be in their correct position, and so will not function effectively (with the help of the pelvic floor muscles) to stop leakage of urine. Surgery aims to lift the neck of the bladder and the urethra, and secure them in their anatomically correct position. The commonest operations are as follows.

- The tension-free vaginal tape (TVP) sling operation is now very popular. It is possible to do it under a local anaesthetic or spinal block (that is, without a general anaesthetic). Working through the vagina and two small incisions in the abdomen, the surgeon places special polypropylene (prolene) tape beneath the urethra, and adjusts the tension on the tape until it is just right. One study showed that it cures almost 70% of people (*British Medical Journal* 2002;235:67–70).
- Sling operations involve passing a piece of tissue or artificial material (such as silastic or nylon) under the urethra and bladder neck, to support them like a hammock, and attaching it to the wall of the abdomen and the pelvic bones on each side. The success rate is about 85%, but later problems (such as an urgent need to pass urine, or damage to the urethra from the tightness of the support) can occur.
- In the Burch colposuspension, the surgeon attaches the top of the vagina to ligaments that lie close to the pubic bones, thereby supporting the bladder neck. This is a more major operation than the tension-free tape operation. The cure rate is approximately 80–90%, but problems (such as an urgent need to pass urine) can occur later.

Bulking injections (for stress incontinence) use collagen, fat or particles of silicone rubber to bulk up the tissues around the urethra and bladder neck. The collagen given in these injections comes from the hides of freshly slaughtered cattle. These cattle are bred and live in closed herds in the US, and never receive any animal protein in their diet. It is therefore very unlikely that collagen injections could transmit mad cow disease (BSE). Some people are allergic to collagen, so every candidate is given an allergy test 4 weeks beforehand.

A newer option is a gel made from non-animal stabilized hyaluronic acid (NASHA) and dextran, both of which are natural substances.

The material is injected by inserting a needle alongside the urethra, or into the urethra and through its wall. A local anaesthetic is given to prevent pain. Most women need 2 or 3 injections, given at weekly intervals. They have to be given by an expert, and you will need urodynamic tests first to measure how your bladder is working.

About 60–70% of women find their symptoms are cured or improved by the treatment. However, the effect may not last. After 3 years only 50% remain cured, and after 5 years only 26%. For this reason, bulking injections are not often used in Europe, but they may be suitable for people who are not fit enough for a surgical operation.

Electrostimulation. An electrode in the vagina, attached to a battery, makes the pelvic floor muscles contract. The electrical current is tiny, so there is no need to worry. The apparatus is used for 30 minutes a day. This normally has to be arranged through a hospital clinic, because it is suitable only for women with severe incontinence who cannot be treated by other methods.

The future. A number of possible new treatments are being investigated.

- The new technique of 'sacral neuromodulation' is being investigated for patients with very severe symptoms. A small electrode is placed close to the nerves in the lower back that control urination. The electrode is connected to a battery and is used to stimulate the nerves. It somehow 'resets' the control of the bladder. It is expensive (the aparatus costs over £10,000 in the UK) and so it is being tried out on only a few patients.
- Drugs based on chilli peppers are being investigated for urge incontinence. Substances in chilli peppers have a numbing effect on nerves in the bladder wall, so could calm the bladder, but the treatment is painful. A similar treatment derived from the cactus-like plant *Euphorbia resinifera* is more promising, because it is not painful.
- *New Scientist* magazine (9 June 2001) reported research at the University of Pittsburgh, USA, that suggests that incontinence might be curable in the future using stem cells taken from the person's own muscles and then grown in a laboratory. The cells would then be injected into the bladder muscle to strengthen it and restore control.

IN MEN

Incontinence (leakage of urine) is not just a women's problem – plenty of men have difficulty controlling their urine.

- 5–7% of men *under* 64 years of age have urinary incontinence.
- 10–20% of men *over* 64 years of age have urinary incontinence.
- In men, incontinence can take various forms.
- If you have the most common form, you have to rush to the toilet (urgency), and perhaps leak on the way (urge incontinence). This is often worse in cold weather or if you hear the sound of running water. You may notice some dribbling after you have passed urine. These problems are most common in older men. They are often partly related to a blockage at the outlet of the bladder, caused by enlargement of the prostate gland – benign prostatic hypertrophy (BPH).
- Some men have had bladder problems all their lives, such as bed-wetting, urgency, urge incontinence or having to pass urine frequently.
- Difficulty in holding urine sometimes results from a previous prostate operation.

Why prostate enlargement causes incontinence

Enlargement of the prostate gland tends to occur with ageing. At 60 years of age, about 40% of men have enlarged prostates, but this rises to 75% by the age of 80. The reason is not known, but it is not a cancerous condition.

A normal adult prostate is about the size of a chestnut and weighs 20–25 g, but in benign prostatic hypertrophy (BPH), it can increase to 60 g or more. As it expands, the prostate wraps itself round the neck of the bladder like a collar, restricting the outlet, and the bladder muscle has to work harder to push the urine out.

- Because of the obstruction, you notice that you have a poor stream or that starting the stream is difficult or that urine seems to flow in stops and starts.
- The strain makes the bladder muscle misbehave so that it often starts to contract before the bladder is full, causing urgency. Because the bladder tends to contract before it is full, you will pass urine frequently in small amounts and often have to get up in the night to urinate.
- The bladder has difficulty in emptying completely, because the outlet is restricted, and there is always some urine left inside. Gradually, more and more urine is left inside and, in severe cases, eventually overflows without any feeling of urgency. This is called 'overflow incontinence'.

What you can do

Try to work out if your prostate is enlarged. If you can answer 'yes' to any of the following questions, it is quite likely that you have an enlarged prostate.

- Do you have difficulty in starting to pass urine?
- Do you think it takes you too long to pass urine?
- Do you pass urine in stops and starts?
- Do you dribble urine without full control when you have tried to stop?
- Do you have a sensation of not having emptied your bladder completely?
- Do you have to get up more than twice a night to pass urine, but only pass small amounts?

If you do think that your prostate may be enlarged, then you should arrange to see your doctor to check that this is the cause of your symptoms. If the problem is really troubling you, your doctor may decide to try medication. A drug (finasteride) is available to shrink the prostate, but when you stop taking it the prostate starts to grow again. Other drugs (alpha-blockers) relax the bladder neck and the prostate itself, but have side effects in some people. You may need a prostatectomy operation to remove the enlarged prostate.

Decide whether urgency is your main symptom. If you have urgency, you could try 'bladder retraining' (see page 290). Some men find this helps, but generally it is not as effective in men as in women. Discuss the problem with your doctor, because there are various medicines (see page 291) that are very effective in calming an overactive bladder.

Dribbling after passing urine. If you dribble after passing urine, try running your finger along the underside of your penis to force out any remaining liquid.

Bed-wetting. If you have always had bladder problems, including wetting the bed at night as an adult, look at the section on bed-wetting (see page 39) and then discuss it with your doctor.

Other approaches. Even if your incontinence cannot be cured completely, there are ways of getting over problems.

LIVING WITH URINARY INCONTINENCE

Even if your incontinence cannot be cured completely, it need not make your life a misery. There are lots of equipment and services (see Useful contacts on page 297) that can help. Your doctor, practice nurse or continence adviser can give you more information.

- Many types of disposable pads and absorbent underwear are available to suit different needs. For example, a bulky pad might be best at night, and a less obtrusive pad or absorbent panties preferable during the day.
- If you have leakage at night, look at the section on bed-wetting (see page 39). In the UK, you can obtain bed protection from the Enuresis Resource and Information Centre (ERIC; see Useful contacts on page 297), and a district nurse can arrange a supply of disposable or washable pads for the bed. If you are incontinent, some local authorities in the UK will collect bedlinen from your house, launder it and return it.
- Urine becomes smelly when it has been exposed to the air for a while. You may become used to the smell and not notice it yourself. Change wet clothes and bedlinen as soon as you can, and keep them in a bucket with a lid until they can be washed. Open your bedroom window to air it thoroughly every day. Put wet, disposable pads or panties into a plastic bag, seal it firmly with a rubber band and put it into an outside dustbin as soon as possible.
- Wear clothes that are easy to manage when you go to the toilet in a hurry. For example, stockings or 'stay-ups' are easier than tights. Tight skirts, or trousers with a tricky fastening, can cause delays.
- Perhaps your toilet could be made easier for you, especially if you are elderly. 'Grab rails' fixed to the wall, or free-standing round the toilet, will help you to balance. If you have arthritic hips, a raised seat to the toilet will help.
- Do not endanger yourself by rushing to the toilet if you are unsteady. Research has shown that elderly people who need to rush to the toilet are more likely to fall and fracture a bone than those who do not have a urine problem. Better to have wet underwear than a broken hip.
- If you are a man, a plastic urine bottle (urinal) by your bed is very helpful. It can also be used when you are sitting in a chair, though this may seem difficult at first. Plastic urinals are also available for women, but are more awkward to use. Make sure that you empty and rinse out the urinal as soon as possible.
- Consider a commode if you cannot reach your toilet easily. This is a special chair that contains a bucket in its seat. Some designs have a lid, so they look like a normal chair.
- A very few people will require a catheter. This is a small tube passed into the bladder through the urethra. The urine empties down the catheter into a disposable bag that is secured to the thigh and hidden under skirts or trousers.

Useful contacts

The Continence Foundation of Australia (CFA) is the national peak body for continence management, promotion and advocacy. It has a national helpline, which offers free, confidential advice about bladder and bowel control. Its website offers a range of fact sheets on incontinence disorders.
www.contfound.org.au

Health*Insite* is an Australian government initiative aimed to improve the health of Australians by providing easy access to quality information about human health. Follow the link \ to topic pages on urinary incontinence.
www.healthinsite.gov.au/topics/Incontinence

The Continence Foundation is a UK non-profit organization that gives advice and information. Their website is first-rate, full of excellent information. Look in the 'Clinics' section of the website to find a local continence advisor, or contact their helpline.
www.continence-foundation.org.uk

Incontact (Action on Incontinence) is a non-profit organization providing information and support for people with bladder and bowel incontinence problems through its publications, website and local groups in the UK. The website has lots of excellent advice in its 'Treatment review' section. It also has an 'Ask an expert' facility. Incontact can also tell you how to get in contact with a local continence advisor.
www.incontact.org

National Association for Continence (NAFC) is a US non-profit organization that aims to improve the quality of life for people with incontinence. Its website has helpful information.
www.nafc.org

The Enuresis Resource and Information Centre (ERIC) is a UK non-profit organization that provides information on all aspects of bed-wetting in children, teenagers and adults. Their excellent website has a special section for teenagers. ERIC also sell useful aids, such as bed protection, as well as providing a range of very helpful publications.
www.trusteric.org (for teenagers)
www.eric.org.uk

National Kidney and Urologic Diseases Information Clearinghouse is a very informative website provided by the US Public Health Service. It has clear and accurate information about all aspects of incontinence, and is well worth a look. Its Bladder Council for Women link gives access to several useful leaflets, including 'Exercising your pelvic muscles'.
http://kidney.niddk.nih.gov/kudiseases/pubs/uiwomen/index.htm
http://kidney.niddk.nih.gov/kudiseases/pubs/bladdercontrol/index.htm

The American Academy of Family Physicians has a web page explaining incontinence and pelvic muscle exercises, and a link to a more detailed article written for doctors; some of the drugs mentioned in this article are not available in other countries. The article was written in 2000, so does not have the latest information.
www.aafp.org/afp/20001201/2447ph.html
www.aafp.org/afp/20001201/2433.html

Help the Aged produces an advice booklet on incontinence, which has useful information for people of any age. The advice booklet is available on their website.
www.helptheaged.org.uk

Prostate Research Campaign UK is a non-profit organization that aims to increase awareness and sponsor research into prostate disorders. If you think you might have a prostate problem, look at their website for unbiased and up-to-the-minute information.
www.prostate-research.org.uk

PromoCon is a UK non-profit organization that provides information on products to prevent and manage incontinence, and on incontinence advisory services and local support groups.
www.promocon.co.uk

Aquaflex vaginal cones are available in the UK from larger branches of Boots. TENA and Poise are some of the many absorbent pads that are available for women with incontinence.
www.tena.co.uk
www.poise.com

Urinating during sex

Passing urine during intercourse, and being unable to control it, happens to many women. No one seems to talk about this, so a sufferer thinks she is the only one with the problem.

Is it common?

A doctor did a survey of women attending his urogynaecology clinic (many of whom of course already had an incontinence problem) and found that 24% had incontinence during intercourse (*British Journal of Obstetrics and Gynaecology* 1988;95:377–81). Most had felt too embarrassed to mention it to their doctor.

- In about two-thirds, the leakage occurs when the penis enters the vagina (penetration).
- In about one-third, the leakage occurs only at orgasm.

What causes it?

The reason is not understood, but it is likely to be partly due to an irritable bladder or a weakness at the neck of the bladder (see page 284). If you have difficulty holding urine during the day, you may experience leakage during intercourse. However, many women have leakage of urine during intercourse but not at any other time.

Could it be 'female ejaculation'?

In 1950, a Dr Grafenberg described what he called 'female ejaculation ... the expulsion of large quantities of clear transparent fluid at the height of orgasm'. Some sex manuals still talk about this 'female ejaculation' as if it were some kind of discharge of sexual glands. They claim it comes from Skene's glands, which are supposed to be similar to the prostate gland in men.

People who believe in 'female ejaculation' say that analysis of this fluid reveals high levels of an enzyme called acid phosphatase that is made by prostate-type gland tissue. In fact:

- a study in six women showed that their 'female ejaculate' fluid contained the same amount of acid phosphatase as their urine
- a study of just one woman did find high levels of acid phosphatase in the fluid she released at orgasm, but the method used to analyse it was unreliable.

The facts have been reviewed in the US medical journal *American Journal of Obstetrics and Gynecology* (2001;185:359–62), and it now seems clear that this fluid is just urine.

What can be done

- Empty your bladder before sex.
- Cut down on caffeine-containing drinks and alcohol.
- Do not drink excessive amounts of fluid – not more than 1.5 litres (2.5 pints) over 24 hours.

- Discuss the problem with your doctor, especially if you have leakage at other times.
- Your doctor may prescribe oxybutynin or a similar drug (see page 291) for you. You should take this about an hour before sex (if you can plan that well ahead!).
- Alternatively, your doctor can prescribe imipramine, to be taken in the evening. This is normally given as an antidepressant, but it also has effects on the bladder (which is why a similar drug is used to treat bed-wetting in children). If your doctor suggests it, it is because of its bladder effects, not because he or she thinks you are depressed. The dose will be lower than given for depression.
- If none of these deals with the problem, it would be worth asking for a referral to a gynaecologist, preferably one who specializes in urogynaecology. If you have leakage at other times, as well as during sex, an operation (see page 293) to strengthen the bladder neck is sometimes recommended. Unfortunately this operation is successful in controlling leakage during intercourse in only two-thirds of people.
- In the end, you and your partner may simply have to come to terms with the problem, and enjoy your sex life in spite of it. If it is causing a real problem in your relationship, or affecting your feelings about yourself, a few sessions with a psychosexual counsellor can be very helpful.
- You can also contact a number of organizations (see pages 297–8) for help and advice.

Urination shyness

Some men find it difficult to urinate in the presence of other men. They cannot urinate in a public toilet if anyone else is there. The muscles that control urination tighten up, stopping the flow. This is called 'parauresis' or 'bashful bladder syndrome'. According to doctors in the armed forces – who know about servicemen living in open barracks – it is quite common and possibly 1 in 10 men is affected. It can be distressing, because it can limit your activities if you are unable to urinate away from home. And some people worry that others might assume they are gay because they are spending so long at the urinal.

What causes 'bashful bladder'?

There is nothing physically wrong. It does not mean that there is anything amiss with your bladder or urethra. No one knows what causes it, but it seems to be an exaggeration of something that most men experience slightly. Research has shown that when a stranger is nearby, most men take slightly longer to start their urine flow, and pass urine for a shorter length of time.

A doctor writing in the medical journal *The Lancet* (1999;354:78) has a suggestion about the cause of bashful bladder. He points out that many male mammals mark their territory by urinating to leave their scent. He wonders if modern men with the problem are subconsciously thinking 'If I urinate in this other male's presence, I am asserting my supremacy over his territory – am I really ready to challenge this male to a fight', and this prevents them from urinating.

What you can do

- Try doing a series of mathematical calculations in your head. This activates the cortex of the brain and blocks the inhibiting impulses to the bladder. A report in *The Lancet* as long ago as 1981 suggested this as an effective remedy.
- Breathe in deeply and tighten your pelvic muscles, as if you are pulling your anus (back passage) inwards. Then relax and breathe out. Repeat until you start to pass some urine.
- If it is really affecting your life, you could get help from a behaviour therapist, who would teach you anxiety-reducing techniques and gradually help you to get used to passing urine when others are nearby.

Vaginal and vulval problems

What are the vagina and cervix?

The vagina is a tube connecting the uterus (womb) to the outside. At the top is the cervix, which is the base of the uterus. The cervix has a hole in the middle to allow menstrual blood to pass out from the uterus into the vagina. If you put two fingers into the vagina and push upwards, you will be able to feel the cervix. It feels quite large and round, and has a firm consistency (similar to the end of your nose).

During penetrative sex, the penis is in the vagina and sperm are squirted out over the cervix at orgasm (cum). Many of the sperm find their way through the hole in the cervix and up through the uterus. At the top of the uterus, there are two Fallopian tubes, which carry eggs from the ovary to the uterus. The sperm swim up into the Fallopian tubes. If an egg is there, one of them will fertilize it and a baby has begun.

The vagina is about 7–9 cm long, but it is very, very stretchy. It has to be stretchy to allow a baby to pass along it during childbirth. During childbirth the hole in the cervix enlarges to allow the baby to pass through.

What is the vulva?

The vulva is the area that surrounds the vaginal opening.

- On the outside, there are the outer lips, which are usually fleshy and covered with hair and skin.
- If you spread the outer lips apart, you will see the inner lips. These are usually thin. Like all parts of the body, they come in all shapes and sizes. In some women, the inner lips are completely enclosed by the outer lips. In other women, the inner lips hang down further than the outer lips; this is absolutely normal.
- The area inside the inner lips round the vaginal opening and the urethra (pee hole) is moist and pink. The medical name for this area is the 'vestibule'.
- The clitoris is at the top, where the outer lips meet.

What is the clitoris?

If you feel forwards from the opening of the vagina, you will feel the clitoris just before the inner lips join together. It feels like a small, soft pea. Its name comes from the Greek word *kleitoris* meaning 'little hill'. Anatomically, its structure is somewhat similar to the male penis. It has a sensitive surface (rather like the end of the male penis) sheltered by a hood of skin (rather like the foreskin of the male penis, but not extending all the way round). Most of the time the clitoris is soft and hidden under the hood but, during sexual arousal, it swells with blood (similar to erection of the male penis) and sticks out.

Research from the University of Melbourne, Australia (*Journal of Urology* 1998;1892: 159), has now shown that the clitoris is much larger than most people realize. It extends quite a long way inside, hidden by fat and bone. The main part is about the size of the end section of your thumb, and only the tip is visible externally. The part that extends inside divides into two arms (rather like a wishbone) surrounding the urethra (pee hole) and reaching towards the vagina. When the clitoris swells during sexual arousal, the whole structure can become quite large.

The clitoris is very sensitive and sexual pleasure is one of its main functions. However, the Australian researchers have found another function. The swollen 'arms' probably squeeze the urethra closed to prevent germs being sucked into the bladder during orgasm. They may also support the walls of the vagina so that sex is easier.

Getting help for a vaginal or vulval problem

If you have a problem in the vulval or vaginal area, such as itching or pain or discharge, you may feel too embarrassed to get help. (Of 100 women attending a clinic for vulval problems in Oxford, UK, five had suffered for over 20 years before plucking up the courage to see their family doctor.) To get help, you must overcome that anxiety. Remember that:

- most vaginal and vulval problems can be dealt with easily
- if you do have an infection, it needs to be treated promptly
- doctors are used to examining the genital area – it's like any other part of the body to them
- if you do not want to see your family doctor, you can go to your local sexual health clinic (see page 335), or talk to the nurse at your doctor's surgery.

Thinking about the problem

Before seeing the doctor, think carefully about what the actual problem is. Is it pain or is it itching? Do you have a discharge? Are you worried that someone could have given you an infection? Are you worried that your vulva does not look normal? Remember, your doctor cannot help you if he or she does not know what the problem is!

PAINFUL VULVA

Any of the causes of vulval itching may cause actual pain if they are severe; trichomoniasis (see page 144), for example, can make the vulva very sore. But if what you are feeling is rawness and burning, not itching, there are three main possibilities: genital herpes, 'vulvodynia' or 'vulval vestibulitis syndrome'. If your main problem is pain on intercourse, look at the section on painful sex on page 228.

Genital herpes

Genital herpes results from infection with the herpes simplex virus. Small blisters form on the genital area and these burst to form small ulcers that take about 10 days to heal. If you have not had herpes before and this is your first episode, it can be quite severe. Your vulva may be very sore, especially when you pass urine, like very bad cystitis. The lymph glands in your groin will probably be swollen, and you may have flu-like symptoms (tiredness, aching muscles, fever), and feel very miserable and tearful.

You may feel angry with your partner for giving you this infection, but it is unlikely that he knew he had it. And you should not feel bad about having it yourself – research has shown that about half the population has been exposed to the virus, but usually it is passed on without causing any symptoms. You were just unlucky to have the pain and discomfort.

If you think that you have herpes, take a look at the section on herpes on page 131 to find out what you should do.

Vulvodynia

Vulvodynia is a very unpleasant burning or aching feeling. The sensation is unremitting and is often worse at night. It is more common in older women. It is diagnosed only when other causes of pain, such as a skin disease, have been ruled out. The vulva looks perfectly normal, but the pain is real.

What can be done about vulvodynia? First, look at the common-sense dos and don'ts for vulval problems on page 314.

- Try applying some ice – some women find this is the best way of relieving the pain.
- Aloe vera gel, Calendula and Dr Bach Rescue Cream are remedies for sore and painful skin. You can buy them from health food stores. Try each separately. You may also be able to soothe the area by applying vitamin E oil (which you can squeeze out from capsules of vitamin E).
- Aqueous cream is a plain, soothing, perfume-free cream that you can buy from pharmacies. Many women with vulvodynia find that aqueous cream helps by soothing and rehydrating the skin. Use it cold, by storing it in the fridge. Unlike steroid creams, you can use it as often and for as long as you like.
- Aveeno (oatmeal) baths are a useful treatment for severe attacks of pain. You can buy the sachets from health shops. Put a sachet in the bath and bathe for 20 minutes. Repeat up to four times.
- Talk to your family doctor, because tricyclic antidepressant medication often helps. This is not because you are depressed (or imagining the condition), but because these drugs suppress transmission in nerves of the skin. Another medication, gabapentin, is sometimes used (*The Lancet* 2004;363:1058–60).
- Your local hospital may have a 'vulval clinic' that your family doctor could refer you to. Vulval clinics are usually part of the hospital dermatology department, and doctors at these clinics are experts in painful vulvas.
- Other organizations that can offer further information and support are listed in the Useful contacts on page 315.
- The good news is that many women with vulvodynia eventually become pain-free, and are able to stop their medication.

Vulval vestibulitis syndrome

With vulval vestibulitis syndrome, you experience severe pain when the opening of the vagina (the 'vestibule') is touched. The syndrome usually comes on quite suddenly, and is most common in women in their 20s or 30s. It is very distressing because, as well having to cope with the pain, your sex life is probably zero and it can even prevent you using tampons, wearing jeans or riding a bike. It may affect 1 in 20 women at some time (*British Medical Journal* 2004;328:1214–5).

The cause of vulvar vestibulitis is not known. Some experts think the nerves of the genital skin become oversensitive. Research from Sweden (*British Journal of Obstetrics and Gynaecology* 2001;108:456–61) suggests that women with vulvar vestibulitis tend to be oversensitive and worry about things that may never happen. So perhaps your brain is over-alert to signals from the nerves of the vulval skin.

What can be done about vulval vestibulitis syndrome? First, look at the common-sense dos and don'ts for vulval problems on page 314.

- Do not feel too discouraged, because the problem often improves with time.
- Teabags (Indian or Earl Grey tea) contain tannic acid, which is a local anaesthetic and can calm the burning sensation of vulval vestibulitis. Put teabags in the bath, or put a cold, damp teabag on the sore area at night.
- You may be able to soothe the area by applying vitamin E oil (which you can squeeze out from capsules of vitamin E).
- Aqueous cream is a plain, soothing, perfume-free cream that you can buy from pharmacies. Many women with vulval vestibulitis find that aqueous cream helps by soothing and rehydrating the skin. Use it cold, by storing it in the fridge. Unlike steroid creams, you can use it as often and for as long as you like.
- 5% lignocaine ointment contains a weak amount of the local anaesthetic lignocaine. It numbs the nerves in the skin and can be used safely on a regular basis. Although it does not cure the problem, it will allow you to have sexual intercourse comfortably if you apply it 15 minutes beforehand.
- You could try a diet that is low in oxalate, a plant chemical. The evidence that this works is scanty, but some women find it helpful. This means avoiding beetroot, chocolate, cola drinks, cranberries, nuts, rhubarb, soya foods, spinach, strawberries, tea and wheat bran.
- As with vulvodynia, tricyclic antidepressant medication often helps. This is not because you are depressed (or imagining the condition), but because these drugs suppress transmission in nerves of the skin. So talk to your family doctor.
- As with vulvodynia, ask your family doctor if your local hospital has a 'vulval clinic' that you could be referred to. Some clinics use a technique called 'electromyographic feedback from pelvic floor muscles', which is a method of training your nervous system to stop sending the pain signals.

VULVAL ITCHING

Itchiness of the vulva is almost never caused by a sexually transmitted infection, but is usually a result of thrush or a skin condition. The 'lips' of the vulva (the labia) are covered by ordinary skin, so the area can be affected by conditions such as eczema and psoriasis. And sometimes only the vulval skin is affected, so the diagnosis may come as a surprise.

The usual mistake with vulval itching is to assume that you have thrush, and keep on applying anti-thrush creams that you have bought from a pharmacy. This may actually worsen the condition, because you can become allergic to some of the ingredients. If an anti-thrush cream does not deal with the problem within a few days, or if the itching comes back, see your doctor. If you have a skin condition, and not thrush, you need the appropriate treatment.

This section explains the most common causes of vulval itching and what you can do about them. And you can find more information about thrush and trichomoniasis in the section on genital infections on page 126.

Thrush is a fungal infection caused by *Candida albicans*. About 1 woman in 5 has Candida in her vagina without it causing any symptoms. Hormones in the vaginal secretions and the 'friendly' vaginal bacteria keep it at bay. But problems can arise when this natural balance becomes upset, and the Candida multiplies.

Thrush does not always cause a discharge – the main symptom is itching or soreness, and this gets worse in the week before a period. If there is a discharge, it is usually only slight, does not smell and looks like cottage cheese.

Trichomoniasis infection (see page 144) can be itchy.

Psoriasis is a skin condition that can be extremely itchy when the genitals are involved. The skin usually becomes bright red, often with painful cracks. The affected area may extend to the groin and to around the back passage (the anus) and between the buttocks. Psoriasis on other parts of the body is scaly (check your scalp, knees and elbows), but in the vulval area it tends to be smooth. You can have psoriasis on the vulva without having it anywhere else on your body.

Lichen sclerosus is another extremely itchy skin condition affecting the vulva. The itching is often so bad that it can affect a sufferer's sleep. It is most common around the menopause and in girls just before puberty, though it can occur at any age. Its cause is a mystery. The skin looks thin and pale, and the area around the anus may also be affected. If it is not treated, the lips of the vulva eventually shrink, the vaginal opening narrows and sex becomes painful. Treatment of this condition is simple, and your doctor can prescribe a special steroid cream.

Allergies and sensitivities can cause redness and itching. The vulval area seems to be very sensitive to chemicals, probably because the vulva is moist and warm – conditions that favour the absorption of chemicals by the skin. It is possible to develop an allergy to almost any chemical substance that comes into contact with the vulva, such as may be present in:

- skin creams
- perfumes in soaps, bubble baths, shower gels and shampoos
- disinfectants
- washing powders and fabric softeners
- deodorants (including 'intimate' ones).

Excessive washing can irritate the vulval area. Older women who may find it difficult to get into a bath may worry about personal hygiene, with the result that they wash the area too much. There is no need to wash several times a day – once is sufficient.

Stress or anxiety can cause itching. When you are stressed or anxious, your nervous system is on alert, and small sensations can become amplified into unpleasant itching or even pain. So it is not imaginary, it is real.

What you can do

- Start by trying to eliminate anything that could be causing an allergy or sensitivity – look at the common-sense dos and don'ts for vulval problems on page 314. Avoid swimming while you have the irritation – the chlorine may make it worse.
- If you have been applying cream from the pharmacy for more than 1 week, and you still have the problem, stop using it. You may have developed a sensitivity to one of the ingredients.
- If the itch is really bad, you may be scratching in your sleep, causing more damage. Keep your fingernails short and wear cotton gloves when you go to bed (you can buy them from a pharmacy).
- If you think thrush is a possibility, look at the information on thrush in the genital infections section on page 139.
- If itching is disturbing your sleep, antihistamine medication at bedtime may help. Ask your pharmacist for a 'sedating' antihistamine.

FISHY SMELL

If your vulva smells fishy, it is almost certain that you have bacterial vaginosis (also known as 'anaerobic vaginosis'). This is an imbalance in the bacteria in the vagina. All women have harmless bacteria in their vaginal passage. In bacterial vaginosis, some of the bacteria multiply so that more are present than is normal (it is usually the *Gardnerella* and *Mobiluncus* bacteria that are the culprits). In other words, bacterial vaginosis is not an infection caught from your partner, it is due to bacteria that are normally present in the vagina.

Bacterial vaginosis is treated with an antibiotic, metronidazole, from your doctor. You will find more information on bacterial vaginosis on page 126.

VAGINAL DISCHARGE

What's normal

It is normal to have some vaginal discharge, because the vagina stays moist as part of its self-cleansing mechanism. The normal moist discharge clears dead cells and bacteria from the vagina. It comes mainly from glands in the cervix (the neck of the womb), and is slightly acidic, which helps to keep infections at bay. The acidity results from lactic acid, formed by 'friendly' bacteria as they break down sugars.

The amount of normal discharge varies from woman to woman, and with the menstrual cycle. Many women notice that, during the week following a period, there is hardly any discharge, and what there is has a thick consistency. Towards the middle of the cycle (about 2 weeks after the start of a period) the amount increases and it becomes thin, slippery and clear, like uncooked egg white. When this discharge is exposed to the air, it becomes brownish-yellow, so it is normal to find a yellowish stain on your knickers in the middle of the monthly cycle. There may also be a feeling of moistness and stickiness. Normal discharge does not smell, and does not cause any irritation or itching.

Discharge also increases during pregnancy. And during sexual excitement, vaginal discharge becomes very profuse because two glands near the vaginal opening (Bartholin's glands) secrete additional slippery mucus, which acts as a lubricant for intercourse.

What's not normal

A discharge is likely to be abnormal if:

- it smells fishy
- it is thick and white, like cottage cheese
- it is greenish and smells foul
- there is blood in it (except when you have a period)
- it is itchy
- you have any genital sores or ulcers
- you have abdominal pain or pain on intercourse
- it started soon after you had unprotected sex with someone you suspect could have a sexually transmitted infection.

Causes of abnormal discharge

Type of discharge	Possible causes
Thick and white	Normal in some women Thrush (Candida infection)
Itchy	Thrush (Candida infection) Trichomoniasis
Smelly	Bacterial vaginosis Trichomoniasis Gonorrhoea Forgotten tampon

Bacterial vaginosis is a very common cause of vaginal discharge. The discharge smells fishy. You will find more information about bacterial vaginosis in the section on genital infections on page 126.

Thrush is caused by the yeast *Candida albicans*. The main symptom of thrush is itching, but it can cause a thick, whitish discharge. You will find more information about thrush in the section on genital infections on page 139.

Forgotten tampons. 'Lost' tampons are quite a common cause of discharge. It is easy to forget to remove the last tampon at the end of a period. After a week or two, the tampon begins to fester, and there will be a foul-smelling discharge.

If you have an old tampon in place, remove it as soon as possible. If your discharge continues for more than a couple of days, see your doctor or visit a sexual health clinic.

Gonorrhoea is one of the most infectious sexually transmitted infections. It is caused by infection with the *Gonococcus* bacterium. If a woman has unprotected sex with a man who has it, she has a 60–90% chance of catching it. It is serious because if it is not treated, it can spread upwards to the Fallopian tubes. These tubes carry the egg from the ovary to the womb (uterus), so damage to them can cause infertility. About one-fifth of women with gonorrhoea have a foul-smelling, greenish-yellow discharge. About one-fifth have vague symptoms, such as a slight increase in discharge, pain on intercourse or lower abdominal discomfort. About one-fifth have no symptoms at all. (Most men with gonorrhoea notice an obvious discharge from the penis – see page 206.) You will find more information about gonorrhoea in the section on genital infections on page 138.

Trichomoniasis is caused by a tiny amoeba-like (protozoan) organism called *Trichomonas vaginalis*. It used to be common, but for mysterious reasons is becoming less so; over the last 10 years the number of cases in England and Wales has fallen from 17 000 to 5000 a year. It causes a discharge that is often frothy and yellowish-greenish, but it may be thin and scanty. The discharge is smelly, and the vulva is often itchy and sore. It may also be painful to pass urine. It is caught from a man who has it, but he may be unaware of his condition as most men with trichomoniasis do not have any symptoms. It is not dangerous, though some doctors think it could possibly spread to the Fallopian tubes. You will find more information about trichomoniasis in the section on genital infections on page 144. If you think you have this infection, you should visit a sexual health clinic (see page 335) for treatment and to be checked for other infections.

What to do if you have vaginal discharge

- For any vaginal problem, you must take care to avoid substances that may cause more irritation. These are the same as those that can cause vulval irritation, so look at the list of common-sense dos and don'ts for vulval problems on page 314.
- During a period, change tampons or sanitary pads frequently (at least two or three times a day), and do not use tampons when you are not having your period.
- Talk to your partner. Ask if he has any discharge from the urethra (the opening at the end of the penis) or any soreness or irritation of the penis. If his answer is 'yes', or if there is any reason to think that he might have a sexually transmitted infection, he should go to a sexual health clinic (see page 335) for a check-up. Do not have sex until the problem has been sorted out.
- If your discharge is thick and white and itchy, it may be thrush, so you could try an anti-thrush cream or tablet from a pharmacist. However, do not persist with an anti-thrush cream from the pharmacist if it does not resolve the problem in a day or two, or if the

discharge returns. Look at the information about thrush in the genital infections section on page 139, then see your doctor or go to a clinic to get a proper diagnosis.

- The best plan is to see your family doctor or go to a sexual health clinic (see page 335) for a check-up. The clinic can do on-the-spot-tests for most causes of vaginal discharge, and you can attend without being referred by your family doctor. You should definitely go to a sexual health clinic if you think that you might have a sexually transmitted infection (for example, if you have had unprotected sex with a new partner, or if your partner has discharge or soreness of his penis).

How your doctor or the clinic can help

Usually, the doctor will look at the vulva for any signs of thrush, and will then insert a hollow plastic or metal tube (speculum) into the vagina, in order to look at your vagina (rather like having a smear). Samples of the discharge can be taken by wiping with cottonwool swabs.

A family doctor will usually have to send the swabs to a laboratory, so it may be some days before the result is available. A sexual health clinic can look at the samples under the microscope straight away, and can usually tell you the diagnosis within half an hour, though they are also sent to the main laboratory for confirmation. Do not be surprised if you see the doctor or nurse testing the acidity of the discharge with litmus paper, or mixing some of it with a liquid (potassium hydroxide) on a glass slide and then sniffing it; these are tests for bacterial vaginosis.

Each cause of vaginal discharge has its own proper treatment, which could be a cream or tablet, and it is important to follow the treatment instructions from your doctor or the clinic very carefully. If you are asked to return for another check-up, it is important that you do so, even if the discharge has gone. The clinic may be checking for gonorrhoea, which can damage your Fallopian tubes and infect a future sexual partner without you having any further symptoms.

CHANGE IN COLOUR

The vulva is usually slightly darker than the rest of your skin – dusky pink or brownish. There are two conditions in which it becomes white in colour.

Lichen sclerosus

Lichen sclerosus is a condition in which the vulva is usually itchy as well as pale. It needs treatment, so see your doctor.

Vitiligo

In vitiligo, the normal skin pigment is lost from patches of the skin, so those patches look milky white. If your skin is naturally dark, the vitiligo will be very obvious. The texture of the skin is normal, and the condition is not painful or itchy. It may affect other parts of your body as well, or the vulva may be the only site. Vitiligo often runs in families, and usually appears in the teens. It is probably an 'autoimmune' disorder in which the body makes antibodies against its own pigment cells. It is not known why it affects some parts of the body (such as the genitals, face, hands and feet) more than others.

Vitiligo on other parts of the body can be treated with ultraviolet light, usually two or three times a week for at least 6 months. This usually produces some repigmentation of the area and the effect is usually permanent. When it affects only the genital area, it is not usually treated, but if you are very distressed by it, ask your doctor for a referral to a dermatologist.

DRY VAGINA

Vaginal lubrication

The natural moistness of the vagina prevents its sides from rubbing against each other as you move about during the day. The vaginal moisture is also slightly acidic, and this helps to keep infections such as thrush at bay. This acidity is caused by the 'friendly' bacteria that live in the vagina and help to keep it healthy.

Vaginal moisture is mainly produced by the cervix (neck of the womb) at the top of the vagina and eventually oozes out of the vagina – some vaginal discharge is normal. This means that there is a very slow flow of moisture through the vagina, and this keeps it clean, as it moves dead cells and the remains of the menstrual period to the outside. On average, a woman discharges 2 g of dead cells and 3 g of mucus through the vagina each day.

During sex. When you are sexually excited, two special glands at the entrance of the vagina, called Bartholin's glands, produce extra secretions. The moisture from these glands is more slimy than the moisture from the cervix, because its purpose is to provide good lubrication during intercourse. Its musky smell is the result of millions of years of evolution to increase female attractiveness to the male of the species, and signals that the woman is ready for sex.

Dryness before the menopause

Vaginal dryness before the menopause is mostly a problem during sex. It may mean that you are not sufficiently aroused – which can occur for all sorts of reasons such as inadequate foreplay, feelings of guilt, fear or relationship problems. Also remember that men generally get aroused sooner than women, so your partner may be attempting penetration before you are ready, before good lubrication has occurred. Lack of lubrication is also common in breastfeeding women, because oestrogen levels are low, and in women with diabetes.

Dryness during or after the menopause

Vaginal dryness can be a particular problem at and after the menopause, because of a lack of oestrogen (the female hormone). Oestrogen is responsible for the plumpness of the lining of the vagina, for the elasticity of the tissues round the vagina and for the production of the moisture from the cervix.

Oestrogen levels fall at the menopause, so the vagina loses some of its elasticity, its lining becomes thinner and it feels dryer. Because there is less moisture, there are fewer of the 'friendly' bacteria that help to keep the vagina acidic. When the vagina becomes less acidic, infections such as thrush can take hold, which cause further irritation and discomfort.

All these changes can make intercourse uncomfortable. Another factor is that after the menopause, the Bartholin's glands are less efficient – they take longer to produce the lubricating juices for sex, and produce less than in younger women. The American sex researchers Masters and Johnson showed that whereas younger women may become sufficiently aroused for penetrative sex in as short a time as a few seconds, menopausal women may take 5 minutes or more.

What to do about dryness before the menopause

A dry vagina can be lubricated easily. For additional lubrication for intercourse, use a water-soluble, starch-based lubricant (e.g. KY jelly) or a vaginal moisturizer (e.g. Sylk, Replens or Senselle) rather than a petroleum-based product like Vaseline, which may interfere with your natural secretions. Apart from Sylk (see Useful contacts on page 315), which is available by mail order and from some stockists, these products can all be bought from a pharmacy – you do not need a prescription. Sylk is a lubricant derived from an extract of kiwi fruit; obviously you should not use it if you are allergic to kiwi fruit. It has a non-sticky texture very similar to natural vaginal lubrication. Some lubricants damage condoms; Sylk, KY jelly, Replens and Senselle do not.

Sylk and KY jelly are used just before intercourse. Smear the product liberally over the vulval area, particularly round the opening of the vagina.

Replens and Senselle are moisturizers that you use two or three times a week. They coat the inside of the vagina with a non-hormonal moisturizer, which lasts for a day or two, so they do not have to be used immediately before intercourse.

What to do about dryness during and after the menopause

Leisurely sex with lots of foreplay. Taking time during sex is particularly important for the older woman. This allows the Bartholin's glands to produce the maximum amount of lubrication before penetration.

Simple lubricants, such as KY jelly, or moisturizers, such as Replens or Senselle, can be used if you need additional lubrication for intercourse.

Hormone replacement therapy (HRT) will increase vaginal lubrication and thicken the vaginal lining, but has risks. Therefore, HRT is not appropriate if vaginal dryness is your only problem; there are safer ways of dealing with dryness.

Vaginal oestrogen creams can be prescribed by your doctor if you prefer not to take HRT. For the first 2 or 3 weeks you use it every night, and it may be a week or two before you notice any improvement. After that, twice a week will be enough.

The creams can be messy. Some come with a special syringe (applicator) to help you insert the cream into the vagina. In fact, the applicators are more trouble than they are worth, because they have to be washed in warm soapy water after each use. More importantly, they tend to give you too much cream. Some of the oestrogen will then be absorbed through the vaginal wall into the bloodstream, where it could be harmful. It is better to smear the cream inside your vagina with your fingers, and not to be over-lavish. If you are not used to touching the inside of your vagina you may find this peculiar at first, but you will very soon become quite relaxed about doing so.

Unless you have had a hysterectomy, oestrogen in the bloodstream needs to be balanced by progesterone tablets, otherwise there is a slight risk of cancer of the uterus (womb). Hormone replacement tablets provide both oestrogen and progesterone, but vaginal cream contains only oestrogen. Some of the oestrogen from the cream will enter the bloodstream through the walls of the vagina. Therefore, to be on the safe side, some doctors prescribe progesterone tablets for women using oestrogen vaginal cream.

Because some oestrogen from a vaginal preparation (whether it is a cream, tablets or ring) may enter the bloodstream, there have been worries that it could cause health risks like HRT. So far, there is no evidence for this (Cochrane Database Systematic Review 2003:CD001500), but research is ongoing.

Vaginal oestrogen tablets are another possibility. They need a doctor's prescription. Each tablet comes in an applicator, which is about the size of a pencil. You insert the applicator into the vagina and press the end to release the tablet into the vagina. For the first 2 weeks you use 1 tablet a day, but later only 2 a week are needed.

Oestrogen-containing vaginal ring. This type of ring may be suggested by your doctor. The ring gradually releases oestrogen into the vagina. It has to be replaced every 3 months, and you must not use it for more than 2 years in total. It is not painful or uncomfortable, but you might feel a slight irritation at first. Some people find that it gets in the way during intercourse, in which case you can remove it beforehand and put it back afterwards. It is easy to take in and out – your doctor will show you how.

Black cohosh capsules can be bought from health food stores. Black cohosh comes from the root of a plant. It is commonly used for menopausal symptoms in Germany. A study in 1987 in Germany found that black cohosh had an oestrogen-like effect on the lining of the vagina, which might translate into better vaginal lubrication. However, this study has been criticized because, surprisingly, it also showed that oestrogen had little effect; scientists therefore think that the study may not be reliable. Black cohosh may cause liver damage; more research is needed.

VAGINAL LIPS
What's normal

To be wholly accurate, the vaginal lips should be called 'vulval lips'. The outer lips are usually fleshy, and the inner lips are usually thin but, like every other part of the body, they come in all shapes and sizes. In some women, the inner lips are completely enclosed by the outer lips. In other women, the inner lips (labia minora) are larger than the outside lips. This is perfectly natural and normal, but many women worry about it. It is a shame that pictures in men's top shelf magazines and articles in womens' magazines are making women feel abnormal when they are not. But, if the inner lips are so large that they are upsetting you, it is possible to have them trimmed by a surgical operation.

See a doctor

It would be best to start by visiting a sexual health clinic (see page 335). These clinics mainly test for genital infections, but deal with other problems as well. Explain to the doctor that you have not come for tests, but because you have another worry. You can then ask the doctor to examine your vaginal lips, and tell you whether or not they are abnormally large. The advantage of going to the sexual health clinic is that the doctors in these clinics examine dozens of women every day, so the doctor you see will be able to give you a good opinion. If the clinic doctor says that you are unusual, you can then ask your family doctor to arrange for an operation if you wish.

Surgery

The operation to reduce the labia minora is simple. It can be done by a gynaecologist or a plastic surgeon. There are two ways of doing it.

- The surgeon may simply trim the edges of the labia, in which case you may be left with a scar running along the edges of the labia.
- The other method is to remove a fan-shaped portion of each lip, and then stitch the cut edges together. This reduces the size of the lip without much scarring.

This is a cosmetic operation, so you would probably not be able to have it done under the NHS in the UK. You would have to have it done privately. Try to pluck up courage to ask your doctor to refer you to a suitable private gynaecologist or surgeon. Explain how troubled you are feeling. This is a better course of action than trying to find a good one yourself, which can be difficult.

COMMON-SENSE DOS AND DON'TS

- Do not use bubble bath or shower gel.
- Do not put disinfectant in the bath.
- Do use an unperfumed soap, such as Simple.
- Do not shampoo your hair in the bath or in the shower where the shampoo could run down and become trapped in the vulval skin folds. Wash your hair in the sink, or by leaning forward into the shower.
- Do not use 'intimate' deodorants or apply deodorant to sanitary towels.
- Do not squirt soapy solution or antiseptic into your vagina to clean it (douching) – the vagina cleans itself very efficiently, so douching in this way is not necessary, and may be harmful.
- Do use a detergent labelled 'for sensitive skin' for washing your underwear, and avoid fabric softeners.
- Do add two handfuls of ordinary salt to your bath water, or bathe the area with salted water (a heaped tablespoon of table salt in a sinkful of warm water).
- If you are so sore that passing urine is very painful, do pee in the bath, or wash the urine away from the vulval area using a jug of warm water while you are on the toilet.

Useful contacts

myDr is an Australian healthcare website compiled by a team of experienced Australian healthcare writers, with contributions from practising Australian healthcare practitioners and recognized Australian health organizations. The website has a 'Women's health centre' section with information on vaginal and vulval problems under 'Women's health A–Z'.
www.mydr.com.au
www.mydr.com.au/default.asp?Section=women%60shealth

Sylk vaginal lubricant. The website has a list of UK stockists or you can buy it by mail order.
www.sylk.co.uk

National Lichen Sclerosus Support Group (UK) has information about lichen sclerosus on its website. www.lichensclerosus.org

Vulval Pain Society is a UK organization with an excellent website that gives information about different types of pain, frequently asked questions and links to similar organizations. They publish a *Vulval Pain Handbook* that gives information about vulval pain, possible treatments, and ways of coping. www.vulvalpainsociety.org

National Vulvodynia Association is a US organization that provides clear information about vulval pain.
www.nva.org

VulvarHealth is a good US website that provides information about vulval disorders, self-examination, self-care and current research. (Americans use the adjective 'vulvar', while the British use 'vulval'.) www.vulvarhealth.org

Oxalate information. If you want to try a low oxalate diet, a list of low-, medium- and high-oxalate foods can be found on the following website.
www.branwen.com/rowan/oxalate.htm

The Vulvar Pain Foundation is a US website that has an 'Oxalate section', which gives advice about a low oxalate diet.
www.vulvarpainfoundation.org

Other useful contacts can be found at the end of the genital infections section on page 145.

Veins

THREAD VEINS

Thread veins are tiny veins that appear most commonly on the cheeks, nose and legs. Small thread veins are red, but larger ones look purplish. They have many names, including:

- spider veins
- broken veins (not an accurate name, because they are not actually broken)
- capillary veins.

Normally, the tiny veins in the skin are invisible, but in some people they expand and show through the skin. One cause of this is too much exposure to the sun over the years. Another is pregnancy or oestrogen treatment. They may also be inherited. Thread veins can sometimes be a sign of rosacea (see page 217), a skin condition, or can result from overuse of steroid creams. Thread veins are more obvious after mid-life, when the skin becomes thinner and loses some of its collagen.

After the menopause, hormone replacement therapy (HRT) improves thread veins in some women (because it strengthens the skin slightly), but worsens them in others (because the oestrogen in HRT encourages veins to dilate).

What you can do

Find a good concealer (see Useful contacts on page 323) and use it under your make-up. Using an artificial suntan preparation will make leg thread veins less obvious.

Avoid alcoholic drinks, very hot drinks and spicy foods if you find these make the veins more obvious.

Horse chestnut cream (available from health food stores) is said to strengthen the tiny veins in the skin. Apply gently to avoid traumatizing the skin.

Treatments

The two main treatments are micro-sclerotherapy and laser treatment. In general:

- laser treatment is best for thread veins on the face
- micro-sclerotherapy, possibly combined with laser, is best for thread veins on the legs.

Micro-sclerotherapy involves injecting the veins with a chemical using tiny needles. This makes the walls of the veins stick together. You need to wear compression stockings for a week, and the veins disperse naturally over the following 2–3 weeks. Several treatments may be needed. If the therapist misses the tiny vein, and injects the surrounding skin by mistake, there can be a skin reaction. Some darkening of the skin (hyperpigmentation) may occur. Overall, the results are variable. It is better for thread veins on the legs than on the face. The veins may come back, but the treatment can be repeated.

Laser treatment gets rid of the veins very successfully and is the best treatment for thread veins on the face, but it does have drawbacks. It cannot be used on dark skin because the pigment in the skin blocks the laser beam, and the pigment may be lost afterwards. It causes bruising, which is at its worst in the first 48 hours, but can last up to 10 days. After treatment, you will have to protect your skin from sunlight. Laser treatment can change the texture of the skin, and sometimes leaves little white scars. It does not work very well on the legs, probably because the thread veins lie deeper in the skin. Some people find it painful, or notice a flicking sensation during the treatment. It is more expensive than sclerotherapy.

High-intensity light treatment (Photoderm) heats the veins to make them coagulate. It can cover a bigger area than laser treatment – areas measuring 2 cm by 0.5 cm can be treated by a single flash. Scientific studies of the treatment have produced contradictory results.

- One study concluded that at least 75% of the veins were cleared in 80% of patients, and that after treatment the skin may look a little red and there may be some tiny blisters, but usually no scarring.
- In another study, patients found the treatment uncomfortable and described each light pulse as being like a burn. There was scarring and thinning of the skin in 21% of patients, and 42% had blistering and peeling. Only 9.5% of patients had complete clearance of the thread veins and there was no change in appearance in 56%.

So, this technique appears to be more risky and less effective than laser treatment.

Electrolysis is cheap, and offered by many beauty clinics. It is less effective than the other treatments, and there is a greater risk of scarring.

Getting treatment

It may be difficult to get treatment for the thread veins through your doctor, because it comes into the 'cosmetic' treatment category. However, if you are very self-conscious about them, and find cover-up creams inadequate, it is worth asking your doctor. If you are in your 20s and notice thread veins, do not think that you are too young to go for treatment – this is the ideal age for laser treatment. About a third of people with thread veins on the legs have varicose veins (see below); in this situation the varicose veins must be treated first.

You may have to use a private clinic. Clinics advertise persuasively, and it is difficult to know which provide good treatment. The best policy is to ask your doctor to find out the name of a good clinic from the local vascular surgeon (blood vessel expert). Some hospitals in the UK are now running private cosmetic laser clinics (to generate money for the purchase of equipment to be used for NHS patients). These clinics have a doctor in charge and their standards are high. You could telephone the dermatology department of your nearest large hospital to find out if it runs one of these clinics or look in the Useful contacts section on page 323.

Before committing yourself to treatment, find out exactly what method the clinic uses, how many sessions will be needed and what the cost will be. Ask about problems, such as scarring. If laser is to be used, make sure it is not an older type – tunable dye or YAG – because they cause more scarring. The pulsed dye laser and KTP laser with variable pulse width are the most satisfactory types for the face.

VARICOSE VEINS

A bulging section of blue, twisted vein on the back of a person's calf or thigh is a common sight – 10–15% of men and 20–25% of women have visible veins. A varicose vein is actually a vein that has lost its elasticity. Its wall has become flabby, so that it easily becomes swollen with blood.

Recent research has found that varicose veins are more common in men than in women

Who gets varicose veins

- Varicose veins affect both men and women.
- You can get varicose veins at any age (even as a teenager), but they are more likely as you get older. They tend to run in families.
- Varicose veins may first occur during pregnancy because of hormonal changes that relax the wall of the vein and because of pressure in the veins from the expanding uterus (womb). After the baby is born, there will be a general improvement in the veins, but they often become worse again in later pregnancies.
- The contraceptive pill makes varicose veins more likely.
- Obesity and repeated abdominal strain (e.g. from heavy lifting) may contribute.
- Long periods of standing or sitting with the legs bent and crossed makes varicose veins worse.
- Sometimes varicose veins occur after a serious thrombosis (blood clot) in the deep veins, because this may damage the valves at the main junctions.
- It has been suggested that a diet low in fibre increases the likelihood of varicose veins (because if we are constipated we have to strain to open our bowels, which puts pressure on the veins), but this is unproven.

How normal veins function

Veins carry blood to the heart. The veins in the leg have a particular problem in getting the blood back to the heart, because they have to carry the blood uphill, against the force of gravity. But the body has a mechanism to deal with the situation, consisting of the following two elements.

- Some of the leg veins are deep in the muscle. These are called the deep veins. The contractions of the leg muscles during walking squeeze these veins, forcing blood along; this is called the muscle pump.
- To prevent the blood going backwards and away from the heart, veins have one-way valves. Not all the veins in the leg lie in the muscle like the deep veins; some are nearer the surface of the leg, in the skin and fatty tissue outside the muscle. These are called superficial veins. There are connections between the deep veins and those outside the muscle. Each connection has a valve, which ensures that blood flows from the vein outside the muscle into the deep vein, and not back the other way.

How varicose veins form

It is the veins that lie outside the muscle, not the deep veins, that become varicose. There are two theories about how varicose veins form and perhaps both are true.

The old theory says that the basic cause is failure of the valve at the connection with the deep vein in the muscle. Over time, the superficial vein will swell to cope with the extra blood, lose its elasticity and become a lumpy, blue, varicose vein. The swelling means that the next valve below will eventually be unable to close, because its edges will no longer meet each other in the closed position. So there is a domino effect, with each damaged valve eventually producing damage to the one below it. As it does so, more of the vein will swell and become varicose. This would happen very slowly over years.

A newer theory, gaining ground among experts, says that the vein wall is inherently weak in people who get varicose veins. The vein swells and so the valves do not work properly.

Symptoms of varicose veins

Varicose veins are a problem for three reasons.

- They look ugly, because the affected veins are just below the skin, and the enlarged and twisted portions are very obvious.
- The pools of non-circulating blood cause symptoms.
- Bad varicose veins over many years can damage the skin near the ankle, causing eczema – the skin becomes stained brownish-black, and ulcers may occur which are difficult to heal.

Lots of symptoms, such as swelling, restless legs (see page 220), cramps, tingling and aching, have been linked to varicose veins. A study in Edinburgh tried to find out the truth, by asking 1566 people about their symptoms (*British Medical Journal* 1999;318: 353–6). They discovered that, in women, varicose veins can cause a heavy feeling in the legs, aching and itching. In men, however, itching seems to be the only symptom. A feeling of swelling of the legs, cramps, tingling and restless legs are probably not actually caused by varicose veins, but may have other causes (such as ageing).

'Varicose' simply means swollen

How you can help yourself

Ordinary 'support tights' are probably a waste of money except during pregnancy. If you think that you are developing varicose veins, see your doctor. If varicose veins run in your family, there is not very much you can do to prevent them.

- If you are overweight, try to lose a few kilos.
- Take regular walks. Walking is the best exercise to improve the flow of blood in the legs, but avoid exercises that use weights and high-impact exercises, such as jogging.
- Avoid long periods of standing. If you have to stand in one position for longer than a few minutes, do some ankle movements, such as standing on tiptoe to encourage your calf muscles to pump blood out of your leg veins.

Varicose veins are the price we pay for our upright posture; if we still walked on all fours, we probably wouldn't have them

- Put your feet up whenever you are sitting around at home. This will help the veins to empty and reduce swelling of the feet. Try not to cross your legs or to sit for long periods with your legs bent. On long train or plane journeys, walk around from time to time; and on long car or coach journeys take advantage of any stops to get out and walk for a few minutes.
- Avoid falling asleep in a chair. If you are tired, go to bed.
- Extract of horse chestnut (conker juice) is very popular in Germany as a remedy for varicose veins. The active ingredient, aescin, is said to strengthen blood vessels. In fact, as varicose veins are a mechanical problem due to leaky valves in the veins, there is no way that horse-chestnut extract could make them close properly. However, some people find that it helps to relieve aching, so it might be worth a try if that is your main problem. It can cause nausea in some people. Some horse-chestnut preparations also contain a plant extract called Butcher's Broom, which should be avoided if you have high blood pressure.
- Do not wear garters or tight 'stay-up' stockings.
- Wear lace-up shoes, which give better support and allow your leg muscles to move more naturally.
- Eat a healthy diet with lots of fruit and vegetables to avoid constipation. Some people think that onions, berries and grapes are especially helpful for varicose veins, but there is no scientific evidence for this.
- If you have varicose veins, take extra care of the skin on your legs, because the blood stagnates and the circulation to the skin is poor. The skin can become deprived of oxygen and any damage will take longer to heal. Use a moisturizing lotion, do not scratch any itchy areas, try to avoid knocks and do not toast your legs in front of a fire.

One person in five has varicose veins or is likely to get them

When to ask for treatment

Do not feel you are wasting your doctor's time if you request treatment for veins that are not too bad. The longer you have them, the worse they get, so surgeons prefer to deal with early cases, because they are easier and the results are better. Colour changes in the skin caused by varicose veins never completely reverse after surgery.

It used to be said that women who develop varicose veins after pregnancy should not be treated if they intend to have more children. Most surgeons now believe it is best to treat after the first baby, rather than wait until the woman's family is complete.

Treatments for varicose veins

Special elastic stockings (compression stockings) are a very effective treatment. They support the veins, stop them from getting worse, and relieve discomfort. They produce maximum pressure at the ankle, and the pressure diminishes up the leg. They are particularly useful if your main symptom is aching or ankle swelling, or if the varicose veins are likely to be temporary (e.g. during pregnancy).

- You must wear your elastic stockings all the time, except when you are in bed.
- You must put them on immediately after you get up in the morning, before blood and fluid have pooled in your feet and ankles.
- Of course they are tight and difficult to put on; if this causes you problems, ask your pharmacist about devices that will help (such as Medi Valet) and request open-toed stockings.
- You will need new elastic stockings every 6 months.

Modern compression stockings are much lighter and look nicer than the old types. In the UK, compression stockings (though not support tights) are available under the NHS; however, for a pair, you have to pay two prescription charges. For men, there are ribbed, below-the-knee stockings that look more like ordinary socks.

How to put on elastic stockings

- Dust your leg with a little talc.
- Put your hand into the stocking until you can feel the seam at the heel.
- Pinch the heel and turn the stocking inside out until you can see the inside of the heel.
- Put your foot in, making sure that the stocking heel is in the right place.
- Pull the rest of the stocking over the foot and up your leg.
- Wearing rubber gloves may help you to grip the stocking and prevent snagging.

60 000 people in England have hospital treatment for varicose veins every year

The usual surgical operation involves tying off the vein (ligation) above the varicose section, usually just before it joins the deep vein. The vein can be removed by 'stripping'; this involves attaching one end of a tiny wire to the varicose section and threading the other end through the vein to a small incision at the calf or ankle where the wire, along with the varicose section of vein, is pulled out. Alternatively, the vein can be removed in small pieces through tiny incisions.

The body does not miss veins that are removed by surgery. The legs have many other veins for the blood to flow through.

Varicose vein surgery used to cause horrendous bruising, but now that doctors use fine instruments that need only tiny incisions, there should be little bruising. However, some surgeons still make big cuts in the legs, so ask about this before you decide to have the operation. You can usually leave hospital on the day of operation or the following morning and then go back to work 1–2 days later (unless your work involves standing, in which case you would need a week off). The leg is bandaged for the first 12 hours, and then a heavy elastic stocking is worn. You may need painkillers for a few days after the operation.

After surgery, there is a 1 in 5 chance that you will develop more varicose veins within the next 5 years.

Newer types of operation have been developed, but only time will tell whether they produce a long-lasting cure (*British Medical Journal* 2002;324:689–90).

- VNUS (named after the US company that developed the technique) is a 'keyhole' treatment. It involves inserting a narrow tube up through the length of the vein from a tiny cut in the ankle, guided by an ultrasound scanner. As the tube is pulled out, high-frequency radio waves are then sent along it, causing the vein to close down. There is no bruising or discomfort afterwards. This technique is not available under the NHS in the UK.
- With 'powered phlebectomy', the surgeon inserts a light through a tiny incision in the skin, around a cluster of veins. This enables the surgeon to see clearly which veins need removing. Then a suction device is inserted through another incision to remove the veins. There is some bruising and discomfort after this technique.
- Laser treatment involves passing a laser tube up the length of the vein. The laser is then slowly pulled out, and its heat blocks the vein.

Sclerotherapy consists of injecting a solution into the varicose vein (*Cochrane Database Systematic Review* 2002;1:CD001732). The solution causes irritation, inflammation, and eventually scarring, which permanently blocks the vein. The body absorbs the accumulated blood from the varicose vein, and the lumps flatten out over time. It used to be a common treatment, but it is not used much now because the results are not long-lasting.

A newer type of sclerotherapy uses a foam that spreads rapidly along the vein after it is injected, and also fills the adjoining smaller veins. This is a hospital procedure, because it need to be guided by an ultrasound scanner.

Varicose veins usually develop slowly over 10–20 years

How easy is it to get an operation?

In the UK, varicose vein operations are performed under the NHS, though some hospitals are rationing this surgery and operating only on people who are developing eczema-type skin changes at the ankle or other problems. This is because a varicose vein operation can take 2–3 hours, using a lot of surgeon and operating theatre time. If the main reason is that you are conscious of the appearance of the veins, you may have to have the operation done privately.

Varicose veins are more common in Wales than anywhere else in the world

Useful contacts

Health*Insite* is an Australian government initiative aimed to improve the health of Australians by providing easy access to quality information about human health. Follow the link to find information relating to varicose veins.
www.healthinsite.gov.au/topics/Varicose_Veins

myDr is an Australian healthcare website compiled by a team of experienced Australian healthcare writers, with contributions from practising Australian healthcare practitioners and recognized Australian health organizations. The website has a 'Women's health centre' section with information on varicose veins under 'Women's health A–Z'.
www.mydr.com.au
www.mydr.com.au/default.asp?Section=women%60shealth

Laura Mercier's Secret Camouflage Concealer is an effective disguise for thread veins. It is supplied as two shades that you mix on the back of your hand. It is available from department stores including Harrods, London, UK.

Lasercare is a chain of private UK skin laser clinics, some of which are attached to NHS hospitals. Its website has an informative page on thread veins. It also lists by name the medical staff (qualified doctors) who work at its clinics, and the charges are clearly stated.
www.lasercare-clinics.co.uk

Videos of microsclerotherapy being done can be seen on the website of private UK surgeon Mr Mark Whiteley.
www.thread-veins.co.uk

Varicose Veins is a reliable and informative book by a famous UK professor of surgery, Professor Harold Ellis, and Peter Taylor. London: Greenwich Medical Media, 1999 (ISBN 1900151677). It does not describe the most recent treatments, but the basic information is good.

American College of Phlebology provides information about various treatments for varicose veins.
www.phlebology.org/brochure.htm

VNUS. This operation is explained on the website of UK private surgeon Mr Mark Whiteley. The site also has graphics explaining what varicose veins are.
www.veins.co.uk

Warts

FACE AND HANDS

Most people develop warts on their hands at some time in their life. They are harmless, and only matter because of their appearance – in fact, some children seem quite pleased with their warts.

There are two main types of warts on the hands or face.

- The type that many people (especially children) have on their hands starts as a small, flesh-coloured pimple that grows slowly over weeks or months to become a rough, raised lump. They are often called 'common warts'. If you look closely, you will see that the normal tiny lines of the skin (the lines that are used in fingerprints) do not cross the surface of the wart. You may also be able to see tiny black dots in the wart; these are blood capillaries.
- Some warts remain as very small, flat bumps; this type often occurs in clusters on the face, neck and hands. There may be 20–100 at any one time. In men, they are usually in the beard area, and in women they may occur on the legs.

Cause of warts

All warts are caused by a virus, human papillomavirus or HPV (see the section on genital warts on page 134). The virus causes overgrowth of cells at the base of the outer layer of the skin. Warts are entirely on the surface of the skin. They do not have deep roots that penetrate into the deep layers of the skin. Papillomavirus takes hold of damaged skin more easily, which is why warts are particularly common in children who bite their nails or pick at the skin round the nail. It also explains why warts tend to occur in the shaved beard area in men.

Folk remedies for warts

There is no scientific evidence that any of these remedies is effective. The reason people believe in them is because warts disappear by themselves.

- Tape the inner side of a broad bean pod over the wart.
- Every day, rub the wart with a raw potato.
- Squeeze radish juice onto the wart.
- Mix castor oil into a paste with baking soda. Apply the paste twice a day.
- Rub the wart with a piece of raw meat. Bury the meat in the garden. Wait for the wart to drop off as the meat rots.

What you can do

It is important to be sure that what you are dealing with really is a wart. If you have even the slightest doubt, ask your doctor to have a look.

- Something that looks like a wart, but which grows rapidly or does not go away with a remedy from the pharmacist, should definitely be checked by a doctor. There have been rare cases in which people have mistaken a skin cancer, such as a melanoma, for a wart and tried to treat it themselves.
- Do not treat warts at the side of your fingernail by yourself, because you may damage the nail.
- If you have warts on the genitals or round the anus, do not try the following remedies. Look at the section on genital warts on page 134 for advice.

Doing nothing is one option, and is the sensible choice for young children, because wart treatment can be painful. Although some warts may last for years, this is unusual. Normally the body's immune system will eventually recognize the wart and get rid of it. A wart has a 50% chance of disappearing within a month or two without treatment, and two-thirds will have gone within 2 years. This is the reason so many people are convinced that folk remedies work – the wart would probably have disappeared anyway. An advantage of doing nothing is that there will be no scarring after the wart has gone.

Duct tape is a simple method of treating warts on the hands. You can buy duct tape at a hardware store, or you can use any strong, sticky, waterproof tape. According to one study (*Archives of Pediatric and Adolescent Medicine* 2002;156:971–4), duct tape is as effective as other treatments, such as freezing.

- Cut a piece of tape the same size as the wart and stick it on.
- Leave it for 6 days, then remove it in the evening.
- After removing the tape, soak your hand in warm water and then gently rub the wart with an emery board. Leave the tape off overnight and then apply a new piece for another 6 days.
- If the skin under the tape becomes red and soggy, stop using the tape for a few days.
- Continue this routine for 2 months.

In the study, 85% of the warts disappeared with this treatment and most did so within 4 weeks.

Wart paint for hand warts. For hand warts, buy some wart paint from a pharmacy. Wart paints are *not* suitable for using on the face (or genital area), or if you are pregnant. Most contain salicylic acid; some also contain lactic acid. The acid does not attack the virus, but simply removes some of the warty tissue, so that the body's natural recovery process has less to do. Therefore the result is very unpredictable. In one person, the wart may disappear in days, while an identical-looking wart in a different person may take weeks and weeks, so this treatment does need patience. Overall, salicylic acid wart paint cures about 75% of warts (*British Medical Journal* 2002;235:461–4).

- The instructions will tell you to rub the wart with a pumice stone or an emery board before applying the paint. Do not overdo it – if you rub too hard, you may encourage spread of the virus onto nearby skin. In fact, this rubbing down needs to be done only twice a week, not every time you apply the paint.

- Before applying the paint, soak the wart in warm water for 2 minutes; this will encourage the paint to penetrate the wart. Then dry it thoroughly using your own towel.
- Then apply a tiny drop of the paint to the centre of the wart using a cocktail stick, matchstick or the applicator from the bottle. Take care to avoid getting the paint onto the skin nearby; you could protect the normal skin with Vaseline.
- Allow the paint to dry and then cover it with a sticking plaster.
- If the skin becomes sore, you have probably been rubbing it down too enthusiastically. Stop the treatment for a few days until the skin recovers.

Other types of wart paint or gel are worth trying if you have been using the salicylic acid wart paint for 3 months and the wart has not gone. Ask your pharmacist for glutaraldehyde (which may stain your skin brown) or formaldehyde paint or gel. However, some people are over-sensitive to these substances, so it might be better to ask your doctor for advice.

Silver nitrate (caustic) pencil is another possibility. In the UK, you can buy these pencils from pharmacies without a prescription. The silver nitrate gently burns the wart and therefore should be used carefully according to the directions on the packet. A study showed that 3 applications of silver nitrate, 3 days apart, had cleared 43% of warts a month later. Do not use silver nitrate on the face and do not use it more than 6 times on the hands. It can cause staining of the skin and clothes.

Freezing aerosol. An aerosol is available from pharmacies that works in a similar way to the liquid nitrogen used by doctors, but does not reach the very low temperatures that their equipment achieves. Only one application is used and you should follow the manufacturer's instructions. Do not use it on your face. If you have dark skin, freezing may not be a good idea, because it can sometimes remove pigment from the skin, leaving a white patch.

What your doctor can do

Freezing the wart with liquid nitrogen (also known as cryotherapy) can deal with warts on the face as well as on the hands. Some doctors are specially trained, and have the equipment to do this; otherwise, you can be referred to a hospital dermatology clinic. Freezing for a few seconds gives the wart frostbite. A blister may form under the wart, and then the roof of the blister, including the wart, falls off. It is painful and sometimes feels sore for several days after each treatment, so it is not suitable for children under the age of 10. You will probably need several treatments and, like all wart treatments, it is not always successful. In one study (published in the *British Journal of Dermatology*), several treatments over 12 weeks got rid of 45% of warts, and treatment every 3 weeks was just as effective as weekly treatments. Some research suggests that freezing is no more effective than wart paints.

Other treatments, such as injecting the drug bleomycin into the wart, are sometimes used in hospital clinics. Laser treatment is another possibility, but it is not better than other treatments; there may be scarring and it is painful. Cutting the wart out might be appropriate for troublesome single warts, but is not a realistic option if you have several.

VERRUCAS

A verruca (plantar wart) is a wart on the sole of the foot. It is the same as a common wart (see above), but the weight of the body presses it into the foot, which can be painful.

Verrucas are slightly raised and circular in shape, with a thickened rim of surrounding skin. The surface may have black dots ('pepper-pot' appearance). There may be several verrucas or just one.

Sometimes verrucas form clusters of small warts, called 'mosaic warts' – these are usually painless. In children, verrucas tend to come and go quite quickly, but in adults they can persist for several years if they are not treated.

How verrucas spread

Like other warts, verrucas are caused by strains of papillomavirus. There is lots of papillomavirus around, and many people carry it on the surface of their skin. It does not cause any harm unless it penetrates into the skin, where it can take hold and cause a wart. This is most likely to happen if the surface of your skin is already damaged, with tiny cracks.

Most people believe that verrucas are caught in the changing rooms of swimming pools and the pool surrounds, but only one scientific study has shown that people who use swimming pools regularly are more likely to get verrucas. Other studies have shown no link.

There is probably plenty of papillomavirus around swimming pools, particularly in the shower area. However, you are very unlikely to get a verruca if your skin is undamaged. If you want to minimize the risk, wear flip-flops in the shower area.

What you might do

Decide whether it really is a verruca. They are easily confused with corns and calluses, which are thickened areas of skin caused by friction. Corns are often seen over hammer toes and where shoes press on the little toe, but they can occur on the sole of the foot just below the toes. Look closely at the verruca, using a mirror and a magnifying glass if possible. Corns and calluses have normal skin lines (like the lines used in fingerprints) over them, but the surface of a verruca is slightly lumpy without lines. If you are not sure, see a chiropodist or ask your doctor.

Do nothing. Just covering the verucca with a plaster and doing nothing might be the best option, for the following reasons.

- Without treatment, verrucas almost always disappear within 2 years. Some go within a month or two. Treatments are inconvenient and can be uncomfortable.
- It is possible that letting verrucas disappear naturally helps the body to build up immunity, making you less likely to have them in the future.
- Most treatments involve rubbing the wart with pumice or an emery board. Some experts think this helps the virus to spread into nearby skin.
- You do not need to worry too much about infecting other people in swimming pools and similar places, because the virus is probably already there.

Decide who should treat it. Decide whether you should treat the verruca yourself, or whether you should see a chiropodist. Do not try to treat it yourself if you have diabetes, or if you already have a skin problem such as eczema. Most chiropodists advise against do-it-yourself treatment, and prefer to be consulted when the verruca is small and easier for them to deal with.

Keep your feet as dry as possible. Papillomavirus can spread through wet, soggy skin to form a patch of mosaic warts.

Relieve the discomfort. Stick a ring-shaped foam pad round the verruca to take the pressure off it. You can buy these from pharmacists and they are sometimes labelled 'for corns'.

Salicylic acid paint, gel or 'verruca plasters' can be bought from a pharmacist. Before using the paint or gel, soak your foot in warm water for 5 minutes, and then rub the surface of the verruca with a pumice stone. Do not overdo it. Carefully apply the paint and let it dry. Cover with a large sticking plaster. Repeat this treatment every evening until the verruca disappears, which may take 12 weeks. If it becomes painful, stop the treatment for a few days.

Verruca plasters are convenient. They are discs soaked in salicylic acid that you stick over the verruca and change every day. Some have built-in padding to deflect pressure from the verruca. Before applying the plaster, soak your foot and use pumice to rub some of the wart away. Put a piece of wide adhesive bandage over the plaster to make sure it stays in position.

Silver nitrate (caustic) pencil. If salicylic acid does not work, you can try a silver nitrate pencil. In the UK, you can buy this from pharmacies without a prescription. It gently burns the wart. Use it carefully according to the manufacturer's instructions.

A freezing aerosol is now available from pharmacies. It works in a similar way to the freezing treatment used by chiropodists and doctors, but does not reach the very low temperatures that their equipment achieves. Only one application is needed. Follow the manufacturer's instructions carefully.

Soaking the verruca in formaldehyde solution is another treatment worth trying if salicylic acid does not work or you have several verrucas. Buy the solution from a pharmacist and dilute it according to the instructions. Smear Vaseline over the normal skin of your foot to protect it, and soak the warty area for 15 minutes a day. After each soaking, you can pare away some of the softened wart. Some people are over-sensitive to formaldehyde, so stop the treatment if the area becomes sore.

Try a herbal remedy from a health shop. It is difficult to know whether these are effective, because most have not been fully investigated in scientific trials. Tea-tree oil, applied twice daily on its own or mixed with garlic juice, is said to have an effect. A tincture made from Chelidonium (the Greater Celandine) is said to be antiviral and to damage wart cells.

What you should never do

Do not try scraping it away with a corn knife. You could damage your skin and cause an infection. Also, the verucca will come back and others may occur nearby in the damaged skin.

What a chiropodist or your doctor can do

Chiropodists can check that you have a verruca and not some other problem, and they offer a range of treatments, including freezing (cryotherapy – see page 326). Freezing tends to be less effective for verrucas than for common warts, and can be painful. It may be a good idea if you have mosaic warts, because these do not respond very well to salicylic acid. If you have a really troublesome verruca, your doctor might refer you to a hospital dermatology department for treatment.

Useful contacts

Health*Insite* is an Australian government initiative aimed to improve the health of Australians by providing easy access to quality information about human health. Follow the link on skin diseases to find a range of information on warts.
www.healthinsite.gov.au/topics/Skin_Diseases

The American Academy of Dermatology has a warts fact sheet on its website.
www.aad.org/public/Publications/pamphlets/Warts.htm

Freezing aerosol. The Wartner aerosol is available from pharmacies. You can also buy it from several websites.
www.wartner.co.uk

The Society of Chiropodists and Podiatrists can help you find a state-registered chiropodist. Their website has information about verrucas and other foot problems, and has a 'Find a local chiropodist' facility.
www.feetforlife.org

Wind

- Methane is one of the most potent 'greenhouse' gases in the atmosphere. Cows' and sheeps' wind is responsible for almost a third of the methane in Europe that passes into the atmosphere. A single sheep typically produces 25 litres of methane a day, while a cow can produce an amazing 280 litres a day (*New Scientist* 15 June 2002).
- In the 1960s, NASA was worried that a build-up of hydrogen from astronauts' wind might accidentally explode in the spacecraft. This stimulated a lot of research into bowel gas.
- At any one time, there is about 200 mL (a mugful) of gas in each person's gut.
- Most people expel about 600 mL of gas per day, but some people produce up to 2 litres.
- Gut gases are 90% nitrogen; the remainder is carbon dioxide, hydrogen, methane and sometimes hydrogen sulphide.
- Healthy young men break wind 14–25 times a day and women half as often.
- Women produce stronger smelling flatus than men, but men produce a greater volume.

There are three main sources of wind.

- Everyone's gut contains gas because we cannot help swallowing air when we swallow food, when we drink and when we swallow our saliva.
- Carbon dioxide is produced by chemical reactions within the gut: saliva contains bicarbonate, which reacts with acid in the stomach to produce carbon dioxide gas; and stomach acid releases carbon dioxide when it reacts with pancreatic digestive juices in the upper part of the intestine.
- About 500 types of bacteria live in our intestines. Some of them act on food residues in the lower gut, releasing hydrogen, methane and carbon dioxide gases.

What happens to the gas in the gut?

Some of the intestinal gas is absorbed into the bloodstream and is eventually exhaled by the lungs. In social situations, we try to hold gas in and more passes from the gut into the bloodstream and then into the lungs; researchers have found that, in social situations, our breath contains increased amounts of hydrogen.

Most intestinal gas, however, has to be got rid of through the mouth (belching, eructation) or through the anus (flatulence, farting, breaking wind).

Why wind smells

The main gases in wind – nitrogen, oxygen, carbon dioxide, hydrogen and methane – have no smell. The unpleasant smell of a fart is due to very tiny amounts of sulphur-containing gases, which have a smell disproportionate to their volume.

Farting and belching may be healthy – or can they spread germs?

Some experts believe that our attempts to hold gas in are an unnatural result of our enclosed lifestyles and the build-up of pressure is responsible for bowel diseases, such as diverticulosis; when we lived mainly in the open air, farting was not a problem and no one was worried about letting wind pass out naturally. In the early 1990s, a publicity campaign was launched in Holland (by the National Liver and Intestine Foundation) to encourage people to break wind at least 15 times a day.

Wind is never serious, except as a cause of embarrassment, unless there are other gut symptoms as well, such as abdominal pain, constipation, loss of weight, pale faeces that are difficult to flush away, or blood in the faeces.

No one knows whether wind can spread germs. The magazine *New Scientist* (30 June 2001) reported an experiment in which a volunteer was asked to lower his trousers and break wind very close to a special dish (blood agar plate) used by laboratories to grow bacteria. The next day, there were lots of gut bacteria growing on the plate. At the edge, there were some skin bacteria that must have been blown onto the plate by the wind.

Reasons for farting and belching

Foods that cause flatulence. Onions, tomatoes and mints actually relax the muscle at the lower end of the gullet, allowing air from the stomach to escape by belching.

Farting is more to do with bacteria in the lower bowel, which are particularly partial to carbohydrates. The carbohydrates in some foods can not be broken down and absorbed in the intestine; they pass straight through to the bowel, where they are fermented by the bacteria to produce gas that comes out as farting. Beans are famous for containing large amounts of 'unabsorbable carbohydrate', but other foods can have the same effect.

Some slimming chocolate contains sorbitol or fructose instead of sugar. Most of this is not absorbed (which is why these products are marketed for slimmers), but can be acted on by the large bowel bacteria to cause wind. Consumption of fruit juices is increasing and, because they contain a lot of fructose, they can cause gas and bloating.

Foods with a high proportion of unabsorbable carbohydrate that cause flatulence

- Beans
- Peas
- Broccoli, cauliflower
- Jerusalem artichokes and other root vegetables such as parsnips
- 'Slimming' foods that contain sorbitol or fructose
- Raisins, prunes
- Apples
- Fruit juices (because of the fructose they contain)

Overeating, as we all know, leads to belching. This is because the stomach normally contains some air. When we overeat, the stomach attempts to relieve the discomfort and distension by expelling the stomach air upwards. This is a reflex over which we have no control.

Fizzy drinks and gulping hot drinks introduce gas into the stomach.

Habit. Some people suck a small amount of air into the oesophagus (gullet) or stomach by swallowing to make themselves belch, without realizing they are doing so (*Gut* 2004;53:1561–5). This habit often starts if there is a period of indigestion, when belching may temporarily relieve the discomfort.

Smoking, chewing gum and sucking on pen tops makes you produce more saliva, which has to be swallowed. Each time you swallow the saliva you also swallow air. Also, chewing gum contains sorbitol.

Tight clothing, such as Lycra shorts, constricting belts and 'hold-in' underwear increase the pressure on the abdomen and make it more difficult for wind to pass along normally, resulting in trapped wind and belching.

Acarbose (Glucobay) is a drug for diabetes. It prevents enzymes in the gut digesting carbohydrates such as starch and sucrose. Because they are not digested, these carbohydrates are not absorbed (which is how the drug helps to lower the blood sugar). Instead, they pass down to the lower bowel, where they are fermented by the bacteria. Most people taking acarbose experience flatulence, tummy rumbles and a feeling of fullness.

Intestinal diseases are occasionally responsible. In lactase deficiency, for example, the enzyme that breaks down lactose, a carbohydrate found in milk, is lacking. The undigested lactose produces hydrogen and carbon dioxide when it reaches the large bowel, causing frothy diarrhoea, griping pains and flatulence.

Constipation can cause farting. Normally, most of the intestinal gas is expelled out of the anus as small puffs which we are not aware of. When we are constipated, the gas becomes trapped behind the faeces and then suddenly emerges as a noticeable amount. Also, when we are constipated, the food residues stay in the bowel for longer, and have more time to ferment and give off gases. (For more information, look at the section on constipation on page 79.)

Anxiety and tension seem to make wind worse. This is partly because when we are anxious we are hyper-alert, and notice body functions that we would otherwise ignore. Another factor is that when we are anxious we tend to swallow more air. Also, our guts become more active because of increased adrenaline levels and they expel the gases more forcefully.

Childbirth. After childbirth, the muscles of the anus or the nerves nearby can be damaged, making it difficult to hold wind in. This is much more common than many people realize. A study in Sweden found that 25% of women were unable to control wind 5 months after giving birth, particularly if they had a long labour. The problem did improve a few months later. Sometimes, there may also be some leakage of faeces (for more information, look at the section on faecal incontinence on page 123). If your problem started after having a baby and does not get better, see your doctor because an operation may cure the problem.

Ageing may make gas worse, because as we get older we do not produce digestive juices, such as saliva, as efficiently. This means that more carbohydrate foods pass untouched to the lower bowel, where they are fermented by the bacteria.

Keep a diary

If you really want to get to grips with the problem, keep a diary of what and when you eat for a week. Also note when you pass wind, and whether it is mild, moderate or severe each time. This may help you to pinpoint foods or drinks that are responsible.

Minimizing belching

- Avoid fizzy drinks and hot drinks.
- Do not rush your food. When you gulp food you swallow more air.
- Do not overeat. To avoid gas, it is better to eat little and often.
- Chew your food properly. This helps the saliva to work on it so it is properly digested, and you are less likely to swallow air with food that is chewed small than with large lumps.
- Do not use chewing gum, and try to avoid sucking on pen tops.
- Stop smoking.

Minimizing flatulence

- Pay attention to the advice for minimizing belching to reduce swallowed air. Some swallowed air may be passed as flatulence instead of belching.
- Try to avoid large quantities of the particular gas-forming foods listed on page 381, but make sure you eat enough fruit and vegetables to avoid constipation and give yourself a balanced diet. The carbohydrates in many foods (such as potatoes, rice, corn and wheat products) are well absorbed so will not worsen flatulence. Dietary fibres, such as bran and cellulose, are also innocent, because they are not converted to gases by gut bacteria.
- Do not suddenly increase the amount of fibre in your diet; the gut needs to get used to increased fibre gradually.
- Avoid 'slimming' foods containing sorbitol. Some people find that reducing their intake of ordinary sugar helps.
- Remove 80% of the most troublesome carbohydrates from dried beans by covering them with water, bringing them to the boil and boiling for 10 minutes, turning off the heat and letting them soak for 4 hours. Drain off the water, replace with fresh water and cook the beans according to your recipe. Or use tinned beans.
- Take plenty of exercise. This helps to keep the bowel moving normally.
- Avoid tight clothing.
- Try taking a charcoal tablet (available from pharmacies), or eating a charcoal biscuit (available from health stores) before a meal.
- Your doctor might be willing to give you a course of broad-spectrum antibiotic. This can sometimes help by changing the balance of bacteria in the gut.

- Anti-wind products can be bought from pharmacies. They disperse bubbles of trapped wind by creating larger bubbles that can pass out of the system. They may relieve your discomfort, but may make you fart and belch even more.
- Beano (see Useful contacts below) is a product containing the enzyme galactosidase, which is said to improve the digestibility of gassy carbohydrate foods. It is made from a mould, so avoid it if you are allergic to moulds or penicillin. You take it just before your first bite of food. It is available from some pharmacies and health-food stores.

Disguising wind

If you make a smell in the toilet, light a match – this makes the smell disappear as if by magic. Considerate people keep a box of matches by the toillet for this purpose.

In the US, a cushion that filters flatulence is available. The Flatulence Filter is covered in grey tweed fabric and looks like an ordinary chair cushion, but is packed with charcoal. It lasts about 12 months, and the manufacturers claim 'It makes a great gift'.

Useful contacts

Health*Insite* is an Australian government initiative aimed to improve the health of Australians by providing easy access to quality information about human health. You can find resources on digestion, stomach and other gastrointestinal disorders by following the link below.
www.healthinsite.gov.au/topics/Digestion_and_Stomach_Disorders

The American Gastroenterological Association is an organization for doctors who specialize in the gut. Look in the 'Patients/Public' section of its website for excellent information about various gut problems, including 'Gas in the digestive tract'.
www.gastro.org/clinicalRes/brochures/gas.html

The Flatulence Filter can be ordered from Ultratech Products Inc. in the US via their website.
www.flatulence-filter.com

www.smellypoop.com tells you more than you ever wanted to know about intestinal wind.
www.smellypoop.com

Beano. More information about Beano can be found on the manufacturer's website, which also has a list of gassy foods.
www.beano.net

Other sources. Look at the Useful contacts for anal problems (see page 29).

Getting help

TALKING TO YOUR DOCTOR

Initiating the discussion

If you say something like, 'I have a problem which I want to discuss with you, but I find it difficult to talk about,' the doctor will immediately be on your side. Another possibility is to write a few lines about your problem, take the note with you to your appointment and ask your doctor to read it. Or print a page from this website (www.embarrassingproblems.co.uk), and take it with you and use it as a starting point. (Or take this book with you and use it as a starting point.)

Do not worry if talking makes you nervous or tearful – doctors are used to people being upset.

Confidentiality

You may be concerned about confidentiality. The best way of dealing with this is to ask the doctor about it. Say, 'I have a rather embarrassing or personal problem that I want to discuss with you, but I am worried about confidentiality. How confidential is our discussion? Who will see the notes you make?'

What if you do not like your doctor?

You may dislike your doctor, or you may like him or her but feel he or she would be unsympathetic to your particular problem. If you genuinely do not like your doctor, you should change.

In the UK, some practices will let you change to another doctor within the practice, or will let you make all your appointments with other doctors within the practice without officially changing. Some practices do not allow this, so your only option if you do not like your doctor is to change to another practice. However, in Australia, you are free to choose the doctor you want to.

VISITING A SEXUAL HEALTH CLINIC

Sexual health clinics deal with sexually transmitted infections and many other genital and sexual problems. Most people are worried about attending a clinic for the first time, but they usually find it all right.

The following is some general information about sexual health clinics.

Why go to a sexual health clinic?

- Staff at sexual health clinics are specially trained and experienced in genital problems. They also have a reputation for being kind, sympathetic and non-judgmental.

- As well as doctors and nurses, sexual health clinics usually have special counsellors who can help you with worries, and give you additional information you may need.
- Sexual health clinics have facilities for doing tests for all genital infections. For many tests, they will be able to give you the results straightaway, and the appropriate treatment.
- You do not need a letter from your family doctor to attend a sexual health clinic – you simply phone the clinic and make an appointment.
- Sexual health clinics are very confidential. They will ask if they can send the result of your tests to your family doctor, but if you refuse, they will not do so.

What sort of problems can the clinic help with?

You can attend a sexual health clinic for tests if you think you might have a sexually transmitted infection, whether or not you have symptoms (such as a discharge). You can attend the clinic to be tested for HIV. The clinic could also help you if you think something is wrong with the shape or appearance of your genitals.

Finding a sexual health clinic and making an appointment

There are several ways of finding your nearest clinic.

- The telephone number is probably listed in the 'Business and Government' section of your telephone directory. Alternatively, you can search for 'Sexual health clinics' in the white pages on the internet.
- You could telephone your local hospital and ask for information about the nearest sexual health clinic.

When you have located the clinic, phone to make an appointment. You do not need a doctor's referral.

Before attending the clinic

- Make sure you know where the clinic is, and leave plenty of time to get there.
- If it is your first appointment, allow at least an hour and a half for it.
- Women should work out the date of their last menstrual period and when they last had a smear test, and jot them down – you will probably be asked for this information.
- Especially for a first appointment, men should try not to pass urine for 2 hours beforehand. This is because samples may be taken for infection at the urethra (pee hole), and if you have passed urine recently, the evidence could be washed away so the test might be inaccurate.

  If you are in the waiting room and feel you must pass urine before seeing the doctor, tell a nurse so the urine sample can be taken.
- Switch off your mobile phone.
- Resolve to be completely honest. The questions you will be asked are simply to help make an accurate diagnosis. If you lie slightly, because of embarrassment, it will be less easy for the doctor to diagnose and treat your problem.

What happens at the clinic

If it is your first visit, you will see a doctor. The doctor will talk to you in private, and will ask you about your symptoms (if any), your recent sexual contacts and various medical questions. The doctor will then examine you, and then the doctor or nurse will take samples for testing. Before taking the samples, the doctor or nurse will talk to you about them, and make sure that you are happy for them to be taken.

- A urine sample is always needed.
- In men, samples are usually taken from the opening of the urethra, from the anus and from the throat.
- In women, samples are usually taken from the vagina, the cervix (neck of the womb at the top of the vagina), throat and sometimes the anus. To take a sample from the cervix, a speculum is put into the vagina (like having a smear).

All these samples will be examined under the microscope in the clinic by an expert technician, who will look for signs of infection. The samples will then be sent to the laboratory for further, more complicated tests. In most cases, the doctor will be able to tell you what is wrong, and give you treatment there and then. The treatment is free.

Blood samples are usually taken, after discussion with you, to test for syphilis and/or hepatitis. If you wish, the clinic can also test you for HIV. You will also be given an opportunity to talk to the health counsellor, who will give you more information about your problem.

Worries about the clinic

It will be embarrassing. Sexual health clinics are not at all embarrassing. The staff deal with genital problems all the time – it is their job. To them, the genital area is just an ordinary part of the body.

The waiting room will be full of seedy people. The other people in the waiting room are just like you – ordinary people who are worried and trying to sort out a problemt.

I do not want to talk about my sex life. They will think I have had too many partners. The staff are not at all judgmental about people's lifestyles. They are more interested in making a diagnosis of your problem, and giving you the right treatment.

The tests will be painful. For women, the tests are not painful (unless you count a blood test as painful). For men, taking the sample from the opening of the urethra (pee hole) is uncomfortable, but it takes only a moment.

They will do an HIV test and I'm not sure if I want one. You will probably be asked if you would like an HIV test, and it will be explained to you properly. If you are not sure, no one will try to persuade you – you can always go back and have it done another time.

They will send a letter to my family doctor telling him or her things about my sex life that I don't want him/her to know. The clinic will ask you if you want the results of tests to be sent to your family doctor. Often this is a sensible thing to agree to, but if you do not wish it, they will not do so. The letter will not go into details about your sex life – it will probably be a short letter explaining the results. If you are worried, ask the doctor to tell you what information will be in the letter.

There will be medical students there. Clinics sometimes do have medical students, because they have to learn about genital problems in order to become useful doctors. There will be one or two, not a huge group. They are bound by the same rules of confidentiality as everyone else in the clinic. The students are usually exceptionally sympathetic to people attending sexual health clinics, and may in fact make your visit nicer. However, if you would prefer not to have students there just say so.

SEEING YOUR DOCTOR ABOUT AN ANAL PROBLEM

Almost everyone is embarrassed about seeing the doctor about an anal problem, such as anal pain, wind or anal itching. It is important that you get over this worry, so that you get treatment for the problem. Value your own health and think of your doctor simply as someone who is helping to maintain your health. Bowel or anal symptoms, such as constipation or bleeding, can sometimes be serious. People are literally dying of embarrassment because they do not see their doctor when bowel symptoms start, often because of a fear of examination of their back passage (rectal examination). Therefore they may reach their doctor only when bowel cancer is quite advanced. Although bowel cancer is much less common than piles, it is always a possibility and can be treated very successfully at an early stage.

Take control

Remind yourself that you are in charge of the consultation with your doctor. He or she can not examine you without your permission. Therefore it is perfectly OK for you to visit your doctor and say, 'I have such-and-such a problem. At the moment I just want to discuss it. I don't want to be examined.' When you have got over the hurdle of talking about the problem you may later feel quite all right about being examined, but it is your decision.

Think the problem through

What do you think will be going on in your doctor's mind while you are being examined? Are you imagining your doctor will be mentally rating and criticizing your appearance? In fact, in this situation your doctor is interested in your insides, not your outsides. By the time he or she becomes a family doctor, your doctor will have seen literally thousands of backsides and is not interested in their appearance. In fact, he or she will be thinking about the symptoms that you have described, and whether they match up with the findings on examination.

Take a friend?

Would it help to have a friend with you? You might feel this would make it worse, but the right person can be reassuring, perhaps someone who has had a lot of medical treatment themselves and so is matter-of-fact about being examined.

What is involved in the examination

If you are a female and the doctor is male, he will ask a female nurse to be present during the examination. Like any other part of the examination, examination of the back passage is methodical, and all doctors are taught the following procedure.

The patient is asked to lie on the left side with the knees drawn up to the chest; this position helps to relax the muscles around the back passage. If you are feeling tense, breathe slowly and deeply with your mouth open. The doctor puts on a pair of gloves and separates the buttocks slightly to look for abnormalities such as piles, cracks in the wall of the anus (anal fissure), skin tags or warts.

The doctor then puts some lubricant on the gloved finger, and places the fingertip on the anus, pressing slightly. When the anal muscle relaxes, the finger is inserted slowly and the tip is rotated gently to feel for lumps and bumps, and specific structures (such as the prostate in men). The finger is withdrawn slowly and then the doctor inspects the glove for blood or pus. It is not painful, so if you experience any pain, tell your doctor. You may just experience a feeling of rectal fullness during the examination, as if you wish to have your bowels open.

Your doctor might suggest inserting a short hollow instrument (proctoscope) to separate the walls of the bowel so that they can be seen clearly as the instrument is withdrawn. Again, this is not painful and your doctor will not do this without your permission and explaining it to you.

CHOOSING A COSMETIC SURGEON

Cosmetic surgery is booming. In the US, the number of women having cosmetic surgery increased by 11% in 2003 compared with the previous year. The increase was even greater for men – 22% more in 2003 than 2002 (data from the American Society for Aesthetic and Plastic Surgery).

Overall, Americans spent $9.4 billion on cosmetic surgery and non-surgical procedures such as Botox in 2003. And the UK is catching up fast; the cosmetic surgery industry is worth more than £225 million a year.

It is not surprising that some clinics use aggressive marketing techniques and advertise persuasively. This means that you have to be very careful.

What do the words mean?

- **Cosmetic surgery** is surgery to improve appearance.
- **Aesthetic surgery** is another name for cosmetic surgery. It comes from the Greek word for beauty.
- **Plastic surgery** is surgery to change the shape or form of the surface and sometimes the deeper structures of the body. The word 'plastic' comes from the Greek word for moulding. Plastic surgery includes cosmetic surgery, repair operations after burns and

other injuries, correction of inherited deformities, breast reconstruction after operations for breast cancer, and removal of skin tumours.

Before undergoing any cosmetic procedure, it is essential to do a lot of homework. The following advice is mainly about the UK with some specific references to Australia. If you live elsewhere, find out about surgeons' qualifications in your country.

Do not rush into anything. Read as much as you can about cosmetic surgery, and note down the names of surgeons who are mentioned or quoted. Remember that all surgery has risks. Think carefully about why you want the procedure done. For example, cosmetic surgery is unlikely to improve a relationship that is going nowhere. If you are going through a life crisis, do not make any decisions about cosmetic surgery.

Do not be pressured by anyone else. You will be the one undergoing surgery, so do it only if you want it for yourself.

Be very clear what you are hoping to achieve. For example, if you want your breasts enlarged, what size do you want them to be? Having a clear idea is essential for a proper discussion with the surgeon.

Find out as much as you can about the procedure itself. Even a simple-sounding procedure such as liposuction requires a lot of skill. Look at the good cosmetic surgery websites (see Useful contacts below). Various cosmetic procedures are also discussed elsewhere in this book: for example, breast reduction on page 58, breast enlargement on page 60, thread veins on page 316, ageing skin on page 21 and ears on page 101.

Locate a good, reputable surgeon. Do not just answer a persuasive advertisement in a magazine or on the web. At present, in the UK, any doctor can claim to be a 'plastic surgeon'. However, this is changing. Doctors are to be banned from carrying out cosmetic surgery unless they have had at least 5 years training in the relevant specialty and have passed appropriate exams.

In Australia, any doctor can be a cosmetic surgeon but he or she is required to undertake further studies and a special exam in order to become a plastic surgeon.

The best plan is to ask your own doctor for a referral. If you think your doctor would be unsympathetic, contact the British Association of Aesthetic Plastic Surgeons or the Australian Society of Plastic Surgeons (see Useful contacts on page 324) for a list of their members and their different specialities.

- Check your surgeon's qualifications in the Medical Directory (see Useful contacts on page 324). In the UK, the letters MRCS or FRCS mean that that he or she is a Member or Fellow of the Royal College of Surgeons, having had several years' experience and passed a stiff exam in general surgery. In Australia, the letters FRACS mean that he or she is a Fellow of the Royal Australasian College of Surgeons. They do not signify special training in cosmetic surgery. Younger surgeons may have the more recently-introduced qualification 'FRCS (Plast)' or 'FRACS (Plast)', which means that the surgeon has additional experience in plastic or reconstructive surgery and passed an extra examination. However, many experienced cosmetic surgeons do not have FRCS (Plast) or FRACS (Plast) because they trained before it was introduced.

- In the UK, most cosmetic surgeons will be members of BAAPS, the main organization responsible for maintaining high standards in cosmetic surgery. However, membership of BAAPS is not an absolute guarantee. To join BAAPS, surgeons have to have had 6 years' training in plastic surgery and provide a log book of operations they have done, and other members have to testify to their experience. Once he or she has joined, there is nothing to stop the surgeon doing other cosmetic operations in which he or she is less experienced.
- Some surgeons are members of the British Association of Cosmetic Surgeons (BACS). This organization represents mainly surgeons in private clinics. To join BACS, they do not need to be qualified plastic surgeons, but have to show they have cosmetic surgery experience. Many BACS surgeons have good experience with certain procedures, but BACS membership is not a guarantee of anything.
- In Australia, plastic surgeons will be members of the Australian Society of Plastic Surgeons. All members are Fellows of the Royal Australasian College of Surgeons (FRACS), the benchmark standard for surgical training within Australia, or its equivalent. Each has a record of accomplishment in their field and a commitment to high ethical standards.
- The General Medical Council has a list of specialist plastic surgeons who are eligible to work in the UK as NHS consultants in plastic surgery.

Make sure you have a proper consultation with the actual surgeon who will be operating on you. New UK government regulations insist on this. Be suspicious if you are not charged a fee for this consultation – a good surgeon's time is valuable. A 'free' consultation will probably be with a counsellor, nurse or salesperson.

- Take a good friend with you.
- Write down a list of questions beforehand. Make sure you ask them all (even if it feels embarrassing). If the answers are not absolutely clear to you, say so and ask for a further explanation. Do not just think you are being stupid. Remember that you are paying for this consultation.
- Ask about any preparations you will need to make, what aftercare is provided, and what the risks are. Does the clinic have resuscitation equipment and doctors actually in the building 24 hours a day? Who will you be able to contact if you need advice after the operation?
- Find out about the recovery period. How much pain and bruising should you expect? How long will you need off work? When will you have stitches out? What will the scar be like?
- Ask how long the results will last.
- Ask the surgeon how many of these procedures he/she has done before. If you are shown 'before-and-after' photographs, ask if the operation was done by your surgeon personally. (You could be shown pictures of operations done at the clinic by a different surgeon.)
- Make sure you know how much the procedure will cost.

Do not ignore the pitfalls. All surgery has risks. If you are really keen on a procedure, it is tempting to disregard possible problems, but this is a big mistake. Weigh up all the pros and cons carefully before making your decision.

Shop around. Do not just go to the first clinic that you contact. Make a short-list of several surgeons and clinics, and have a consultation with more than one. Although this will cost you, it is money well spent.

Consider location. It is tempting to travel overseas for cheaper surgery, but do not do so unless you are sure about follow-up arrangements and what would happen if there were problems.

Allow yourself a 'cooling off 'period of about 2–3 weeks after the initial consultation, so that you can think clearly about the procedure before making the decision to go ahead. A respectable clinic will encourage this, and will not hassle you into making an immediate decision. UK government regulations from the National Care Standards Commission (set up to regulate private clinics) ban having the surgery within 2 weeks of the consultation, but you could still be pressured into making the decision too quickly. Go ahead only if you feel you can trust the surgeon, and that he or she has explained everything properly to you and understands what you are hoping to achieve.

Remember you can always change your mind. You can cancel right up to the moment you go to sleep for surgery.

Most popular operations

In the UK, 16 000 cosmetic surgery operations are done each year. The most popular operations requested by women are:

1 breast enlargement
2 breast reduction
3 facelift.

In the US, the most popular operations are:

1 liposuction (384 626 in 2003)
2 breast enlargement (280 401 in 2003)
3 eyelid lift (267 627 in 2003)
4 rhinoplasty or 'nose job' (172 420 in 2003)
5 breast reduction (147 173 in 2003).

In addition, more than 2.5 million chemical peels and antiwrinkle injections (such as Botox) were done in the US in the year 2000.

(Information from the British Association of Aesthetic Plastic Surgeons and the American Society for Aesthetic and Plastic Surgery.)

Useful contacts

British Association of Aesthetic and Plastic Surgeons (BAAPS) has a fact sheet on cosmetic surgery on its website, as well as a list of their members. The website also gives details of the common cosmetic surgery procedures, and tells you the risks and limitations of each, and has a list of points for you to think about beforehand.
www.baaps.org.uk

Australian Society of Plastic Surgeons (ASPS). The Australian Society of Plastic Surgeons can give you advice and post you a list of your State's members. Society members are all fully qualified in both reconstructive and cosmetic surgery. All members are Fellows of the Royal Australasian College of Surgeons (FRACS). Each has a record of accomplishment in their field and a commitment to high ethical standards.
www.plasticsurgery.org.au

The Medical Directory is a two-volume book listing UK doctors and their qualifications. It is published every year, and should be available in your local library. Look up your surgeon, and check his/her qualifications. The Directory may also mention that he or she is a member of the BAAPS.

General Medical Council. The website gives details of UK doctors, and if a doctor is a specialist in plastic surgery (if they were appointed as an NHS consultant since 1997).
www.gmc.org

British Association of Cosmetic Surgeons (BACS). The association provide a forum for the exchange of expertise and to maintain standards in this specialist area of cosmetic surgery. The website contains details of the association's constitution, code of practice, and membership, including contact information and links to members own websites. There is also information on a cosmetic surgery book, which can be ordered from the association.
www.b-a-c-s.co.uk

Health Which? October 2002 (no longer published, but back copies are available in most local libraries) contains a report on cosmetic surgery and a useful checklist to help you make an informed decision.

The American Society for Aesthetic Plastic Surgery (ASAPS) can provide the names and qualifications of surgeons in all areas of the US. Its website has web pages giving information about various cosmetic surgery procedures. Some of the information may not be applicable to other countries.
www.surgery.org/public/procedures.php

Wendy Lewis is an expert on cosmetic surgery procedures and her website is informative. The 'Ask the beauty junkie' section is a mine of information.
www.wlbeauty.com

First published in 2005 by Health Press Limited
This edition published in 2007 by Murdoch Books Pty Limited

Murdoch Books Australia
Pier 8/9
23 Hickson Road
Millers Point NSW 2000
Phone: +61 (0) 2 8220 2000
Fax: +61 (0) 2 8220 2558
www.murdochbooks.com.au

Murdoch Books UK Limited
Erico House, 6th Floor
93–99 Upper Richmond Road
Putney, London SW15 2TG
Phone: +44 (0) 20 8785 5995
Fax: +44 (0) 20 8785 5985
www.murdochbooks.co.uk

Chief Executive: Juliet Rogers
Publishing Director: Kay Scarlett

Design manager: Vivien Valk
Project manager: Rhiain Hull
Editor: Sandra Davies
Cover design: Reuben Crossman
Internal design concept and designer: Jacqueline Richards
Production: Monique Layt

National Library of Australia Cataloguing-in-Publication Data
Stearn, Margaret.
Warts and all: straight talking advice on life's embarrassing problems.
ISBN 978 1 92125 984 5 (pbk.).
1. Medicine, Popular. 2. Self-care, Health. I. Title. 616.024

A catalogue record for this book is available from the British Library.

Printed by McPherson's Printing Group in 2007.
PRINTED IN AUSTRALIA.